Autism and Child Psychopathology Series

Series Editor

Johnny L. Matson, Baton Rouge, LA, USA

Brief Overview

The purpose of this series is to advance knowledge in the broad multidisciplinary fields of autism and various forms of psychopathology (e.g., anxiety and depression). Volumes synthesize research on a range of rapidly expanding topics on assessment, treatment, and etiology.

Description

The **Autism and Child Psychopathology Series** explores a wide range of research and professional methods, procedures, and theories used to enhance positive development and outcomes across the lifespan. Developments in education, medicine, psychology, and applied behavior analysis as well as child and adolescent development across home, school, hospital, and community settings are the focus of this series. Series volumes are both authored and edited, and they provide critical reviews of evidence-based methods. As such, these books serve as a critical reference source for researchers and professionals who deal with developmental disorders and disabilities, most notably autism, intellectual disabilities, challenging behaviors, anxiety, depression, ADHD, developmental coordination disorder, communication disorders, and other common childhood problems. The series addresses important mental health and development difficulties that children and youth, their caregivers, and the professionals who treat them must face. Each volume in the series provides an analysis of methods and procedures that may assist in effectively treating these developmental problems.

Susan Lowinger · Shiri Pearlman-Avnion
Editors

Collaborative Care and Partnerships in Autism Diagnosis and Treatment

Therapists, Parents, Children

Springer

Editors
Susan Lowinger
Kishurim Clinic
Jerusalem, Israel

Shiri Pearlman-Avnion
Tel-Hai College
Kiryat Shmona, Israel

ISSN 2192-922X ISSN 2192-9238 (electronic)
Autism and Child Psychopathology Series
ISBN 978-3-032-07008-1 ISBN 978-3-032-07009-8 (eBook)
https://doi.org/10.1007/978-3-032-07009-8

This Springer imprint is published by the registered company Springer Nature Switzerland AG
The registered company address is: Gewerbestrasse 11, 6330 Cham, Switzerland

Preface

Collaboration is often defined as the action of working with someone to produce or create something; in short, a partnership. Discussions between therapists and parents can be termed "collaborative consultation". Despite the recognition of the overwhelming importance of collaboration between parents and therapists of children on the autism spectrum, this essential partnership is often not attained. Moreover, there is a scarcity of research as to how this collaboration can be achieved.

It is important to understand that the various partners in a collaborative relationship have different but complementary roles. The following is a synopsis of the difficulties faced by the parents in the collaborative process.

A. Parents begin the collaborative effort feeling overwhelmed by the child's diagnosis of autism spectrum disorder (ASD).
B. The medical community may have been reluctant to offer a diagnosis, which led to difficulties with other system supports.
C. Parents have underlying emotional needs that are linked to their child's difficulties.
D. Parents have competing demands on their time.
E. Parents have less power and control than clinicians in collaborations.
F. Parents suffer from ongoing stigma, which creates barriers to participating in clinical programs.
G. Lack of knowledge in the community about ASD creates difficulties for the families in accessing treatment (Burney et al., 2024).

Therapists and clinicians also face various barriers to working with parents of children with ASD. Therapists often do not know how to establish collaboration with parents or overcome the parents' disengagement from the therapy.

In general, professionals should ask parents what extent of involvement and types of services are most suitable for their child and their family. Therapists should involve the parents in choosing goals and give them a strong sense of engagement in the intervention (An & Palisano, 2014). Below are some of the many recommendations for therapists to improve their engagement with parents.

A. Align family priorities with the purpose of therapy (Klatte et al, 2019).
B. Establish rules of collaboration for the therapists (Klatte et al., 2023).

    1. Invest time in collaboration.
    2. Be aware of your important role in collaboration with parents.
    3. Get to know the family.

C. Optimize collaboration between families and professionals (An & Palisano, 2014).

    1. Shared planning.
    2. Shared implementation.
    3. Shared evaluation.

The growing use of information technologies offers a significant advantage to those who are not familiar with the long-standing efforts to improve and enhance the functioning of individuals on the autism spectrum. However, online research does not offer partnership with professionals or a shared commitment by the therapeutic community to improve responses and treatments. This book delves into collaborative relationships and their potential to promote—and sometimes to hinder—the progress of individuals on the autism spectrum.

Many methods for improving collaboration, from choosing goals through shared planning and implementation, are presented in the chapters of this book. The book is organized into four parts. The first part emphasizes the diagnostic process and the difficulties of the parents in handling the hurdles of diagnosis. This is highlighted in the chapter on Self-Discovery as well as in the chapter on Self-Disclosure of Women, (both by Almog et. al). The chapter on The Parental Journey through Autism Diagnosis (by Dolev), also underscores the importance of this issue.

Successful collaboration between parents and therapists is exemplified in the chapters in part two regarding school refusal (by Zacharia and Pearlman-Avnion), eating patterns (by Peretz and Pearlman-Avnion), educational choices (by Schvarzman-Sinai and Pearlman-Avnion), and sexual education (by Juliusberger and Pearlman-Avnion).

Section three presents chapters highlighting the consistent and meaningful involvement between therapists, parents, and children. The chapter Self-Disclosure and Self-Advocacy (by Dwek and Lowinger) outlines implementation of training procedures for educators and caregivers via a protocol for fostering self-advocacy. The chapter on Identity Development (by Felsenthal-Berger) delineates milestones and challenges over a ten-year period. The chapter Shared Experiences Across Time (by Mizrahi-Zinman) discusses how parents' experiences across past, present, and future time frames impact the autistic child's cognitive, emotional, and social growth.

Part four focuses specifically on the dynamics of collaboration. The chapter on Parent Teacher Collaboration (by Mekayten and Pearlman-Avnion) relates to parental involvement and parent–teacher relationships. The chapter on Enhancing Parental

Involvement (by Moyal and Lowinger) stresses that reaching meaningful collaboration between parent and child requires helping parents overcome their own emotional needs.

This book is designed to serve as a catalyst for transforming the current state of often-unattained collaboration between parents and therapists of autistic children. By meticulously outlining the difficulties faced by parents and by therapists, this book clears the path for meaningful change. It underscores the critical importance of shared commitment and partnership in promoting the progress of individuals on the autism spectrum. Its ultimate vision is to cultivate a future where parents and therapists consistently engage in true partnerships, aligning family priorities with therapy purposes, establishing clear rules of engagement, and optimizing collaboration through shared planning, implementation and evaluation.

Israel Susan Lowinger
Shiri Pearlman-Avnion

References

An, M., & Palisano, R. J. (2014). Family–professional collaboration in pediatric rehabilitation: A practice model. *Disability and Rehabilitation, 36*(5), 434–440. https://doi.org/10.3109/09638288.2013.797510

Burney, V., McCann, C. M., & Arnold-Saritepe, A. (2024). Parent engagement in child-focused interventions: A systematised review of qualitative allied health literature. *Child & Youth Care Forum, 53*(6), 1451–1486. https://doi.org/10.1007/s10566-024-09797-6

Klatte, I. S., Harding, S., & Roulstone, S. (2019). Speech and language therapists' views on parents' engagement in Parent–Child Interaction Therapy (PCIT). *International Journal of Language & Communication Disorders, 54*(4), 553–564. https://doi.org/10.1111/1460-6984.12459

Klatte, I. S., Bloemen, M., de Groot, A., Mantel, T. C., Ketelaar, M., & Gerrits, E. (2024). Collaborative working in speech and language therapy for children with DLD—What are parents' needs? *International Journal of Language & Communication Disorders, 59*(1), 340–353. https://doi.org/10.1111/1460-6984.12951

Contents

About the Editors

Dr. Susan Lowinger is a developmental and clinical psychologist who worked for many years as the Chief Psychologist in Developmental Clinics. She lectured in the Education Department at Bar Ilan University and was head of its adjunct clinic for Children with Autism Spectrum Disorders. In this capacity, Dr. Lowinger oversaw yearly conferences for educators, clinicians, parents and researchers to expand their means of working with children on the spectrum. In addition, she ran a weekly lecture series for the parents and clinicians who worked in the clinic.

In her private practice, Dr. Lowinger works with autistic individuals and their families. In recent years, Dr. Lowinger edited six books about the diagnosis and treatment of autism (the first five were published by Ach Publishers, which focused on children from birth to adulthood). The sixth book, Autism in Adulthood, which she co-edited with Dr. Shiri Pearlman-Avnion, was published by Springer Publishers in 2019, and is about the many facets of autism in adulthood, including diagnosis, employment, residential issues, romantic relationships and sexuality.

Dr. Shiri Pearlman-Avnion is an educational psychologist and lecturer at Tel-Hai Academic College, specializing in autism spectrum disorder, metacognition, theory of mind and social cognition. Her work has been instrumental in advancing the understanding of cognitive and social development among individuals with autism, particularly in the areas of language use, social interaction, and the impact of metacognitive skills on learning outcomes. She held a postdoctoral fellowship (National Alliance for Autism Research, NAAR) at BUMC (Boston University Medical School), Boston, 2002-2005. In addition to her academic role, Dr. Pearlman-Avnion runs a private clinic which focuses on therapy and diagnostics for children, adolescents, and adults with autism. Dr. Pearlman-Avnion has co-edited the book Autism in Adulthood, published by Springer Publishers in 2019, exploring the unique challenges faced by adults on the autism spectrum, and bridging theoretical insights with practical approaches.

Diagnosis and Self-Discovery

Chapter 1
Autism Self-Discovery: Understanding Identity and Building Awareness

Nitsan Almog, Bar Amar - Sahar, Tamir Gabai, and Einat-Haya Keren

Abstract This chapter presents the first empirically derived four-stage model of autistic self-discovery. Our findings reveal four themes that represent the developmental journey beginning long before diagnosis disclosure: (1) early experiences of difference, (2) hidden diagnosis period with intuitive questioning, (3) diagnosis revelation and active meaning-making, and (4) identity integration. The model traces the journey from early, unconscious experiences of difference and a hidden diagnosis period characterized by intuitive questioning, to the transformative process of diagnosis revelation, and finally, the integration of an autistic identity. Analysis identified a two-phase search engine process, where children passively collect clues about their differences before actively investigating following diagnosis disclosure. These findings inform recommendations for clinicians and parents: recognize early signs of difference, provide age-appropriate responses to children's questions, support emotional processing during diagnosis revelation, and facilitate connections with autistic peers during identity development.

Keywords Autism self-discovery · Autism identity · Identity development · Neurodiversity · Diagnosis disclosure · Early autism recognition

Introduction

Identity is a multidisciplinary concept constructed within historical and social contexts that allows individuals to define themselves and others (Bucholtz & Hall, 2005). In recent decades, autistic communities have increasingly conceptualized autism as an identity. Person-first language (a person with autism) was, until recently, widely employed to separate individuals from their autism spectrum disorder (Vivanti, 2020). This linguistic choice reflected the medical model approach adopted by researchers and therapists, who viewed autism as a deficit or disadvantage

N. Almog (✉) · B. Amar - Sahar · T. Gabai · E.-H. Keren
Ono Academic College, Kiryat Ono, Israel
e-mail: nitsan.al@ono.ac.il

S. Lowinger and S. Pearlman-Avnion (eds.), *Collaborative Care and Partnerships in Autism Diagnosis and Treatment*, Autism and Child Psychopathology Series,
https://doi.org/10.1007/978-3-032-07009-8_1

and sought to separate the perceived negative disability from the person (Bury et al., 2023). However, a notable shift has occurred, with autistic individuals reclaiming discourse through identity-first language (autistic person). Jim Sinclair, one of the most influential voices advocating for autism as an identity, asserted as early as 1993 that autism cannot be separated from the person, as it constitutes an essential aspect of their being rather than a removable attribute (Sinclair, 1993).

This philosophical stance has been embraced by autistic individuals, drawing inspiration from two primary socio-political movements. First, the disability rights movement, which, according to the social model, posits that disability results not directly from impairment but from societal constraints (Gil, 2008; Oliver, 2013). Motivated by these principles, autistic individuals worldwide have formed communities characterized by socio-political awareness and shared objectives (Milton, 2014; Owren & Stenhammer, 2013). Second, the neurodiversity paradigm, which proposes a change in attitudes toward autism and divergence in general, acknowledging the wide range of expressions of the human brain, under the view that there are more common and typical brain manifestations, but these are not "healthier" or more "normal" than the less common neurodivergent brain manifestations (Walker, 2014). The terminological shift back to identity-first language represents the autistic attempt to reframe autism as a legitimate neurodivergence and strip it of the tragic, pathologized narrative propagated by the previously unchallenged medical model. In this sense, autistic identity, like other disability identities, is embedded within social context (Dirth & Branscombe, 2018).

Consequently, the discourse surrounding autism as identity has gained attention within the research community. The reconceptualization of autism guided by the neurodiversity paradigm has influenced researchers who explore this topic through their research questions (e.g., Davies et al., 2024), compare autism to other marginalized minority populations (e.g., Shmulsky et al., 2021), or propose alternative terminology such as autism spectrum condition rather than autism spectrum disorder (Mandy & Lai, 2016). Additionally, researchers are promoting these perspectives through qualitative methodologies that provide a platform for autistic voices and collaborating with autistic individuals in research that provides autistic perspectives as well (e.g., Almog et al., 2023; Bury et al., 2023).

Several studies focus specifically on the development of disability identity. Current research indicates that disability identity shapes how disabled individuals perceive themselves and their relationship with the world (Forber-Pratt & Zape, 2017). For disabled individuals, developing a disability identity is associated with self-esteem. It serves as a source of affirmation for personal experiences and has been found to correlate with mental health and well-being (Bogart et al., 2017; Forber-Pratt et al., 2019).

Similar findings apply to autistic identity. Davies et al. (2024) conducted a comprehensive review of autistic identity, identifying studies that address predictors facilitating positive autistic identity development, as well as factors associated with negative attitudes toward autistic identity. Comparable to disability identity, as autistic identity consolidates, it positively influences self-image and psychological well-being (see also Corden et al., 2021).

Although literature regarding the development of autistic identity exists, these studies unanimously reference the moment of diagnostic disclosure as the pivotal turning point enabling autistic identity development. Nevertheless, in multiple studies highlighting autistic voices, the theme of experiencing a sense of difference throughout life, present in early childhood, repeatedly emerges (e.g., Kanfiszer et al., 2017; Mesa & Hamilton, 2022). Moreover, in many cases, autistic individuals' internal search engine activates before parents choose to share with them that they are autistic (Almog et al., 2023). This suggests that while exposure to autism diagnosis represents a significant stage in the development of autistic identity, it is not the first stage.

Autistic individuals approach this stage with certain emotional charge and predispositions regarding autism, their autistic experience, and autistic identity. Some experience self-discovery even prior to the formal autism diagnosis disclosure phase.

Regarding the moment of self-discovery itself, only one relevant academic finding appears in the research literature. Linton's work (2014) references the concept of self-discovery in the context of developing a positive model of autistic identity. In her research, she explains that investigating and learning about autism assisted autistic individuals in these aspects, enabling them to retrospectively analyze their lives and thus view their behaviors and environmental responses in a new light. However, even in this study, the focus on the moment of discovery does not center on reconstructing self-discovery as part of the timeline of autistic identity development. To our knowledge, Mullally et al. (2024) are the only researchers to examine how autistic identity develops among children, yet they too primarily addressed the importance of investigating and learning about autism as predictors of psychological well-being and positive autistic identity formation, without referring to the discovery experience that occurs through investigation and learning.

The current chapter presents a comprehensive analysis of interviews with autistic youth and adults (ages 13–30) and proposes what is, to our knowledge, the first empirically derived four-stage model of autistic identity formation. This model traces the journey from early unconscious experiences of difference, through a hidden diagnosis period characterized by intuitive questioning, to the transformative process of diagnosis revelation, and finally to the integration of an autistic identity.

Research Methods

This study employed a qualitative approach combining grounded theory methodology with emancipatory research principles, positioning autistic individuals as knowledge experts through their lived experiences. The participants included 45 autistic individuals aged 13–30 ($M = 22.37$, $SD = 5.28$), with varying experiences of diagnostic delay between initial diagnosis and discovery. Data were collected through semi-structured interviews, with most conducted by an autistic co-researcher (third author) and the remainder by the first author, creating what Sinclair (2010) describes as an autistic space in those instances where both interviewer and interviewee shared neurotype.

Analysis was performed using MaxQDA24 software, following an inductive coding system developed collaboratively by the research team, which consisted of autistic co-researchers. This approach enhanced both reliability and representation of autistic perspectives throughout the analytical process.

The study received approval from Ono Academic College's Ethics Committee, and participants were allowed to choose whether they preferred to be identified by their real names or pseudonyms.

The full methodological framework, recruitment strategies, interview procedures, and analysis protocols are described in detail in our previous publication (Almog et al., 2024), which presents the broader study from which this chapter derives its findings. For this chapter, only participants who were diagnosed before the age of 18 were included in the analysis.

Participants

The study comprised 45 autistic participants between the ages of 13 and 30 (M = 22.37, SD = 5.28), including 17 females, 26 males, and 2 genderqueer individuals. Participants were diagnosed with autism at a mean age of 7.61 years (SD = 5.37) and discovered their diagnosis at a mean age of 12.17 years (SD = 4.52). A key variable in this study was the diagnostic delay pattern—the temporal gap between receiving a diagnosis and discovering it. Analysis revealed significant group differences. Overall, 42.2% of participants (n = 19) experienced no delay. These are referred to as the immediate disclosure group. Another 6.7% (n = 3) experienced a small delay (1–3 years), 17.8% (n = 8) experienced a medium delay (4–7 years), and 33.3% (n = 15) experienced a long delay of 8 or more years. Together, these are referred to as the delayed disclosure group (57.8%, n = 26). Notably, over a third of participants faced substantial delays of 8 or more years in learning about their diagnosis.

For this chapter, we specifically focused on participants who were diagnosed before the age of 18, allowing us to examine the experiences of autism discovery during childhood and adolescence. This methodological choice distinguishes our study from most existing research on autistic self-discovery, which has primarily concentrated on adult experiences (e.g., Botha et al., 2020; Hens & Langenberg, 2018; Lewis, 2016). By centering on individuals diagnosed during formative developmental periods, we aimed to capture the unique dynamics of identity formation that occur when autism is identified early in life, particularly examining how children and adolescents navigate diagnostic information and integrate it into their emerging sense of self (Table 1.1).

Table 1.1 Interviewee characteristics

Group	Number	Mean Age (SD)	Mean Age at Diagnosis (SD)	Mean Age at Discovery (SD)	Mean Diagnosis-Discovery Gap (SD)
Men	26	22.48 (4.27)	7.00 (4.54)	11.35 (4.26)	4.35 (5.71)
Women	17	21.88 (6.66)	8.50 (6.27)	13.35 (4.85)	4.85 (5.55)
Genderqueer	2	25.00 (2.00)	8.00 (6.00)	12.75 (1.25)	4.75 (4.75)
Total sample	***45***	***22.37 (5.28)***	***7.61 (5.37)***	***12.17 (4.52)***	***4.56 (5.61)***

Self-Discovery Process in Autism: Findings

The process of self-discovery of autism is profoundly personal and private, unfolding within the inner world of the child. This process is shaped by multiple factors: the child's individual characteristics, their surrounding environment (family dynamics, peer relationships, educational settings, therapeutic interactions), and the broader societal discourse about autism and neurodiversity. Self-discovery involves the process of becoming aware of one's own autism, recognizing and understanding personal characteristics, behaviors, and experiences in the context of being autistic.

Based on our analysis of interviews with autistic individuals, we have identified four interconnected stages in this self-discovery journey, though these stages often overlap and individuals may move between them in non-linear ways. These stages include: 1) initial feelings of otherness, where children sense their difference without understanding its source; 2) the hidden diagnosis period, during which children may actively search for explanations for their perceived differences; 3) diagnosis revelation, a transformative process when individuals learn about their autism—a profound experience that goes beyond the initial moment of discovery to encompass deeper understanding, emotional responses, and cognitive reframing of past experiences; and 4) integration of autistic identity, as individuals incorporate their diagnosis into their self-concept and find meaning in their neurodivergent experiences.

As for the self-discovery process of autism diagnosis, it is characterized by early feelings of difference, a period of not knowing and concealment, a gradual process of discovery and understanding, and finally integration of the diagnosis into one's self-identity (Fig. 1.1).

A notable finding emerging from our analysis is the gradual nature of participants' self-awareness regarding their autism. Most participants described a slow, incremental process of understanding their differences through accumulated everyday experiences. This gradual self-awareness often began long before any formal diagnosis, with participants recalling early childhood moments when they first sensed their divergence from peers. As one participant eloquently described, I always felt different, but during adolescence, it began to bother me, and I started asking why

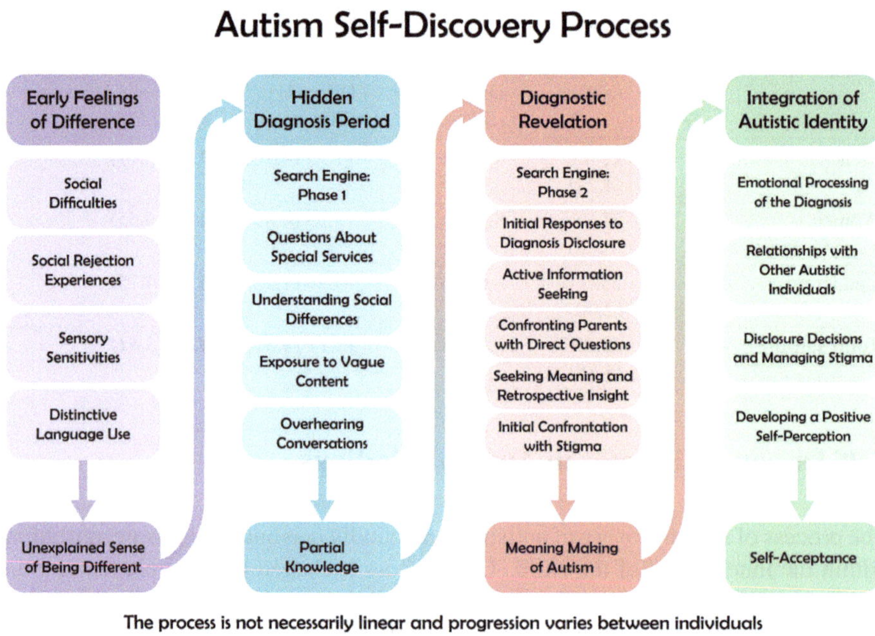

Fig. 1.1 Autism self-discovery process

I feel this way. Many participants expressed that even after the diagnosis revelation, their understanding of how autism manifested in their specific lives continued to evolve over months and years. This ongoing process involved connecting past experiences to new knowledge, reinterpreting social interactions through a neurodivergence lens, and gradually developing language to articulate previously unnamed feelings and perceptions. For many, this cumulative self-awareness represented not just cognitive understanding but an emotional journey that ultimately led to a more coherent and authentic sense of self.The following sections will explore each of the four stages of the autism self-discovery process in detail, examining the specific experiences, challenges, and transitions that characterized participants' journeys toward self-understanding and identity formation.

Early Feelings of Difference

Nearly two-thirds of all participants reported feelings of difference or otherness, prior to discovering their diagnosis, highlighting the centrality of this experience in the narrative of autistic individuals. These experiences provide early indicators of neurodivergence even before formal diagnosis is achieved or communicated. These early experiences of otherness emerge in the form of social difficulties, social rejection experiences, sensory sensitivities, distinctive language use, and an overall unexplained sense of being different from peers. While participants lacked the framework to understand these differences during childhood, these experiences formed the foundation of their self-discovery journey, representing the initial awareness that would later be contextualized through their autism diagnosis.

Analysis of the interviews revealed four key sub-themes within the early experience of otherness, organized below according to their prevalence among participants. Social difficulties were the most prominent characteristic, mentioned by nearly half of the participants (46%). Experiences of social rejection appeared in about one-fifth of the interviews (23%), sensory sensitivities in 16%, and distinctive language use in 7% of participants.

Social Difficulties

Participants consistently identified fundamental challenges in navigating social interactions as primary markers of their early sense of difference. These difficulties manifested as an inherent struggle with the intuitive social understanding that appeared natural to their neurotypical peers. The narratives revealed a developmental pattern wherein social difficulties emerged remarkably early—often during preschool and early elementary years—well before participants possessed the cognitive framework or language to comprehend their autistic identity. As Anthony articulated: "I very much wanted to be friends with people, but I didn't know how to approach them or create interest. Even now, I still don't know how to approach and create interest-it's still difficult for me." This fundamental disconnect between social desire and social capability created significant internal tension. Several participants described their strategic adaptation to social challenges. Thomas demonstrated metacognitive awareness of different social styles within autism: "Among autistic people, it's divided into two types socially- those who really try to make contact in an even quite aggressive way, and those who really avoid it. I belong to the second group. This self-categorization reflects an attempt to understand social differences." Emma highlighted the nuanced distinction between social capability and communication ease: "It's not that I didn't have friends. I did know how to be in social relationships. It's just that the matter of communication came to me less easily in many ways compared to other people." This recognition of comparative difference in social processing emerged as a significant element of pre-diagnostic awareness. These findings suggest that early social difficulties serve not merely as behavioral manifestations of autism but as profound shapers of self-concept and identity formation, with implications for both diagnostic practice and early intervention approaches.

Social Rejection Experiences

Unlike social difficulties, which primarily reflect internal processing challenges, social rejection experiences represent the external manifestation of difference—the concrete instances where neurotypical peers actively excluded, rejected, or marginalized participants. These experiences of social exclusion emerged as powerful early markers of difference, creating formative memories with lasting emotional impact. Kevin described the moment this rejection first became conscious: "In kindergarten, I received the shock of my life… like wow, why don't all these children want to be my friends? What happened?"

This disconnect between social desire and social reality has created profound confusion. Ronald articulated this logical inconsistency: "It was always clear to me that other children treated me differently than they treated each other, and it didn't feel very logical to me, and I didn't understand why." The incomprehensibility of rejection was particularly distressing because participants lacked the conceptual framework to interpret others' behavior without internalizing it as personal failure.

For many participants, rejection extended beyond casual social settings into structured activities. Mark recounted: "It was difficult for me to integrate socially. I was also in a youth movement (Scouts), and it was very, very difficult for me there." His repetition emphasizes the emotional weight of these experiences. The interference with fundamental needs created distress, as Patricia (in the immediate disclosure group) explained: I always loved learning; it was something that always fascinated me. The fact that I would attend school, and the children would prevent me from doing something I really wanted to do, troubled me because I couldn't understand why they were hurting me.

These experiences of rejection created a profound sense of injustice and exclusion that shaped participants' early understanding of themselves as fundamentally different, even before they had words or a diagnosis to explain this difference.

Sensory Sensitivities

Heightened sensory sensitivities emerged as a powerful marker of difference across participants' narratives, with atypical responses to sensory stimuli making ordinary environments challenging or overwhelming. These differences often manifested remarkably early in development, predating linguistic or social markers. In one notable case, Steven, being under 18, was interviewed alongside his mother. During this interview, she noted that her son's sensory difficulties began at seven months, a developmental stage when most parents are just establishing basic routines. This parental perspective demonstrates how sensory regulation difficulties serve as externally observable indicators recognizable to caregivers, often constituting the earliest evidence of neurodivergence. James (in the delayed disclosure group) articulated the multisensory nature of these differences: "Many times, when there's extremely complex noise, or certain types of lighting, or certain smells, or when I feel physical sensations in my fingers, or with something like paper. I have all kinds of different sensitivities." These accounts illuminate how sensory sensitivities directly impacted social participation and created visible markers of difference long before diagnosis. Isabella demonstrated the connection between sensory overwhelm and social limitations: "How do I make a situation stop? If I'm in sensory overload… I can't say 'I need to go for a moment, leave me alone.'" She further crystallized this relationship between sensory processing and unexplained social challenges: "Why doesn't your shirt feel comfortable? Sensory regulation. Why aren't you going to the bat mitzvah? Sensory regulation."

Mary highlighted overwhelming olfactory sensitivities that defied complete articulation: "I'm terribly, terribly sensitive to smells, like any bad smell immediately rises up to my..." Her inability to complete the sentence mirrors the overwhelming nature of the sensory experience itself.

Distinctive Language Use

Language differences emerged as significant markers of autism that participants recognized in themselves prior to diagnosis. Five key patterns were identified: First, advanced or formal language use, exemplified by Abigail: "When I was six, I came back from school. I was at my grandmother's house, and she asked me, 'Hi Abigail, tell me, how was your first day of school?' I told her—she's a pedicurist and had a client—I said, 'I was skeptical.' My grandmother's and the client's mouths dropped open because they were shocked that I spoke like that."

Second, difficulties in understanding social communication or challenges in self-expression, illustrated by Evelyn: "I would say a very confusing sentence and I had to think about how to phrase it so people would understand me." Third, social-communicative barriers despite desire for connection, as Anthony described: "I don't know how to express interest in a person, I don't know how to start a conversation." This highlighted not a lack of interest in others, but rather a gap between his social desires and the communicative tools needed to fulfill them. These shared experiences of difference suggest that the subjective experience of being autistic in a neurotypical world emerges independently of diagnostic knowledge. The sense of otherness appears intrinsic to the autistic experience, although how individuals interpret and integrate these differences into their self-concept varies significantly based on whether diagnostic information is available to them.

The four manifestations of difference described above collectively create a profound yet initially inexplicable sense of otherness in autistic children. These accumulated experiences form a foundation of felt difference that exists prior to diagnosis or conceptual understanding. This awareness of divergence becomes the driving force behind what we term the search engine. As Joseph expressed: "I felt something in me was different, but I didn't know how to call it... It was very difficult to feel I had some kind of difficulty without knowing what to name it." This unnamed difference creates cognitive dissonance and emotional tension that propels children into the first phase of their search for understanding, which will be discussed in the next theme.

Hidden Diagnosis Period—Search Engine: Phase 1

The hidden diagnosis period is characterized by unstructured exploration and attempts to make sense of participants' experiences, involving the operation of what we term the child's search engine first phase. Analysis reveals this critical period of unstructured, often unconscious exploration. This preliminary stage is characterized by a nascent awareness—a subtle recognition that something about their perception, interaction, and experience of the world diverges from their peers or family members, without possessing the language or knowledge to define this divergence.

This first phase operates beneath conscious awareness. Children do not actively seek answers but instead accumulate experiential data—a series of observations, feelings, and partial understandings that gradually construct a mosaic of difference. It is a period marked by intuition rather than explicit investigation, where the individual begins to sense the contours of their unique neurological landscape without yet having the map to navigate it fully. Characteristics of the search engine's first phase include.

Questions about Special Services and Accommodations

Participants described that as children, they noticed their distinctive educational and support experiences, often with a mix of confusion and unspoken questioning. As John wondered, "Why am I in two classes instead of one?" (This is referring to his simultaneous placement in both special education and integration classrooms.) Similarly, William reflected on his unique educational experiences: "I had various tests and needed different...accommodations. I understood that these were not things other children required." Roni recalls her early experiences with personal support: "From age five until the end of elementary school, I was with what I later understood were my personal tutors...as a small child, I didn't know what their role was."

These experiences, though often unaddressed and unexplained by adults, created an unmistakable awareness of difference—a fundamental understanding that their experiences diverged from their peers and siblings, even without the words or framework to comprehend why.

Understanding Social Difference

The landscape of social interaction emerges as a complex terrain of difference and confusion for the participants, for some even before any formal diagnosis. This awareness of social divergence manifests through a nuanced, often unspoken recognition of one's unique social experience.

For many participants, social difference was not a singular moment of realization, but a gradual accumulation of experiences that highlighted their distinctive social processing.Nancy describes this experience: "What happened was that I tried to connect with groups of people my age, and it didn't work out well for me. I found myself alone a lot during breaks, with at most one or two friends, but these connections never lasted long." Her narrative reveals a profound sense of social isolation, where attempts at connection were fleeting and ultimately unsuccessful.

Richard provides an equally stark portrayal of social marginalization: Then came elementary school, from which I have very strong memories—memories of people who didn't like me. His experience illuminates the harsh social hierarchies that often exclude autistic pupils, creating a sense of outsiderness. Michael captures the fundamental nature of this difference more abstractly: I knew I was different. I felt the gap between me and the others; the functioning level was different. This sentiment echoes across many narratives–a deep understanding of social difference that precedes linguistic or diagnostic explanation. These experiences are characterized by a continuous, often painful process of recognizing one's social distinctiveness.

Exposure to Vague Content

The search engine's first phase is marked by seemingly random encounters that trigger moments of partial recognition–fragmentary insights that hint at, but do not fully illuminate, the individual's autistic experience. These encounters serve as cryptic signals, offering glimpses into a broader understanding that remains just beyond comprehension. Thomas provides a quintessential example of this ambiguous exposure: "My mother once told me to watch an Arthur episode with a character with Asperger's...I didn't understand the connection between me and this Carl character." This moment encapsulates the preliminary stage of recognition, yet it remains unclear and undefined. Later, at the age of 10, he described: "My parents told me I have attention deficit and that's why I take Ritalin, but I didn't understand that this was Asperger's."

These encounters are not straightforward moments of understanding, but rather complex intersections of partial information, personal experience, and emerging self-awareness.

John relates: "I was always in a small class and didn't understand what it meant, who knows what. Then, I didn't really care that I was in a small class, I just tried to integrate with everyone, and then some pupil at school asked me: 'Are you from the special ed (therapeutic) class?'"

The exposure to vague content presented from another pupil, outside the family and professional context, yet still containing information regarding John's identity, contributed to participants' questions about their own narratives.

Overhearing Conversations

Fragments of information begin to accumulate, often through inadvertent exposure. Emma recalls a telling classroom moment: "Once in a class, someone in my grade asked why I have a tutor, and the teacher simply said, 'That's not your business'". Such fleeting encounters become subtle markers of difference, offering glimpses into a world not fully understood. When asked in our interview about her early feelings of difference, Mia recalled an experience involving a conversation between her mother and teacher while she was present: "It happened when I was little, in kindergarten, I was already like, the teacher told my mom that…that there were all kinds of instances where I wasn't playing with the children's group and such. This was in the second special education kindergarten I was in. She didn't exactly say autism, but she talked about the characteristics while I was right there listening."

This fragmented conversation exemplifies the ambiguous and confusing nature of autism disclosure, where the information is presented partially and without clear context, leaving the individual bewildered and uncertain about the meaning and implications of the diagnosis. These partial revelations create a landscape of confusion, where children sense something distinctive about themselves without having a clear framework to comprehend their experiences.

In other cases, the confrontation stems from accidental discovery of the diagnosis, as Abigail. recounts: "They didn't tell me. I was diagnosed at 11 and discovered it by accident at 14... My parents were talking about it, and I overheard, so I came and asked."

This pattern of accidental discovery indicates the communication gap within the family regarding the diagnosis and the parents' difficulty in managing open conversation about the topic. Christopher shared a pivotal moment of accidental disclosure: It was during the summer vacation after sixth grade, and there were landline phones, you know, where you could listen in on any conversation. By chance, I came to call my friend to ask if I could come over, and... ummm... I heard my mother saying to another mother that I'm like on the spectrum."

The quote captures a child overhearing a conversation about their own diagnosis, highlighting the often unintentional and indirect ways children first encounter information about their diagnosis. The phrase like on the spectrum is particularly nuanced, suggesting a tentative, not-yet-fully-acknowledged understanding of the diagnosis.

The hidden diagnosis period was described by participants as emotional and sensory–a lived experience of otherness that precedes cognitive understanding. Children collect these fragments of experience, storing them like pieces of a puzzle they cannot yet assemble, waiting for the moment when context, language, and self-awareness will allow them to see the complete picture.

Diagnostic Revelation and Search Engine: Phase 2

The moment of diagnosis revelation is rarely a singular, definitive event, but rather a complex, deeply personal journey of self-understanding. Participants described learning about their diagnosis as a nuanced process that transcends a simple conversation or clinical report. It is a transformative experience that interweaves personal awareness, familial dynamics, professional insights, and individual emotional processing. Each participant's path to understanding is unique —some discover their diagnosis through careful parental explanations, others through accidental encounters with diagnostic documents, and some through conversations with professionals or educational staff.

The revelation is not merely about receiving information but about constructing a new framework of personal identity. Following this revelation and once they receive the right keywords, participants typically enter a second phase of their search engine, characterized by active exploration and meaning-making, rather than the passive observation that marked the first phase.

Initial Responses to Diagnosis Disclosure

Participants exhibited diverse initial reactions to learning about their diagnosis, ranging from immediate relief to complex resistance. These initial responses represent the starting point of an ongoing process of identity integration.

Relief and Validation

For most participants, receiving a diagnosis explanation provided immediate relief and validation of their life experiences. This initial reaction often centered around finally having an explanation for lifelong feelings of difference. Abigail eloquently articulates this sense of immediate relief: "It wasn't about asking questions but rather that I finally understood, I could breathe again, I understood why I felt the way I did. It gave me breathing room to understand - okay, there's something here. I'm not... it's not... it's not weird. There's a diagnosis for this. That's what liberated me, gave me some breathing room, and helped me."

This validation of previous experiences represents a crucial first step in the integration process, as it transforms unexplained feelings of difference into a contextualized understanding of one's autistic identity. George describes a moment of cognitive clarity: "Suddenly 'ah,' and then I saw what it actually meant, and I was like: oh, and it made much more sense." This sentiment of increased coherence in one's life narrative appears consistently across interviews.

Denial and Rejection

In contrast, a subset of participants initially responded with denial or rejection of their diagnosis. This reaction often manifested as an unwillingness to accept the diagnosis as applicable to themselves. Charles describes an immediate rejection: "After the conversation I was very afraid, I was convinced it wasn't true, and then there was a day I went to my mom, wanting to tell her 'Mom, don't believe dad, I'm not really autistic.'" Similarly, Nancy recounts her defensive response: "After checking, I simply threw the papers aside and told myself: no, I'm like everyone else and everything is fine. I went on with my life."

For some, the denial was rooted in concerns about stigma or negative implications. Ronald described a specific fear related to visibility and identification: During this period when I thought autism was something bad, it somewhat made me afraid if it was so easy to identify. Those who know how to identify it can do so very easily because you can't hide it. His reflection reveals the profound vulnerability felt when first confronting the possibility that characteristics previously perceived as personal quirks might now be recognized by others as symptoms of autism.

Active Information Seeking

Following diagnosis revelation, participants typically engage in deliberate, often intensive information gathering about autism, driven by a deep need to understand themselves. This process represents a critical meaning-making endeavor, integrating abstract diagnostic information into personal narrative.

Participants described actively researching autism through various channels, predominantly online resources. Paul explains, "I started searching and discovered, googling what autism is and then understood that I have a condition, Asperger's, various things..." This statement illustrates the transition from receiving a diagnostic label to actively seeking to understand its implications.

Sophia offers insight into the investigative nature of this phase: "I remember reading the diagnosis, but I didn't understand what it meant. I remember entering the internet, reading what it is, what its meaning is, what it says and what the results are and what the difficulties are. Really reading everything." This active yet uncertain searching characterizes the initial phase of diagnosis revelation. In Sophia's case, she discovered her diagnostic documents independently and never had a formal discussion about it with her parents. In a later interview, she described her upbringing as Soviet education due to the lack of information and closed family environment. Consequently, she had to process the information independently and contemplate its implications for her identity.

Confronting Parents with Direct Questions

A significant stage in the active search process that occurs after exposure to diagnosis is manifested in direct confrontation with parents. This stage involves challenging family narratives and demanding transparency about concealed information, revealing emotional complexity in family negotiations. In many cases (25), discovering that parents hid the diagnosis evokes anger and resentment, as Richard describes: "I deeply hated my parents for not telling me earlier. I asked them: How long have you known this? They said they've known for several years." The confrontation represents a turning point in family power dynamics, where the child demands their right to information about themselves and challenges decisions made on their behalf but without their involvement.

Interestingly, not all participants direct their questions toward parents. Some describe seeking information from other trusted adults when family communication channels are limited or uncomfortable. Thomas explains, "I understood this in seventh grade, and then started asking more questions about it. [Who did you ask?] Mostly... also... primarily my teachers who handled my case. With my parents, I think I talked about it less." This redirection of information-seeking behavior highlights two important patterns: first, the child's agency in finding alternative sources of knowledge when parental communication is insufficient, and second, the critical role that those educational professionals can play as informational resources during this sensitive period of identity development.

Seeking Meaning and Retrospective Insight

The diagnosis serves as a powerful interpretive key, enabling participants to reunderstand their personal history through a new explanatory framework. This process represents a crucial cognitive reorganization of autobiographical memory, as individuals systematically reassess their life experiences in light of their newly acquired diagnostic knowledge.

Participants consistently described using their newfound diagnostic knowledge to create an organized understanding of their behaviors, experiences, and difficulties. The diagnosis serves as a conceptual scaffold that brings order to previously disconnected experiences. Emma described this moment of recognition: "It was like–aha! Now many things make sense. Many behaviors, many sensations I experienced over the years suddenly had a clear context." This retrospective reframing represents a profound psychological transformation, as previously fragmented experiences coalesce into a coherent autobiographical narrative.

Participants described moments of profound realization as they began to revisit past experiences through the lens of their autism diagnosis. These revelations often took the form of sudden insight regarding previously puzzling situations or reactions. Isabella described such a moment of recognition during a psychological assessment: There was a moment with my psychologist where she showed me pictures, asking me to understand what's happening there, and I said–I know what I'm supposed to say, but what I see here is different. This statement captures the moment when she recognizes the distinctive nature of her perceptual processing–a recognition only possible after acquiring the diagnostic framework.

The retrospective assessment process facilitates the identification of previously unrecognized patterns that have spanned the individual's life. Participants described suddenly connecting disparate experiences that, when viewed through the autism framework, revealed consistent themes or characteristics. Mia articulated this pattern recognition: "When I looked back at my behaviors, I realized this explains many things." This statement demonstrates how retrospective assessment allows individuals to see continuities in their experiences that were previously invisible to them, creating a more coherent self-narrative.

Initial Confrontation with Stigma

Many participants described experiencing significant internal conflict upon first learning about their diagnosis, predominantly related to concerns about stigma and social perception. These immediate emotional responses precede any cognitive processing or strategic thinking about how to manage the diagnosis in social contexts.

For many participants, these initial responses to potential stigmatization were dominated by fear, confusion, and uncertainty rather than clear strategies. As Charles describes: "After the conversation I was very afraid, I was convinced it wasn't true." Other participants described initial denial or rejection of the diagnosis itself as a form of protection against stigma.

The initial cognitive processing of stigma during diagnosis revelation typically involves black-and-white thinking and immediate associations with negative stereotypes, rather than nuanced understanding. This represents an early, unprocessed response to the social implications of the diagnosis, which will later evolve into more sophisticated identity management strategies during the integration stage.

The second phase of the search engine represents a fundamental shift in the individual's relationship with their autism and themselves. Unlike the first phase characterized by undefined questioning and intuitive sensing of difference, this second phase features focused exploration with a clear objective: to understand the profound meaning of the diagnosis and its implications for identity and life.

Integration of Autistic Identity

The integration of autistic identity represents the fourth and final stage in the self-discovery process. This stage is characterized by a long-term process that may last years or even a lifetime, during which the individual incorporates the diagnosis into their self-concept and develops a consolidated self-perception. Comprehensive analysis of interviews with autistic individuals reveals several key characteristics that define this integration stage, which focus on the ongoing emotional processing and gradual development of a positive autistic identity.

Emotional Processing of the Diagnosis

Following initial reactions, participants described a period of emotional processing characterized by ambivalence and a non-linear movement between acceptance and rejection of the diagnosis. This intermediate phase represents an important transitional period in identity development.

For many, there was an initial resistance or rejection that gradually gave way to acceptance. William articulates this struggle: "I was ashamed of myself, angry at myself, because I didn't understand why this had to happen specifically to me... it's terribly easy to lose yourself and fall into a state of frustration and not think positive things about yourself." This pattern of initial rejection followed by gradual acceptance appeared frequently across interviews, particularly among those who discovered the diagnosis in adolescence (due to a parental disclosure delay or due to late diagnosis).

For some, the denial persisted over extended periods but eventually transformed into acceptance. Mary admits, "I denied the diagnosis for many years... I wasn't willing. I did everything normally, I denied it and didn't like it, and I didn't understand exactly how I was diagnosed." In the same interview, Mary continued to describe how, after years of denial, she eventually came to terms with her diagnosis: "Today I understand that this is part of me."

Robert describes a similar journey from resistance to acceptance: "I wanted to be a normal person, like everyone else. But it doesn't work, and it didn't work. When I learned to accept this label, I felt that it wasn't part of me." This reflection highlights how acceptance is rarely immediate but rather develops gradually through a process of internal negotiation. Robert mentioned that today he gives presentations in schools to promote autism awareness, demonstrating how his relationship with his diagnosis evolved from rejection to advocacy.

This resistance often stemmed from concerns about stigma or negative implications. However, the longitudinal nature of our interviews revealed that most participants eventually developed a more nuanced and accepting relationship with their diagnosis, even when initial reactions were strongly negative.

Relationships with Other Autistic Individuals

Meeting other autistic individuals represents a significant milestone in the process of integrating autistic identity. Our findings show that encounters with other autistics can serve as a powerful catalyst for self-identity development. For many, this is their first opportunity to feel understood, experience belonging, and engage in unmasking—the removal of masks they typically wear in relationships with neurotypical individuals.

Isabella describes a defining moment when she met another autistic friend: "He suddenly said 'Yes, I'm autistic' and I was like 'Me too!!!!' [...] It was a very emotional moment for me- now I didn't have to pretend... I needed to play-act much less with him than I do with others." The expression of removing masks appears in various forms throughout many interviews, reflecting the ongoing effort many autistic individuals invest in camouflaging their autistic characteristics in neurotypical environments.

Many participants emphasized the importance of organized social groups designed for autistic individuals: Most of my friends are from the spectrum. I got to know them in the larger "FRIENDS" group in my hometown city during high school (Roni). David describes a gradual process of connection: "It felt a bit awkward at times but then I met the friend I told you about who was functioning at my level, and I really had a language for how to talk with him." For others, such groups provided a source for meaningful friendships, as Richard described: "Once a week I went to 'FOR YOU' and met...with young people on the autism spectrum, and it was wonderful. [...] That's also where I met my best friend. He's really my best friend."

However, there is also complexity in these relationships. Some participants find it difficult to identify with others on the spectrum, and some even create separation and functional ranking between themselves and other autistic individuals. Anthony describes ambivalence: "With all the pain, I prefer to be friends with neurotypicals rather than autistics, because I haven't met many autistic people whose reaction to everything is as moderate as mine, or at least moderate in my view." James describes a dynamic of distancing from a broader autistic group identity: "I didn't really want to be in the same category as them, and the separate category of Asperger's syndrome kind of gave me satisfaction that there's a separate niche that I belong to."

Linda describes an internal process of hierarchy: "I think sometimes I make a differentiation between people even here at the preparatory program and myself, when I see them functioning at a lower level and I'm functioning at a higher level and I see myself as more elevated, more like... I tell myself I'm almost like normal people. I'm in between, I'm almost not autistic." These testimonies reflect the tension between the need to belong to a community and the desire to distance oneself from stigmas that may be attributed to autistic people.

Disclosure Decisions and Managing Stigma

As individuals progress in their identity integration, they develop more sophisticated approaches to managing disclosure and navigating potential stigma. The process involves complex decisions about when, how, and to whom they disclose their diagnosis, reflecting both their level of self-acceptance and their assessment of potential social responses.

Daniel describes his personal process: "I feel that I'm on the autism spectrum, for example, when I repeat things, when I repeat myself, when I speak in repetitive speech, which is what indicates that I'm on the spectrum... It's actually good to share... because this is who I am and...that's why it's important that people know I'm on the spectrum, to come out of the closet a bit with these things." This approach reflects a level of self-acceptance where disclosure becomes an act of authenticity.

Other participants still hesitate to disclose autism, as Barbara explains: "I felt there are a lot of stigmas about being on the spectrum. I prefer to share as little as possible because I feel there's a lot of aversion toward people on the spectrum." This statement reflects ongoing considerations about vulnerability and self-protection in social contexts where autism remains stigmatized.

Both Peter and Mia demonstrate carefully considered disclosure strategies focused on audience selection. Peter articulates a pragmatic approach: "I would share more with people who wouldn't treat me differently... With professionals who I felt wouldn't have too much prejudice. Similarly, Mia emphasizes disclosing to informed audiences: "I want to tell people who understand these definitions, not people who don't understand these definitions." These participants consciously evaluate potential recipients of disclosure based on their perceived knowledge and attitudes, revealing understanding of how different audiences might respond to information about their autism.

Kevin describes a different approach: "Anyone I don't know how to talk to who wants to enter a relationship with me; I tell them upfront: I'm autistic. If that deters you, you're welcome to leave." This direct approach reflects growing comfort with one's identity and a shift toward placing responsibility for acceptance on others rather than attempting to mask autistic traits.These strategic disclosure decisions represent an important form of self-advocacy and indicate growing agency in how individuals choose to present and express their autistic identity in different social contexts.

Developing a Positive Self-Perception

The journey toward accepting autism as part of one's identity often culminates in recognizing its positive aspects and eventually viewing it as an integral and valuable part of oneself. Many participants developed a positive perception of their autism over time.

Abigail eloquently expresses this perspective: "I see advantages in being autistic. Like, being specialized in things. When I fixate on something, I know it well... it's a gift to me. It's something that represents me, and I love myself... Autism isn't a problem; it's a gift."

Richard frames his autism as "An advantage in a world of people without advantages... I take the benefits of autism, the fact that I'm very genuine and honest—something many people don't have—and I simply express it. People see this and understand there's something special here, and they accept it."

Some participants described autism as an inseparable part of their identity, a fundamental element of how they see the world and how the world sees them. For many of them, this acceptance evolves into seeing autism as simply a different neurological variation, neither inherently positive nor negative. As Charlotte explains: "I talk about it just like I talk about any other part of who I am- it's just another part of my history, my character... it's just one thing out of a million things that I'm part of." Michael articulates a fundamental sense of worth: "Inside, I feel like an equal person".

This final stage of developing a positive self-perception represents the culmination of the integration process, where autism becomes neither something to overcome nor something that defines one's entire identity, but rather an integral and valued aspect of a multifaceted self.Most participants developed a positive perception of their autism over time. The ultimate outcome of the fourth stage is genuine self-acceptance, where individuals embrace their authentic autistic identity as part of their whole, complete, and worthy selves.

Methodological Note

It is important to note that this model is based on retrospective accounts. Participants who contributed to this study have reached an advanced stage of identity integration, which inevitably colors their interpretation of earlier experiences. The emancipatory methodology of this research itself represents a practice of forming and establishing autistic identity—the opportunity to tell one's own story.

Discussion

This study presents the first empirically derived four-stage model of autistic self-discovery process, highlighting the complex interplay between personal experience, familial communication, and broader societal narratives. Our findings significantly expand the existing literature on disability identity development by demonstrating that the process begins long before formal diagnosis disclosure—a critical insight that contradicts previous assumptions in autism research that positioned diagnosis revelation as the starting point of identity formation (Davies et al., 2024; Mullally et al., 2024).

The self-discovery process in autism represents a profound journey that significantly impacts how individuals understand themselves and their place in the world. By recognizing and supporting this process, professionals can move beyond traditional expert-driven models toward truly collaborative partnerships that honor the autonomy, agency, and lived experience of autistic individuals.

The model presented here offers a framework for more developmentally appropriate approaches to diagnosis communication that recognize children as active agents in their own identity development rather than passive recipients of medical information. This aligns with emerging literature on the importance of investigating and learning about autism as predictors of psychological well-being and positive identity formation (Linton, 2014; Mullally et al., 2024).

Our findings highlight the complex interplay between internal self-discovery processes and external disclosure practices, providing crucial insights for more supportive and developmentally appropriate approaches to autism diagnosis communication. The analysis demonstrates that integrating an autism diagnosis into one's identity is a complex, individualized process that unfolds gradually over time, with significant variation in how individuals navigate this emotional terrain.

Unlike most previous studies on autistic identity that focus on adult experiences (Botha et al., 2020; Hens & Langenberg, 2018; Lewis, 2016), our focus on individuals diagnosed before age 18 provides a unique perspective on how autism diagnosis is processed during critical developmental periods. This approach illuminates the experiences of those who must integrate their diagnosis while simultaneously navigating the complex identity formation processes of childhood and adolescence.

When children experience differences without an appropriate explanatory framework, they may internalize feelings of inadequacy and otherness. The model can assist in identifying the early stages and the child's search engine in action and provide reliable, age-appropriate information. Early recognition of these patterns, combined with strengths-based approaches, could potentially transform these early experiences of otherness from sources of distress into foundations for positive identity development and self-understanding.

The analysis reveals a two-phase process of searching for meaning and self-understanding. While the first phase is characterized by intuitive and unconscious searching, where the central question is what is different about me?, the second phase develops after exposure to the diagnosis, when the question transforms into what does this diagnosis mean for me?

During the first phase, children collect clues and signals about their differences through passive observation. This is a stage of vague feelings and internal questions, in comparison to the second stage, which includes active searching and direct questioning. A central part of the second phase is the confrontation with parents, reflecting a deeper process of identity formation and independence. When children confront their parents, they are essentially asking to actively participate in constructing the narrative of their lives, taking ownership of their personal story, and transforming themselves from passive objects of medical and educational decisions to active subjects in the process of shaping their identity.

In the diagnosis revelation stage, time and space are needed for emotional processing and active exploration of the diagnosis's meaning. During the integration stage, professionals can facilitate connections with peer groups and help develop a positive self-perception. It is particularly important to remember that the timing and manner of diagnosis disclosure should be individually tailored, considering the person's psychological readiness and their family and cultural context. An affirmative approach that considers these stages of self-discovery can support the development of a positive and integrated autistic identity.

The analysis suggests that despite the complexity and ambivalence that sometimes accompanies relationships between autistic individuals, meeting similar others provides a unique opportunity for self-understanding and a sense of belonging that is not possible in other spaces. Organized frameworks such as support groups provide an important platform for meetings between autistic individuals, enabling the formation of social connections in a structured and supportive environment.

The integration stage involves complex decisions about when, how, and to whom individuals disclose their diagnosis. These strategic choices reflect both levels of self-acceptance and assessments of potential stigma. As participants progress through the integration process, many develop adaptive skills and the ability to advocate for themselves. Disclosure decisions evolve over time, often becoming less restrictive as individuals develop greater self-acceptance and better strategies for managing potential negative reactions.

The final stage in the self-discovery process is characterized by the development of an integrative autistic identity. In this stage, participants transition from experiencing their differences as arbitrary personal failures to understanding them as coherent manifestations of their autistic identity. For many, this transition provides profound relief—not because it changes their experiences, but because it transforms how those experiences are interpreted and integrated into their sense of self. This process marks the completion of the transformation from vague feelings of difference to contextualized self-knowledge, from disconnected experiences to a coherent autobiographical narrative. It represents the transition from passive experiencing to active meaning-making, from confusion to clarity, and from isolation to potential connection with a broader autistic community.

Recommendations for Parents and Professionals

The findings of this study suggest important clinical implications both for professionals working with autistic individuals and for parents. Understanding the four stages of the self-discovery process can help support this process more effectively.

Our research findings provide practical guidance for parents and professionals seeking to support the self-discovery process of autistic children. These recommendations are based on understanding the four stages of the process and how to support children through transitions between them:

1. Early Experiences of Difference: Identify early signs of otherness and offer positive language to explain these differences. When children express feelings of social difference, sensory sensitivities, or communication challenges, treat these as legitimate expressions of neurodiversity rather than deficits.
2. Hidden Diagnosis Period: Be attentive to the child's search engine that operates even before formal knowledge of the diagnosis. When children ask questions about the services they receive or differences between themselves and others, respond with age-appropriate honesty rather than assuming they are not ready for information.
3. Diagnosis Revelation: Provide reliable, age-appropriate information while allowing time and space for emotional processing. Support the child's active information seeking and need to understand the diagnosis in the context of their life.

4. Integration of Autistic Identity: Encourage connections with others on the spectrum, respect the child's decisions regarding self-disclosure, and support the development of a positive self-perception.

Conclusion: Toward a more Collaborative Model

By understanding and supporting the stages of self-discovery, professionals and families can become more effective partners in the self-discovery journey, moving from models focused primarily on symptom management to holistic approaches that value authentic self-expression, positive identity development, and quality of life as defined by autistic individuals themselves. This approach honors the fundamental premise of both the neurodiversity paradigm and disability rights movement: that autistic individuals should be active participants in shaping not only their personal narratives but also broader societal understandings of autism itself.

References

Almog, N., Kassel, O., Levy, N., & Gabai, T. (2023). Mapping the dilemmas parents face with disclosing autism diagnosis to their child. *Journal of Autism and Developmental Disorders, 53*(10), 4060–4075. https://doi.org/10.1007/s10803-022-05711-y

Almog, N., Keren, E. H., Gabai, T., & Kassel, O. (2024). Autistic people's perspectives on parental diagnosis disclosure: A grounded theory study. *Journal of Autism and Developmental Disorders, 1–15.* https://doi.org/10.1007/s10803-024-06468-2

Bogart, K. R., Rottenstein, A., Lund, E. M., & Bouchard, L. (2017). Who self-identifies as disabled? An examination of impairment and contextual predictors. *Rehabilitation Psychology, 62*(4), 553–562. https://doi.org/10.1037/rep0000132

Botha, M., Dibb, B., & Frost, D. M. (2020). "Autism is me": An investigation of how autistic individuals make sense of autism and stigma. *Disability & Society, 37*(4), 427–453. https://doi.org/10.1080/09687599.2020.1822782

Bucholtz, M., & Hall, K. (2005). Identity and interaction: A sociocultural linguistic approach. *Discourse Studies, 7*(4–5), 585–614. https://doi.org/10.1177/1461445605054407

Bury, S. M., Jellett, R., Spoor, J. R., & Hedley, D. (2023). "It defines who I am" or "it's something I have": What language do [autistic] Australian adults [on the autism spectrum] prefer? *Journal of Autism and Developmental Disorders, 53*(2), 677–687. https://doi.org/10.1007/s10803-020-04425-3

Corden, K., Brewer, R., & Cage, E. (2021). Personal identity after an autism diagnosis: Relationships with self-esteem, mental wellbeing, and diagnostic timing. *Frontiers in Psychology, 12*, 699335. https://doi.org/10.3389/fpsyg.2021.699335

Davies, J., Cooper, K., Killick, E., Sam, E., Healy, M., Thompson, G., Mandy, W., Redmayne, B., & Crane, L. (2024). Autistic identity: A systematic review of quantitative research. *Autism Research, 17*(5), 874–897. https://doi.org/10.1002/aur.3105

Dirth, T. P., & Branscombe, N. R. (2018). The social identity approach to disability: Bridging disability studies and psychological science. *Psychological Bulletin, 144*(12), 1300–1324. https://doi.org/10.1037/bul0000156

Forber-Pratt, A. J., Mueller, C. O., & Andrews, E. E. (2019). Disability identity and allyship in rehabilitation psychology: Sit, stand, sign, and show up. *Rehabilitation Psychology, 64*(2), 119–129. https://doi.org/10.1037/rep0000256

Forber-Pratt, A. J., & Zape, M. P. (2017). Disability identity development model: Voices from the ADA-generation. *Disability and Health Journal, 10*(2), 350–355. https://doi.org/10.1016/j.dhjo.2016.12.013

Gil, R. (2008). Thinking differently about autism: An insider's perspective on society's attitudes and the education system for autism in Israel in the first decade of the 21st century. *Activists of the Autistic Community in Israel.* https://www.acisrael.org/thinkdiff.pdf

Hens, K., & Langenberg, R. (2018). Experiences of adults following an autism diagnosis. *Palgrave Pivot Cham.* https://doi.org/10.1007/978-3-319-97973-1

Kanfiszer, L., Davies, F., & Collins, S. (2017). 'I was just so different': The experiences of women diagnosed with an autism spectrum disorder in adulthood in relation to gender and social relationships. *Autism, 21*(6), 661–669. https://doi.org/10.1177/1362361316687987

Lewis, L. F. (2016). Exploring the experience of self-diagnosis of autism spectrum disorder in adults. *Archives of Psychiatric Nursing, 30*(5), 575–580. https://doi.org/10.1016/j.apnu.2016.03.009

Linton, K. F. (2014). Clinical diagnoses exacerbate stigma and improve self-discovery according to people with autism. *Social Work in Mental Health, 12*(4), 330–342. https://doi.org/10.1080/15332985.2013.861383

Mandy, W., & Lai, M. C. (2016). Annual research review: The role of the environment in the developmental psychopathology of autism spectrum condition. *Journal of Child Psychology and Psychiatry, and Allied Disciplines, 57*(3), 271–292. https://doi.org/10.1111/jcpp.12501

Mesa, S., & Hamilton, L. G. (2022). "We are different, that's a fact, but they treat us like we're different-er": Understandings of autism and adolescent identity development. *Advances in Autism, 8*(3), 217–231. https://doi.org/10.1108/AIA-12-2020-0071

Milton, D. E. M. (2014). Autistic expertise: A critical reflection on the production of knowledge in autism studies. *Autism, 18*(7), 794–802. https://doi.org/10.1177/1362361314525281

Mullally, S. L., Edwards, C. C., Wood, A. E., Connolly, S. E., Constable, H., Watson, S., & Rodgers, J. (2024). "I like being autistic": Assessing the benefit of autistic-led psychoeducation for autistic children. *medRxiv.* https://doi.org/10.1101/2024.07.12.24310317

Oliver, M. (2013). The social model of disability: Thirty years on. *Disability & Society, 28*(7), 1024–1026. https://doi.org/10.1080/09687599.2013.818773

Owren, T., & Stenhammer, T. (2013). Neurodiversity: Accepting autistic difference. *Learning Disability Practice, 16*(4), 32–37. https://doi.org/10.7748/ldp2013.05.16.4.32.e681

Shmulsky, S., Gobbo, K., Donahue, A., & Klucken, F. (2021). Do neurodivergent college students forge a disability identity? A snapshot and implications. *Journal of Postsecondary Education and Disability, 34*(1), 53–63.

Sinclair, J. (1993). Don't mourn for us. *Our Voice, 1*(3), 1–5. https://philosophy.ucsc.edu/SinclairDontMournForUs.pdf

Sinclair, J. (2010). Cultural commentary: Being autistic together. *Disability Studies Quarterly, 30*(1) https://doi.org/10.18061/dsq.v30i1.1075

Vivanti, G. (2020). Ask the editor: What is the most appropriate way to talk about individuals with a diagnosis of autism? *Journal of Autism and Developmental Disorders, 50*(2), 691–693. https://doi.org/10.1007/s10803-019-04280-x

Walker, N. (2014, September 27). Neurodiversity: Some basic terms and definitions. *Neurocosmopolitanism.* https://neuroqueer.com/neurodiversity-terms-and-definitions/.

Chapter 2
The Parental Journey through Autism Diagnosis: Experiences of Acceptance, Support, and Cultural Sensitivity

Smadar Dolev

Abstract Receiving an autism spectrum disorder (ASD) diagnosis is a profoundly challenging journey for parents, often marked by prolonged uncertainty, anxiety, and significant life shifts. This compelling chapter provides an in-depth exploration of this complex process, from initial suspicions to the crucial stage of acceptance. It delves into the dilemma of early versus delayed diagnosis, highlighting the benefits of timely intervention alongside the emotional difficulties parents face. Drawing on the Reaction to Diagnosis Interview (RDI), the chapter distinguishes between "resolved" and "unresolved" parental acceptance, illustrating how this emotional state profoundly impacts the parent-child relationship and overall well-being. Unresolved grief can hinder effective caregiving, while resolution fosters secure attachment and sensitive responses. Crucially, this work reveals the immense influence of professional involvement, emphasizing the need for empathy, clear communication, comprehensive guidance, and ongoing emotional support to navigate this period. The chapter provides vital insights and practical implications to better support parents in fostering a positive, integrated family life following an ASD diagnosis.

Keywords Diagnostic process · Parental acceptance · Resolution of diagnosis · Early intervention · Parental emotions · Professional support

Introduction

Receiving a diagnosis of a significant developmental disorder, such as autism spectrum disorder (ASD), is an immensely challenging experience for parents. ASDs are often diagnosed during infancy or early childhood, and at times only during middle childhood. Consequently, the process of recognizing that there is a significant developmental difficulty, as well as formally diagnosing it, can take several months or even

S. Dolev (✉)
University of Haifa, Haifa, Israel
e-mail: smadar_d@oranim.ac.il

S. Lowinger and S. Pearlman-Avnion (eds.), *Collaborative Care and Partnerships in Autism Diagnosis and Treatment*, Autism and Child Psychopathology Series,
https://doi.org/10.1007/978-3-032-07009-8_2

years (Brian et al., 2019; Hine et al., 2018; Stasik et al., 2024). This process typically begins with parents' initial sense that their child may have a developmental problem, noticing that their child's development is atypical, and recognizing differences in their child's functioning compared to peers. In many cases, it is the parents (particularly the mother) who first notice these difficulties in their child's development. In other instances, it is a relative, a nurse, a preschool teacher, or an occupational therapist who notices the child's difficulties and brings them to the parents' attention.

The process of diagnosing a child with autism varies from family to family and involves significant differences in the time taken to initiate the diagnostic process and the number of professionals involved. During this process parents often experience anxiety, uncertainty, and difficulty in understanding the child's behavior.

In the current chapter, we aim to understand the significance of early vs. late diagnosis for parents of children with ASD. Testimonies from parents regarding their experiences following the diagnosis will be presented, and questions will be raised regarding the recommended approaches to delivering this diagnosis to parents. Subsequently, we will examine the concept of parental acceptance of the diagnosis through studies utilizing the "Reaction to Diagnosis Interview" (Marvin & Pianta, 1996) to assess parents' resolution of the diagnosis. The association between parents' resolution of the diagnosis and the quality of their relationship with their child will be explored. Finally, we will discuss the importance of the quality and nature of professional involvement in supporting and guiding families toward acceptance of the diagnosis.

Early Diagnosis of Children with ASD: Should the Process Be As Short as Possible?

Professionals involved in diagnosing ASD often include developmental pediatricians, neurologists, psychologists, and para-medical professionals. There is frequently a dilemma about whether to share the diagnosis with parents immediately or to wait to observe the child's natural developmental progression to confirm or refute the diagnosis. Both approaches have advantages and disadvantages (Goin-Kochel et al., 2006; Osborne et al., 2008). Delaying the diagnosis allows the diagnostic team to gain more certainty, permitting them to monitor the emergence of autistic symptoms and developmental delays over time. Some professionals believe that delaying the diagnosis provides parents with a more gradual process of exposure to the developmental disorder, thereby contributing to better acceptance when the diagnosis is eventually made. Additionally, delaying the diagnosis allows the child to continue developing without the label of a developmental disorder, reducing the potential for negative reactions based on preconceived notions from their surroundings.

On the other hand, early diagnosis enables timely intervention, which has been shown to improve prognosis for children with ASD (Dawson et al., 2012). However, the timing of the diagnosis significantly influences parental experiences and acceptance of the diagnosis. Reed et al. (2019) found that both actual and perceived speedy diagnostic processes are associated with difficulties in coming to terms with the diagnosis in mothers, emphasizing the need for balancing promptness with sensitivity and comprehensive communication.

Early diagnosis allows for early intervention specifically tailored for children with autism. These treatments are typically more intensive compared to treatments given to children with suspected general developmental delays. Indeed, several studies emphasize the importance of early intervention in improving outcomes, such as better adaptation to daily life and a reduction in the severity of autistic symptoms (Costello, 2005; Dawson et al., 2010; Dawson et al., 2012). Additionally, in many countries, an autism diagnosis often grants families access to financial aid and intervention support from the government, further underscoring the importance of early diagnosis. Finally, professionals emphasizing early diagnosis argue that when parents receive a diagnosis sooner rather than later, they remain in a state of uncertainty for a shorter period, which facilitates the acceptance of the diagnosis and the selection of appropriate treatment programs. This assumption is supported by a Japanese study which found that the child's age at diagnosis correlates with the mother's acceptance of the disorder (Futagi & Yamamoto, 2002): Mothers of children diagnosed at a younger age were found to come to terms with the disorder earlier compared to mothers whose children were diagnosed at an older age.

Despite the advantages of early diagnosis, findings indicate that families wait at least several months and up to four years between their initial consultation with a professional regarding their child's development and receiving a definitive ASD diagnosis (Brian et al., 2019; Hine et al., 2018; Stasik et al., 2024). This prolonged delay is due to several factors, including the parents' emotional process, long waiting times for diagnostic processes (especially in public healthcare), and professionals' attitudes toward the diagnostic process. This long wait contrasts with findings from Makino et al.'s (2021) review that examines parents' attitudes toward receiving a significant developmental diagnosis. The review underscores that timely identification and collaborative deliberations with professionals are crucial for parental satisfaction and better outcomes for children with ASD. Additional support for this stance comes from a study by Goin-Kochel et al. (2006), which found that parents who received an autism diagnosis at a younger age expressed higher satisfaction with the diagnostic process.

Hence, despite the difficulty of giving an ASD diagnosis to a young child still in early development, there are several advantages to attempting early diagnosis, alongside the need for caution and careful consideration. One prominent advantage is ending the period of uncertainty for parents, which many parents describe as the most difficult, as it leaves them in a state of ambiguity and uncertainty, especially regarding intervention and treatment options.

Parents' Experiences and Satisfaction with the Diagnostic Process

Many parents experience the diagnostic process as a challenging and stressful period (Renty & Roeyers, 2006). Parental satisfaction with the diagnostic process, particularly how the diagnosis is communicated, may influence their ability to support and raise their child (Jurin et al., 2022). In a study examining the factors that predicted parents' satisfaction with the diagnostic process, the most important elements were providing written information about the developmental disorder, fostering a positive perspective on the child's future, and assisting in identifying treatment and support services (Hill et al., 2003). Similarly, Anderberg and South (2021) found that maintaining warmth, clarity, and confidence by professionals during diagnostic sessions mitigated negative emotions and improved parents' readiness to act following receiving the diagnosis. Parents were reported to value specific, actionable advice, including resource lists, prognosis details, and guidance on accessing support. Furthermore, Reed et al. (2019) emphasize that mothers who perceive the diagnostic process as coherent and empathetic report greater satisfaction and are more likely to adapt positively.

A review by Sher-Censor and Shahar-Lahav (2022) highlighted the importance of involving parents throughout the diagnostic process, emphasizing that feeling engaged and well-informed enhances parental ability to come to terms with their child's diagnosis. They emphasized that when parents are involved in decision-making, they tend to feel more empowered and effective in supporting their child's progress and daily functioning, rather than feeling helpless in the face of developmental challenges. These feelings may support better adjustment and a greater sense of agency among parents. Finally, the perception of the diagnostician as a professional who understands parents' concerns and communicates effectively was also found to be associated with greater satisfaction with the diagnostic process (Hasnat & Graves, 2000; Moh & Magiati, 2012).

The process of diagnosis for parents of children with ASD includes several unique characteristics that may heighten parental difficulty during and after the diagnostic process. ASD tends to be diagnosed at an older age compared to other developmental disorders, such as cerebral palsy or Down syndrome. Thus, parents are often required to shift their perception of their child from one of typical development to a child with a broad developmental disorder that will affect their entire life course. Research indicates that early diagnosis of ASD, which allows an earlier shift in parents' perceptions of their child, enhances parents' satisfaction with the diagnostic process and improves their coping abilities (Futagi & Yamamoto, 2002). However, doctors and therapeutic professionals do not always promptly refer children for a comprehensive diagnosis, often advising parents to "wait and see" if the issue resolves on its own (Ahern, 2000; Schall, 2000). Additionally, the lack of physical indicators for ASD makes it challenging for both parents and others to comprehend the child's difficulties. Parents often struggle to reconcile their child's appearance of being "a regular child" with their actual abilities and functioning.

In many cases, parents are provided with unclear diagnoses such as "borderline autism" or "autistic traits," requiring them to remain in a state of uncertainty for an extended period. Parents receiving ambiguous diagnoses tend to report lower satisfaction with the diagnostic process (Makino et al., 2021; Watson, 2008). The difficulty in providing an accurate prognosis regarding the child's future developmental trajectory tends to be more pronounced in the case of ASD compared to other developmental disorders. Consequently, the diagnostic process can leave parents feeling confused and may even diminish their hope for their child's future. Therefore, the process of delivering the diagnosis to parents should emphasize professional engagement, emotional sensitivity toward families, and collaborative discussion to prevent adverse parental outcomes (Oppenheim et al., 2024; Sher-Censor et al., 2017).

To gain a more comprehensive understanding of parents' experiences after their child is diagnosed with ASD, parents' descriptions of their emotional experiences and their interactions with professionals during the diagnostic process will be presented.

Many parents report that receiving an ASD diagnosis for their child is accompanied by overwhelming emotions: "It wasn't a surprise for me, and yet when he said it, it was a blow. I was somehow ready for it. But you can't really be ready for it, even though I knew what the answer would be. After that, the real difficulty began. It's very hard to go through... nights... day by day...you deal with it all the time...it's more mentally challenging, but also physically draining, with all the tests and hopes that the results will come out well. Many thoughts ran through my mind, like 'Why do I deserve this?' It was really a very, very hard period." Another mother described receiving the diagnosis as follows: "I can tell you, it was simply a feeling of absolute depression... darkness, like a lightning strike, um... I don't know what."

Other descriptions similarly conveyed the difficult feelings accompanying the receipt of an autism diagnosis: "It was very hard; everything closes in on you. You feel like you're in a dead end... you don't know how you're going to get out of it."

> "I believe every mother feels like me, that the whole world has collapsed on her. Autism sounds like such a bombastic word... I just felt like I couldn't move. I couldn't drive. We took a half-hour break. It was really quite devastating in the beginning."

> "I didn't show it, but inside it felt like I was walking in a bubble, like I was in an unseen space. I didn't even know if I was moving forward or if I was stuck in the present or past. It felt like it wasn't happening to me. You feel like you need to wake up from a dream, saying, 'No, no, this isn't happening to me. It will get better.'"

These descriptions reveal feelings of sadness, helplessness, loss, pain, shock, and crisis. Such emotions frequently accompany parents in the initial period after receiving the diagnosis. This period is crucial, as it is during this time that parents must make decisions regarding the type and extent of treatment for their child and choose an appropriate educational framework. The parents' ability to cope with their feelings about the diagnosis can directly influence this decision-making process. Moreover, the parent's responsiveness to their child is also directly related to their emotional state. In early childhood, adaptive intervention and parental responsiveness are crucial for a child's progress, as this period is marked by significant neural plasticity (Bryck & Fisher, 2012).

Before exploring the process of coming to terms and accepting the diagnosis, we will first try to understand the experiences of parents during their interactions with the diagnostic team. Despite a common ASD diagnosis, parents' experiences vary widely. One example is the case of Jonathan's mother, who described the meeting in which they received the diagnosis:

> "She said it in such a sensitive way. It was hard; I won't say it wasn't hard, but I remember leaving that day without… it wasn't like thunder on a clear day. She somehow managed to convey it gently, gradually… she talked about the difficulties but also about the hopes. It helped a lot. The knowledge that we would meet again the next week was reassuring. She emphasized that we would think about everything together, what was best to do. It helped."

It is evident how the sensitivity of the professional toward the parents helped support the family. In this interview, conducted approximately three years after the diagnosis, the mother recalls the significant meeting and emphasizes the sensitive way in which the diagnosis was conveyed. This approach facilitated the parents' process of understanding and accepting their son as a child with autism. The practitioner's sensitivity also fostered the mother's sense of hope regarding her child's future. This sense of hope is central to the acceptance process, which we will return to later in the chapter.

In contrast, Sophia's mother described a very different and less positive experience:

> "First of all, I think she really wasn't there for us and that if other parents had been sitting there and she had phrased herself the same way, they would have felt similarly… There was no empathy, no sensitivity. There was no recognition that it is not only about giving a diagnosis; she should have thought about our feelings and tried to support and not hinder our understanding of what autism is. I felt a lot of criticism towards her, and I was very angry about her tone. Even if my daughter was supposed to receive some intervention in that place, I knew I wouldn't take her there. Fortunately, we had another place to turn to. But talking with her made it much harder."

The lack of satisfaction with how Sophia's diagnosis was conveyed is evident in the mother's description. The presentation of the diagnosis lacked joint thinking with the parents and was devoid of sensitivity and empathy. In the mother's opinion, this difficult interaction with the diagnostic team made it even harder for her husband and her to cope with the crisis.

Additional negative testimonies regarding the way the child's diagnosis was communicated can be seen in the following examples:

> "She said our son has autistic traits in medical terms. I accepted the diagnosis, but she didn't provide any guidance on what to do next. She scheduled an appointment three months later… she didn't give me any direction on what to do now."
>
> "He wasn't sensitive at all. After two days I went into a deep depression. I wanted to die and called the office there, but they didn't really help me. I think he didn't have time."
>
> "In the diagnosis, they didn't say 'autism' or 'ASD,' but afterward, when I received the letter at home, it said 'ASD'. No one talked about it in the meeting. They only said it could be treated. At home I was so alone; I didn't know what to do."
>
> "In the diagnosis meeting, he didn't give us a clear diagnosis. He only mentioned developmental difficulty and that more observations were needed. They gave us an appointment a month later for occupational and speech therapy. In the end, he looked at us and said, 'You need to give the child a lot of love.' We both left feeling awful; we cried because it felt like we were being blamed for the problem."

From these examples, three central themes of parents navigating the diagnostic process for their child emerge: first, the significance of the diagnostic journey and their relationship with the diagnostic team; second, the necessity for the team's sensitivity, comprehensive and realistic information about the disorder, clear explanations of appropriate treatment methods, and guidance; and third, the value of emotional support from professionals, enabling them to express their feelings openly. When these needs are unmet, the difficult experience of receiving the diagnosis can be even more challenging and linger for years.

With the experiences of parents in mind, we can now focus on what the acceptance of the diagnosis entails.

Acceptance of the Diagnosis

Receiving a diagnosis of ASD, combined with parents' concerns about their child prior to the diagnostic procedure, begins a process during which parents need to adjust their expectations for their child in light of the diagnosis (Siegel, 1996). Acceptance of the child's diagnosis is a deeply personal process influenced by both personal and environmental factors. For most parents, this process bears similarities to the grieving process following the loss of a loved one (Pianta & Marvin, 1993). Parents must let go of the idea of their child as one who will have typical development, but rather developmental difficulties, a process that can be emotionally challenging and has numerous personal implications. Grieving is an essential part of the process of coming to terms with the child's diagnosis. This may lead the parent to retain hope that their child will continue to develop and even meet typical developmental milestones that they always envisioned (Siegel, 1996). However, such hopes, if they dominate the parents' entire perception of their child, may hinder the acceptance process, during which the parent must reconcile their expectations with their child's actual abilities and developmental challenges.

Common emotional reactions to the diagnosis of ASD include a wide range of responses, such as surprise, anger, denial, relief, shame, helplessness, shock, sorrow, despair, and pity (Altiere & von Kluge, 2009; Wachtel & Carter, 2008). Some parents find that the diagnosis confirms their worst fears but brings them to a state where the problem is defined, thereby establishing a path for treatment. Others are completely surprised and cannot fully believe the diagnosis. Many parents go through a multi-stage process of grief and acceptance (Siegel, 1996). Although there is no uniform sequence of progression between these stages, and no fixed time for staying in each stage, some parents may not reach acceptance even years after the diagnosis (Oppenheim et al., 2009). These parents might remain in a state that prevents them from seeking any support for their own needs and adapting themselves and their lifestyle to the fact that their child has a severe developmental disorder. Wayment and Brookshire (2018) identify that mothers who internalize their child's diagnosis as a loss, tend to exhibit chronic sorrow, whereas those who perceive it as unjust may struggle with distress rather than grief. They found that parents with mental health issues and identity ambiguity (i.e., when a parent's self-perception becomes deeply intertwined with their child's diagnosis) may find the acceptance process especially challenging.

Gombosi (1998) argued that even parents who successfully navigate the acceptance process retain a strong sense of trauma, although it may no longer involve the confusion and depression experienced at the beginning of the process. He stated that through the process of coming to terms with their child's diagnosis parents undergo a psychological reorganization that enables them to balance their child's needs with their own capabilities.

Marvin and Pianta (1996) described this process of acceptance among mothers of children with cerebral palsy (CP) as one of changing the mother's internal representations of the child and the parent-child relationship. This approach is grounded in Bowlby's attachment theory (1980), which posits that people who experience a significant loss undergo several stages of grief, including denial, yearning, despair, confusion, and ultimately reorganization. Reorganization represents the optimal outcome, involving a change in internal working models to fit the new reality following the loss.

In the case of grief over the loss of "the typically developing child," changing the internal model regarding the child and their future occurs when the parent successfully reorganizes in response to the child's diagnosis, adapting their view of themselves and their child to fit the reality of the child's diagnosis. When parents see their child as they truly are, they can adapt their behavior to suit the child's unique needs, fostering an emotionally secure attachment.

If parents do not adapt their working model following the diagnosis, there will be a disconnect between their model and the child's actual needs and abilities. This can lead to unresolved grief, manifesting as an inability to adapt and reorganize their views of their child, which may result in insensitive or inappropriate parental behaviors (Marvin & Pianta, 1996; Pianta & Marvin, 1993). Such behaviors can include misunderstandings of the child's cues, unrealistic expectations, feelings of anger or depression toward the child, and avoidance of close interactions, all of which negatively affect the quality of the parent-child relationship.

Reaction to Diagnosis Interview

The Reaction to Diagnosis Interview (RDI) was developed to empirically examine parent's ability to come to terms with their child's diagnosis by assessing their current perception of their affected child and the diagnosis (Marvin & Pianta, 1996). The RDI is a semi-structured interview consisting of five questions aimed at exploring the parents' perceptions of their diagnosed child's condition. The interview seeks to track the emotional process of discovering the problem and accepting the diagnosis. It lasts about fifteen minutes and includes questions asking the parent to recall when they first noticed their child's developmental difficulties and how they felt at that time, how they felt and what were their thoughts upon receiving their child's ASD diagnosis, whether their thoughts and feelings have changed over time from receiving the diagnosis until the present, and whether they have thoughts or ideas regarding the cause of their child's ASD.

The analysis of the interview relies on several characteristics that allow classification of the interview into one of two main patterns: *resolved* or *unresolved*.

Characteristics indicating resolution of the child's diagnosis:

1. Recognition of the emotional change the parent underwent from the time of diagnosis until the present.
2. Description of a challenging emotional period surrounding the diagnosis, followed by an acknowledgment that life must go on, with efforts to do the best for the child.
3. Realistic recognition of the child's abilities.
4. A balanced description of the experience of raising the child—the difficulties and challenges alongside the recognition of the child's abilities and uniqueness.

Characteristics indicating lack of resolution of the child's diagnosis:

1. Presence of cognitive distortions—unrealistic beliefs about the child's abilities.
2. Constant search for reasons for the child's difficulties, which prevents the parent from seeing their child and responding to their needs.
3. Being "stuck in the past"—the parent repeatedly describes the experience of receiving the diagnosis, using the present tense to recount past events.
4. The parent's description is confused and incoherent, making it difficult to understand their narrative.
5. Parental emotional detachment while describing difficult events surrounding the diagnosis.

Based on these characteristics, the interview is categorized into one of two main orientations, further divided into several subtypes:

Parents who accept the diagnosis are considered *Resolved*. These parents have managed to overcome the diagnostic crisis and recognize their emotions about the diagnosis and the changes in those emotions over time. They adapt their internal representations of their child and integrate the diagnosis into their perception. They are currently focused on their child's present and future, without dwelling on the past. They provide realistic descriptions of the child's abilities and traits, demonstrating acceptance, clear and effective communication, and a balanced understanding of the child's condition in relation to themselves. These interviews are consistent, reliable, and well-structured. *Resolution* has three subtypes: Parents who are *feeling oriented* tend to be emotional in their descriptions, acknowledging the need to grieve but also to move forward; *action oriented* parents primarily discuss their actions, highlighting vigorous efforts on behalf of the child, with their grieving process reflected in practical, tailored care for the child; *thinking oriented* parents tend to express their thoughts more than their emotions regarding the process they underwent since receiving the diagnosis.

Parents who have not come to terms with the diagnosis are seen us *Unresolved*. These parents have not successfully navigated the stages of crisis following the diagnosis and therefore have not undergone the emotional process typical of parents showing resolution. These parents do not express acceptance of their child's condition and its impact on themselves. They tend to fixate on the day of the diagnosis, describing it with anger, emotional overwhelm, or a sense of detachment. Some of these parents exhibit denial of the diagnosis, viewing it as incorrect, and tend to describe their child and their abilities unrealistically. There are six subtypes: *emotional overwhelmed* parents express intense sadness or anger during the interview, giving the impression of reliving the time of diagnosis; *angrily preoccupied* parents present significant anger during the interview, attempting to convince the interviewer of their position; *neutralizing* parents do not show emotions during the interview, even when recounting challenging experiences and events; *depressed/passive* parents tend to present passivity and depressed feelings during the interview, offering minimal descriptions, and appear consumed by their sadness, expressing hopelessness regarding the future; in the *cognitive distortion orientation* parents hold unrealistic perceptions regarding the diagnosis and/or their child; finally, in the *disorganized/confused orientation* parents' speech is incoherent, and they appear confused and unsure in their responses.

To illustrate the differences between parents classified as *Resolved* and *Unresolved*, we will present examples from interviews. In the first example, we revisit Jonathan's mother, who was asked during the interview whether her feelings and emotions had changed since receiving the diagnosis. "It took us a whole year to come to terms with it. We always thought, 'It can't be, maybe there's another problem,' and we looked for differences between Jonathan and other children with an ASD diagnosis. We tried very, very hard to convince ourselves it wasn't autism. Then, about a year later, we accepted it—it's autism. And our feelings changed. Today, I have many moments of satisfaction, seeing his progress, seeing how he grows as a child. We're still worried, but things have changed, and we see that he's progressing."

Jonathan's mother, who was classified as showing a *resolved-thinking orientation*, vividly described her evolving thoughts and feelings after the diagnosis. She acknowledged the initial struggle to accept it and the attempts to disprove it. Over time, she and her husband came to understand and accept their child's autism while balancing ongoing concerns with optimism about his progress. This excerpt demonstrates her ability to describe her thoughts and emotions coherently, showing acceptance of her child and his condition.

Other mothers who also demonstrate resolution of their child's diagnosis tend to focus more on actions and finding appropriate treatments for their child, with less emphasis on their own feelings and thoughts. For example:

Mother: "He (the doctor) said he has ASD, and right away we asked many questions, immediately bombarded him with questions-What? What do we do? How?""

Interviewer: "Can you think about how you felt at the time?"

Mother: "That day we cried, but the next day we were ready to take action. We sought treatment options, searching online, asking friends, and reaching out to child development services. We wanted the best, and everyone recommended this specific treatment center. So, we went there immediately and got things moving. We knew time was crucial—early intervention mattered. We decided to help our child progress, and we committed to working intensively with him, even in the afternoons. It was important for us to help him move forward. That's what we did."

Interviewer: "Have your feelings about everything you've described changed from then to now?"

Mother: "They've changed. We've moved past the initial shock. Now, our focus is entirely on helping him move forward—teaching him something new so he can continue to learn and grow. Every small progress motivates us to think about the next step."

In this case, the mother described how she and her husband coped with their child's diagnosis. She acknowledged the emotional difficulty but emphasized channeling their energy into action—finding effective treatment and supporting their child. This mother was classified as *resolved-action orientation.* Parents who adapt their actions to support their child's needs and challenges demonstrate acceptance of the diagnosis. They adjust their daily routines, financial priorities, and interactions to align with the autism diagnosis.

In contrast, the following examples illustrate mothers who struggle to accept their children's diagnoses. Noa's mother vividly described the day she received the diagnosis, highlighting the ongoing emotional impact of that day.

Interviewer: "Can you describe what happened and how you felt on the day you received Noa's diagnosis?"

Mother: "I remember every moment in slow motion. I walked with Noa to the car. We drive. I try to think, but I can't. My husband talks, but I don't hear him. The phone rings, but I can't answer… Earlier, there was a meeting with the social worker. It offended me—implying something might be wrong with me as a mother. Then we met with the doctor. He asked, 'What do you want to ask?' What do I want to ask? I just wanted to know what was wrong with my child. He said: 'I see signs of autism.' In that moment, the sky fell. He answered our questions like a robot—no emotion, hardly any information. He referred us to a treatment center. We left, and I didn't know what to do with myself. I still get so angry remembering it…".

Interviewer: "And how have your feelings about everything you described changed since then until today?"

Mother: "I've moved on; I'm not in the same place. But I think about it a lot. I see other families, some with three children or more, while I have only Noa and all the work I have to do with him. There's no joy. With him, it's just one day after another. It's very hard."

This mother, categorized as having an *unresolved-emotionally overwhelmed orientation*, expresses profound pain regarding the diagnosis. Although the interview took place three years after the diagnosis, her responses reveal significant emotional overwhelm. Her shifts between past and present tense indicate how vividly that day remains in her mind. She struggles to accept the diagnosis and her journey since. Despite initially claiming progress, her sorrow, pain, and difficulty in seeing her child's positive traits are evident. Anger toward the diagnostic system and depressive tendencies also emerge, but emotional flooding remains the dominant element.

In the following example, we encounter a mother exhibiting emotional detachment. Her responses to questions about the period surrounding the diagnosis and her subsequent coping are laconic and devoid of emotional expression:

Interviewer: "When was he first diagnosed with ASD?"

Mother: "About a year ago, he was diagnosed, and they told us it's autism. In the report we received it said Autistic Spectrum Disorder."

Interviewer: "Can you describe how you felt, what you did on that day?"

Mother: "I expected it. So, I wasn't surprised. It was simply a statement of fact, and that's it. I wasn't emotional. It was just an ordinary day. I felt the same as usual. Nothing stood out other than the fact that he has ASD."

Interviewer: "Do you feel that over time, your feelings about the diagnosis have changed?"

Mother: "No. Everything has stayed the same."

The responses in this interview are brief and limited. It appears this mother denies her emotions regarding the process of coping with her child's diagnosis. Her verbal responses convey indifference, likely a defense mechanism against confronting the pain of the diagnosis. She even states that her emotions have not changed since the diagnosis. She does not describe her child, his abilities, or progress, suggesting she struggles to fully see him; therefore, she was classified as having an *unresolved-neutralizing orientation.*

Resolution of the Diagnosis: Research Findings

The question arises whether resolution or irresolution of the child's diagnosis by the parent has any long-term significance. Research findings from the last two decades suggest that resolution contributes to a beneficial relationship with the child and fosters sensitive and appropriate parental behaviors. Some studies have examined parents of children with various developmental disorders, while others specifically examined resolution of the diagnosis among parents of children with ASD.

Studies examining acceptance among mothers of children with various special needs found that between 41% and 69% of parents showed resolution (Lord et al., 2008; Pianta et al., 1996). Among parents of children with ASD 33% to 62% were found to have a resolved pattern (Barak-Levy & Paryente, 2023; Milshtein et al., 2010; Oppenheim et al., 2009; Poslawsky et al., 2014). In a review that explored parents of children with ASD as well as other developmental disorders, the resolution of a child's diagnosis using Marvin and Pianta's model, 18% to 73% of parents remained unresolved following their child's diagnosis (Sher-Censor & Shahar-Lahav, 2022). Thus, indicating a wide range of outcomes among families. In the Sher-Censor and Shahar-Lahav (2022) review, the average rate of unresolved parents was found to be 44%, suggesting that nearly half of all parents struggle to fully come to terms with their child's diagnosis. In another review, Naicker et al. (2023) identified six key factors affecting parental resolution, including: symptom severity, religion and cultural beliefs, knowledge and uncertainty, negative and positive emotions, and social support. Their findings indicated that resolution was positively associated with parental well-being, reduced stress, and improved mental health outcomes.

Research indicates that longer time since diagnosis and greater symptom severity may influence parental resolution of an ASD diagnoses, though findings are mixed. Studies like Yirmiya et al. (2015) show that these factors positively impact maternal resolution. Similarly, Di Renzo et al. (2020) found that symptom severity and time since diagnosis predicted mothers' resolution. In contrast, Milshtein et al. (2010) and Oppenheim et al. (2009) reported no link between these factors and parental resolution. Finally, Poslawsky et al. (2014) observed that while symptom severity influenced resolution, time since diagnosis did not. These findings underscore the complexity of parental resolution, shaped by coping mechanisms and support systems.

Several studies have examined the relationships between resolution and other factors, such as attachment style, interaction quality, and children's communication abilities. Mothers with a resolved pattern tend to develop a secure attachment with their children with ASD, while unresolved mothers are more likely to develop insecure attachments (Oppenheim et al., 2009; Yirmiya et al., 2015).

These attachment patterns tend to be related to the level of sensitivity parents show in responding to their children's needs, even though sensitive caregiving is particularly challenging for parents of children with ASD, as these children often struggle to communicate their desires and needs (Dolev, 2011). Nevertheless, mothers who were found to be resolved regarding the diagnosis demonstrated higher sensitivity toward their children compared to those who did not (Dolev et al., 2009). They responded more accurately to the children's cues, adjusted their behavior to their children's needs, and demonstrated supportive behaviors during play. Consequently, children of mothers who accepted the diagnosis exhibited better communication skills and cooperation during play, as well as higher responsiveness and more frequent eye contact. Di Renzo et al. (2020) also found that mothers and fathers who were both insightful (i.e., able to understand their child's internal states) and resolved regarding their child's ASD diagnosis were more likely to demonstrate attuned behaviors during play, such as responding to their child's signals and adjusting appropriately. Wachtel and Carter (2008), found that mothers of children with ASD who accepted the diagnosis showed more cognitive and supportive involvement during play, and they also provided verbal and non-verbal scaffolding to support children's play. Finally, quality of attachment was also positively associated with maternal sensitivity in this population (Oppenheim et al., 2009). These findings suggest that mothers who accepted the diagnosis were better able to interpret their children's cues and adjust their behavior accordingly, fostering a positive attachment relationship.

It is important to note that resolution is not merely a state, but an ongoing process influenced by cultural, contextual, and interpersonal factors. For instance, parents in traditional societies may face stigma that impedes resolution, whereas supportive professional and familial networks promote it (Sher-Censor et al., 2017; Sher-Censor & Shahar-Lahav, 2022).

Summary and Practical Implications

Coping with a child's autism diagnosis is a multifaceted and challenging process for parents, impacting their perception of the child, their future, family relationships, and their roles both personally and socially. The diagnostic process also requires interaction with various professionals, educational systems, and health and social services. Many parents find this period to be highly challenging, both emotionally and physically. The initial interaction with diagnostic teams may lack sufficient emotional support and guidance, which exacerbates the difficulties parents face. It is crucial to recognize that, upon receiving the diagnosis, parents embark on a long-term journey requiring continuous emotional support and professional guidance.

Accordingly, Sher-Censor and Shahar-Lahav (2022) identified factors that may facilitate acceptance, including access to supportive community resources, professional guidance, and ongoing psychological support. These factors help parents navigate the emotional journey from shock and denial to acceptance. In another review by Ali et al. (2023), the complexity of the parental experience is emphasized as well as the need for better communication and support during and after the diagnostic process. Therefore, improved communication training for healthcare professionals to ensure a more supportive and inclusive environment for families during and after the diagnostic process should be encouraged. In accordance, Aguiar and Pondé (2020) emphasize the need for healthcare providers to receive training to enhance their communication skills, ensuring they can deliver diagnoses with empathy and support. Additionally, they emphasize the importance of providing ongoing psychological support and resources to parents' post-diagnosis, aiding them in coping strategies and adjustment processes.

Although diagnosing ASD requires careful consideration, it is essential to involve parents in the professional team's assessment and decision-making processes. When parents feel involved, they are more likely to mobilize emotional, physical, and financial resources to cope effectively with the situation. Professionals should also acknowledge the emotions parents experience upon receiving the diagnosis and provide opportunities for them to ask questions and express concerns. Scheduling follow-up meetings soon after the diagnosis ensures continued support during this critical adjustment period. It is equally important for professionals to understand the characteristics of the resolution process and to incorporate parental support into their practices to help parents come to terms with their child's diagnosis. Parents need guidance not only during the diagnostic stage but throughout their child's development, as they face new challenges. Since unresolved narratives often reflect ongoing grief and confusion, which can negatively impact a parent's ability to provide consistent and sensitive caregiving, addressing these unresolved emotions through targeted interventions, such as psychotherapy and parental support groups, can improve both parent and child outcomes.

Parents of children with ASD make significant efforts to support their children's development, often leading to meaningful improvements in the child's adaptive abilities. However, parents' own experiences and coping processes are sometimes overlooked. Accepting the child's diagnosis is a profound, challenging, and significant journey that demands appropriate and professional support to ensure the well-being of both parents and their child.

References

Aguiar, M. C. M. D., & Pondé, M. P. (2020). Autismo: Impacto do diagnóstico nos pais [autism: Impact of the diagnosis in the parents]. *Jornal Brasileiro de Psiquiatria, 69*(3), 149–155. https://doi.org/10.1590/0047-2085000000276

Ahern, K. (2000). Something is wrong with my child: A phenomenological account of a search for a diagnosis. *Early Education and Development, 11*, 187–201. https://doi.org/10.1207/s15566935eed1102_4

Ali, A., Rashid, M., Davila-Cervantes, A., Dennett, L., Thompson-Hodgetts, S., & Goez, H. (2023). Parents' immediate reaction and responses to their child's ASD diagnosis: A synthesis review. *Journal on Developmental Disabilities, 28*(1), 1–27.

Altiere, M. J., & von Kluge, S. (2009). Searching for acceptance: Challenges encountered while raising a child with autism. *Journal of Intellectual and Developmental Disability, 34*(2), 142–152. https://doi.org/10.1080/13668250902845202

Anderberg, E., & South, M. (2021). Predicting parent reactions at diagnostic disclosure sessions for autism. *Journal of Autism and Developmental Disorders, 51*(12), 3533–3546. https://doi.org/10.1007/s10803-020-04817-5

Barak-Levy, Y., & Paryente, M. (2023). Diving into the resolution process: Parent's reactions to child's diagnosis. *International Journal of Environmental Research and Public Health, 20*(4), 3295. https://doi.org/10.3390/ijerph20043295

Bowlby, J. (1980). *Attachment and loss: Vol. III. Loss*. Basic Books.

Brian, J. A., Zwaigenbaum, L., & Ip, A. (2019). Standards of diagnostic assessment for autism spectrum disorder. *Pediatrics & Child Health, 24*(7), 444–451. https://doi.org/10.1093/pch/pxz117

Bryck, R. L., & Fisher, P. A. (2012). Training the brain: Practical applications of neural plasticity from the intersection of cognitive neuroscience, developmental psychology, and prevention science. *American Psychologist, 67*(2), 87–100. https://doi.org/10.1037/a0024657

Costello, C. M. (2005). Early intervention in autism. *Infants and Young Children, 18*(2), 74–85. https://doi.org/10.1097/00001163-200504000-00002

Dawson, G., Jones, E. J. H., Merkle, K., Venema, K., Lowy, R., Faja, S., Kamara, D., Murias, M., Greenson, J., Winter, J., Smith, M., Rogers, S. J., & Webb, S. J. (2012). Early behavioral intervention is associated with normalized brain activity in young children with autism. *Journal of the American Academy of Child & Adolescent Psychiatry, 51*(11), 1150–1159. https://doi.org/10.1016/j.jaac.2012.08.018

Dawson, G., Rogers, S., Munson, J., Smith, M., Winter, J., Greenson, J., Donaldson, A., & Varley, J. (2010). Randomized controlled trial of an intervention for toddlers with autism: The early start Denver model. *Pediatrics, 125*(1), e17–e23. https://doi.org/10.1542/peds.2009-0958

Di Renzo, M., Guerriero, V., Zavattini, G. C., Petrillo, M., Racinaro, L., & Bianchi di Castelbianco, F. (2020). Parental attunement, insightfulness, and acceptance of child diagnosis in parents of children with autism: Clinical implications. *Frontiers in Psychology, 11*, 1849. https://doi.org/10.3389/fpsyg.2020.01849

Dolev, S. (2011). Ineteraqtsiyyah ben immahot liladim im otizm: Khashivutah shel regishutah shel haem leitute hayyeled [interaction between mothers and children with autism: The importance of maternal sensitivity to the child's signals]. *Ketav Et Yisreeli Lerippuy Beissuq [Israeli Journal of Occupational Therapy], 20*, 93–109. https://www.jstor.org/stable/23469949

Dolev, S., Oppenheim, D., Koren-Karie, N., & Yirmiya, N. (2009). Emotional availability in mother-child interaction: The case of children with autism spectrum disorders. *Parenting: Science and Practice, 9*(3–4), 183–197. https://doi.org/10.1080/15295190902844332

Futagi, Y. A., & Yamamoto, Y. U. (2002). Disclosure of a diagnosis of childhood autism and parents' acceptance of the disability. *No to Hattatsu = Brain and Development, 34*, 336–342.

Goin-Kochel, R. P., Mackintosh, V. H., & Myers, B. J. (2006). How many doctors does it take to make an autism spectrum diagnosis? *Autism, 10*(5), 439–451. https://doi.org/10.1177/1362361306066601

Gombosi, P. G. (1998). Parents of autistic children: Some thoughts about trauma, dislocation, and tragedy. *The Psychoanalytic Study of the Child, 53*(1), 254–275. https://doi.org/10.1080/00797308.1998.11822486

Hasnat, M. J., & Graves, P. (2000). Disclosure of developmental disability: A study of parent satisfaction and the determinants of satisfaction. *Journal of Pediatrics and Child Health, 36*(1), 32–35. https://doi.org/10.1046/j.1440-1754.2000.00463.x

Hill, V., Sahhar, M., Aitken, M., Savarirayan, R., & Metcalfe, S. (2003). Experiences at the time of diagnosis of parents who have a child with a bone dysplasia resulting in short stature. *American Journal of Medical Genetics Part A, 122*(2), 100–107. https://doi.org/10.1002/ajmg.a.20201

Hine, J. F., Herrington, C. G., Rothman, A. M., Mace, R. L., Patterson, B. L., Carlson, K. L., & Warren, Z. E. (2018). Embedding autism spectrum disorder diagnosis within the medical home: Decreasing wait times through streamlined assessment. *Journal of Autism and Developmental Disorders, 48*(8), 2846–2853. https://doi.org/10.1007/s10803-018-3548-3

Jurin, A., Šimleša, S., & Cepanec, M. (2022). Parental perception of the process of communicating a diagnosis of autism spectrum disorder in the Republic of Croatia. *Clinical Child Psychology and Psychiatry, 27*(4), 1006–1018. https://doi.org/10.1177/13591045221105191

Lord, B., Ungerer, J., & Wastell, C. (2008). Implications of resolving the diagnosis of PKU for parents and children. *Journal of Pediatric Psychology, 33*(8), 855–856. https://doi.org/10.1093/jpepsy/jsn020

Makino, A., Hartman, L., King, G., Wong, P. Y., & Penner, M. (2021). Parent experiences of autism spectrum disorder diagnosis: A scoping review. *Review Journal of Autism and Developmental Disorders, 8*(3), 267–284. https://doi.org/10.1007/s40489-021-00237-y

Marvin, R. S., & Pianta, R. C. (1996). Mothers' reactions to their child's diagnosis: Relations with security of attachment. *Journal of Clinical Child Psychology, 25*(4), 436–445. https://doi.org/10.1207/s15374424jccp2504_8

Milshtein, S., Yirmiya, N., Oppenheim, D., Koren-Karie, N., & Levi, S. (2010). Resolution of the diagnosis among parents of children with autism Spectrum disorder: Associations with child and parent characteristics. *Journal of Autism and Developmental Disorders, 40*(1), 89–99. https://doi.org/10.1007/s10803-009-0837-x

Moh, T. A., & Magiati, I. (2012). Factors associated with parental stress and satisfaction during the process of diagnosis of children with autism spectrum disorders. *Research in Autism Spectrum Disorders, 6*(1), 293–303. https://doi.org/10.1016/j.rasd.2011.05.011

Naicker, V. V., Bury, S. M., & Hedley, D. (2023). Factors associated with parental resolution of a child's autism diagnosis: A systematic review. *Frontiers in Psychiatry, 13*, 1079371. https://doi.org/10.3389/fpsyt.2022.1079371

Oppenheim, D., Koren-Karie, N., Dolev, S., & Yirmiya, N. (2009). Maternal insightfulness and resolution of the diagnosis are associated with secure attachment in preschoolers with autism spectrum disorders. *Child Development, 80*(2), 519–527. https://doi.org/10.1111/j.1467-8624.2009.01276.x

Oppenheim, D., Koren-Karie, N., Slonim, M., Mottes-Peleg, M., Sher-Censor, E., Dolev, S., & Yirmiya, N. (2024). Maternal and paternal insightfulness and reaction to the diagnosis in families

of preschoolers with autism spectrum disorder: Associations with observed parental sensitivity and inter-parent interaction. *Attachment & Human Development, 26*(1), 22–40. https://doi.org/10.1080/14616734.2024.2326416
Osborne, L. A., McHugh, L., Saunders, J., & Reed, P. (2008). A possible contra-indication for early diagnosis of autism spectrum conditions: Impact on parenting stress. *Research in Autism Spectrum Disorders, 2*(4), 707–715. https://doi.org/10.1016/j.rasd.2008.02.005
Pianta, R. C., & Marvin, R. S. (1993). Manual for classification of the reaction to diagnosis interview. *University of Virginia.*. https://education.virginia.edu/documents/ehdmanual-classification-reaction-diagnosis-interview1993pdf
Pianta, R. C., Marvin, R. S., Britner, P. A., & Borowitz, K. C. (1996). Mothers' resolution of their children's diagnosis: Organized patterns of caregiving representations. *Infant Mental Health Journal, 17*, 239–256. https://doi.org/10.1002/(SICI)1097-0355(199623)17:3<239::AID-IMHJ4>3.0.CO;2-J
Poslawsky, I. E., Naber, F. B., Van Daalen, E., & Van Engeland, H. (2014). Parental reaction to early diagnosis of their children's autism spectrum disorder: An exploratory study. *Child Psychiatry & Human Development, 45*(3), 294–305. https://doi.org/10.1007/s10578-013-0400-z
Reed, P., Giles, A., White, S., & Osborne, L. A. (2019). Actual and perceived speedy diagnoses are associated with mothers' unresolved reactions to a diagnosis of autism spectrum disorder for a child. *Autism, 23*(7), 1843–1852. https://doi.org/10.1177/1362361319833676
Renty, J., & Roeyers, H. (2006). Satisfaction with formal support and education for children with autism spectrum disorder: The voices of the parents. *Child: Care, Health and Development, 32*, 371–385. https://doi.org/10.1111/j.1365-2214.2006.00584.x
Schall, C. (2000). Family perspectives on raising a child with autism. *Journal of Child and Family Studies, 9*(4), 409–423. https://doi.org/10.1023/A:1009456825063
Sher-Censor, E., Dolev, S., Said, M., Baransi, N., & Amara, K. (2017). Coherence of representations regarding the child, resolution of the child's diagnosis and emotional availability: A study of Arab-Israeli mothers of children with ASD. *Journal of Autism and Developmental Disorders, 47*(10), 3139–3149. https://doi.org/10.1007/s10803-017-3228-8
Sher-Censor, E., & Shahar-Lahav, R. (2022). Parents' resolution of their child's diagnosis: A scoping review. *Attachment & Human Development, 24*(5), 580–604. https://doi.org/10.1080/14616734.2022.2034899
Siegel, B. (1996). *The world of the autistic child: Understanding and treating autistic spectrum disorders.* Oxford University Press.
Wachtel, K., & Carter, A. S. (2008). Reaction to diagnosis and parenting styles among mothers of young children with ASD. *Autism, 12*(5), 575–594. https://doi.org/10.1177/1362361308094505
Watson, S. (2008). "Something you have to do"–why do parents of children with developmental disabilities seek a differential diagnosis? *Developmental Disabilities Bulletin, 36*(1/2), 168–198.
Wayment, H. A., & Brookshire, K. A. (2018). Mothers' reactions to their child's ASD diagnosis: Predictors that discriminate grief from distress. *Journal of Autism and Developmental Disorders, 48*(4), 1147–1158. https://doi.org/10.1007/s10803-017-3266-2
Yirmiya, N., Seidman, I., Koren-Karie, N., Oppenheim, D., & Dolev, S. (2015). Stability and change in resolution of diagnosis among parents of children with autism spectrum disorder: Child and parental contributions. *Development and Psychopathology, 27*(4, Pt. 1), 1045–1057. https://doi.org/10.1017/S095457941500067X

Chapter 3
Autism Disclosure for Girls and Women: Perspectives from Parents and Autistic Individuals

Nitsan Almog, Tamir Gabai, Einat-Haya Keren, and Orit Kassel

Abstract This chapter explores the complex issue of autism diagnosis disclosure, focusing specifically on girls and women on the autism spectrum. It combines insights from two key sources: a focus group with parents of autistic girls, and interviews with autistic women reflecting on their own diagnosis disclosure experiences. The parental perspective reveals the unique dilemmas and considerations faced when deciding whether and how to disclose an autism diagnosis to their daughters. Complementing this, the firsthand accounts from autistic women provide valuable retrospective insights and recommendations for parents navigating this process. By juxtaposing these viewpoints, the chapter offers a comprehensive examination of the disclosure journey, highlighting potential gaps between parental concerns and the expressed needs of autistic girls.

Keywords Female autism · Gender · Diagnosis · Parental disclosure · Masking

Introduction

This investigation into autism disclosure practices for girls was initiated following a consultation request in October 2018 from Linda (pseudonym), the mother of a recently diagnosed 9.5-year-old autistic girl. While my research had extensively examined invisible disabilities and disclosure, I had limited knowledge of how these dynamics manifested specifically in autism. I suggested to Linda that we approach this challenge systematically: by convening a focus group of parents to explore their experiences while simultaneously interviewing autistic individuals to understand their perspectives. The first parent focus group on autism disclosure filled up

N. Almog (✉) · T. Gabai · E.-H. Keren · O. Kassel
Ono Academic College, Kiryat Ono, Israel
e-mail: nitsan.al@ono.ac.il

T. Gabai
e-mail: tamir.g.c.p@gmail.com

S. Lowinger and S. Pearlman-Avnion (eds.), *Collaborative Care and Partnerships in Autism Diagnosis and Treatment*, Autism and Child Psychopathology Series,
https://doi.org/10.1007/978-3-032-07009-8_3

instantly—all with parents of boys (Almog et al., 2023). This unexpected gender homogeneity led to a promise to Linda that we would create a group dedicated to girls exploring their unique experiences. The following year, Linda joined this group, whose insights and outcomes form the foundation of this chapter's examination of the distinctive challenges in autism disclosure for girls.

Parental Disclosure Delay in Autism Disclosure

Autistic individuals report that their parents delayed disclosing their diagnosis during childhood (Huws & Jones, 2008; Riccio et al., 2020; Smith et al., 2018). Studies examining parental attitudes toward autism disclosure similarly highlight a tendency to postpone informing children of their diagnosis. This delay is often linked to concerns that the child may not fully understand the diagnosis, might find the label distressing, or could face social stigma, potentially negatively affecting their self-esteem (Camarena & Sarigiani, 2009; Huws & Jones, 2008). However, in a society where autism stigma persists, withholding a diagnosis may hinder a child's ability to develop essential skills like self-advocacy (Duek-Huri, 2014). Despite parental concerns, research shows that disclosure helps autistic children better understand themselves and develop coping strategies (Kiely et al., 2020). Parents further report that disclosure enhances their child's self-awareness and self-advocacy skills.

Autistic adolescents may experience intensified conflicts and internal struggles as they develop their self-identities (Browning et al., 2009), and delays in diagnosis disclosure render autism an "absent presence" during a critical period in their lives. Before being diagnosed, many autistic individuals report feeling different and struggling to fit in. For most, receiving a diagnosis contributed to the validation of their identities and helped them understand themselves better (Harmens et al., 2022). DePape and Lindsay (2016) emphasize the importance of recognizing subjective experiences in early development to facilitate the transition to adulthood. Thus, early recognition of the diagnosis and self-understanding before adulthood may facilitate a more gradual identity formation with fewer conflicts and difficulties, as the diagnosis becomes an integral part of one's self-identity.

In addition to the parental disclosure delay, another factor that can delay disclosure and hinder self-understanding for autistic individuals is a late diagnosis. Since autism diagnosis relies on behavioral evaluation, cases of "atypical autism" manifestations—meaning those with characteristics that differ from the ones described in older diagnostic manuals (DSM IV and ICD-10)—can sometimes make it more difficult for diagnosticians to identify autism (Loubersac et al., 2021). In such cases, the delay in disclosure can be more significant and have a larger impact on the identity formation of autistic individuals.

The Gender Bias in Autism

Autistic girls are typically diagnosed later than boys due to insufficient recognition of their distinct autism presentation, which differs from the more commonly recognized male presentation or the "classic" stigmatized manifestation of autism (Driver & Chester, 2021; Eckerd, 2020). Late autism diagnosis is more common among autistic girls and women due to gender biases in autism. Historically, diagnostic criteria were based on male presentations, leading to an under-recognition of the unique characteristics of female autism (Cammuso & Knapp-Ines, 2024; Tsirgiotis et al., 2024). From the earliest documented cases of autism by Leo Kanner (1943) and Hans Asperger (1944/1991), the male-to-female ratio was 4:1, establishing the foundation of gender bias in autism. This male-centric framework has led to systemic biases in diagnosis and support, affecting both genders (Lockwood-Estrin et al., 2021; Werling & Geschwind, 2013). Existing diagnostic tools often reflect this male-centric perspective, creating significant barriers to timely diagnosis and intervention for girls (Cammuso & Knapp-Ines, 2024; Lockwood-Estrin et al., 2021). Even when girls and women exhibit "classic autism" characteristics, they are often undiagnosed or misdiagnosed with other conditions, such as social anxiety, regulatory challenges, learning disabilities, attention deficit disorders, or personality disorders (Lockwood-Estrin et al., 2021).

Gender Differences in Autistic Behaviors and Their Impact on Diagnosis

Autistic girls often exhibit autism differently than autistic boys. Their autistic behaviors tend to be more subtle, with fewer RRBIs, special interests that are generally more mainstream and socially acceptable, and a greater willingness to engage in social interactions. As a result, they are more likely to form successful social relationships compared to autistic boys (Lockwood-Estrin et al., 2021; Mandy et al., 2011; Werling & Geschwind, 2013; Young et al., 2018). The perception of autism characteristics as more socially acceptable in girls may contribute to delays in identification and support (Corscadden & Casserly, 2021). At the same time, social pressures, particularly during adolescence, compel girls to hide or internalize their autism characteristics. They are often expected to be shy and introverted, leading to their social difficulties being dismissed as typical shyness. Additionally, girls experience greater pressure to conform socially, with different upbringings and expectations for increased social engagement. These factors can exacerbate anxiety and hinder early diagnosis (Bargiela et al., 2016; Corscadden & Casserly, 2021; Dolović, 2024; Lockwood-Estrin et al., 2021).

Autistic women report that their autistic difficulties were misunderstood during childhood. They describe experiencing mental health challenges that led them to professionals who failed to recognize their symptoms as autism related (Bargiela et al., 2016; Harmens et al., 2022; Lockwood-Estrin et al., 2021). Many report high levels of anxiety, depression, self-harm, and suicidality (Cassidy et al., 2020).

The Psychological Toll of Late Diagnosis in Autistic Girls

Another phenomenon associated with autistic girls is masking or camouflaging—deliberately concealing their difficulties and mimicking typical peers' behaviors to conform to social norms (Corscadden & Casserly, 2021; Young et al., 2018). These efforts have a negative long-term impact on their well-being and mental health (Goodall & Mackenzie, 2019; Sedgewick et al., 2018; Tierney & Burns, 2017; Tomlinson et al., 2020). As a result, autistic females are often undiagnosed, late diagnosed, or misdiagnosed with non-autistic conditions. There is an urgent need for clinicians to understand the distinct presentation of autism in girls and non-binary people to prevent misdiagnosis and ensure appropriate support (Dolović, 2024; Harmens et al., 2022; Young et al., 2018). This highlights the importance of a nuanced and careful approach to the diagnostic process.

The Role of Parental Diagnosis Disclosure for Autistic Girls

While some autistic women express regret over not receiving an early diagnosis, believing it could have improved their lives, others suggest that an early diagnosis might have led to negative labeling and assumptions about their capabilities, potentially hindering their growth (Seers & Hogg, 2022). Delays in diagnosis and disclosure can have profound implications for access to support, as individuals who experience these delays often face negative judgments from others, leading to social isolation (Cridland et al., 2014).

An in-depth exploration of adolescent autistic girls' experiences highlights their unique challenges, including stigma, social isolation, and the complexities of navigating their diagnosis. Research indicates that autistic girls feel ambivalent about their autism label and that post-diagnosis support is often inadequate (Josefsson & Johansson, 2024). This may explain the post-parental disclosure process in which autistic individuals frequently seek additional information about autism through media, support groups, family, professionals, and other autistic individuals (Corden et al., 2021; Kiely et al., 2020). This process plays a crucial role in shaping an inclusive self-identity, fostering acceptance, and embracing autism as an integral part of one's sense of self.

However, in the absence of a diagnosis, this entire process is significantly hindered. For autistic girls, a late diagnosis can further complicate parental decisions regarding when and how to disclose the diagnosis. While the benefits of disclosure are widely recognized, research on effective disclosure strategies for children and adolescents remains limited (Kiely et al., 2020; Riccio et al., 2020; Smith et al., 2018). Notably, existing studies have yet to address the unique aspects of autism disclosure to girls.

Developing post-diagnosis guidance tailored to autistic girls and their parents is crucial for fostering self-understanding and supporting social navigation. Without adequate guidance, many struggle to process their diagnosis and face difficulties managing disclosure decisions later in life (Milner et al., 2019). As awareness of gender biases in autism increases, diagnostic practices are adapting to better recognize and support the diverse experiences of autistic individuals, particularly women and girls.

The Current Study

This chapter has two primary objectives. First, to examine the unique characteristics and dilemmas faced by parents when considering diagnosis disclosure and sharing with their daughters. Second, to illuminate these parental diagnosis disclosure dilemmas through the retrospective lens of autistic women's lived experiences.

The parental perspective allows us to understand the complex decision-making process and specific concerns that arise when sharing an autism diagnosis with girls, revealing gender-specific challenges that may differ from general autism disclosure experiences. Equally critical is the perspective of autistic women, whose retrospective accounts of their diagnosis disclosure journeys provide invaluable insights into the impact of different disclosure approaches. By integrating these two complementary viewpoints, this study seeks to develop more nuanced, gender-informed guidance for parents and professionals supporting autistic girls through the disclosure process.

Research Methods

This study employs both grounded theory (Glaser & Strauss, 1967) and emancipatory research approaches (Barnes, 2003; Oliver, 1992) to examine the unique dynamics of autism diagnosis disclosure to girls. The grounded theory methodology enabled us to develop integrated theoretical concepts directly from our empirical data, while the emancipatory approach focused on identifying and addressing societal barriers that affect autistic individuals. Specifically, we explored how concealing an autism diagnosis from girls can potentially hinder their personal development and self-understanding.

The analysis presented in this chapter draws from a broader ongoing research project (Almog et al., 2023, 2024) on autism diagnosis disclosure delay. We collected data from two complementary perspectives:

1. Parental perspective: focus groups with parents of autistic girls (n = 14) who had not yet shared the diagnosis with their daughters. These sessions provided insights into parental decision-making processes, concerns, and approaches to managing diagnostic information.
2. Autistic perspective: interviews with autistic women (n = 18, all diagnosed before age 18) about their experiences of learning about their diagnosis and their recommendations for how parents and professionals should approach diagnosis disclosure with young girls.

By integrating these dual perspectives, our analysis highlights the different viewpoints and experiences from both sides of the disclosure process. This methodological approach allows us to examine the complex interplay between parental intentions and the lived experiences of autistic women who have navigated this journey. Given the limited research on parental disclosure decisions, particularly regarding autistic girls, this study's findings are essential for developing evidence-based resources to support both parents and daughters through this critical developmental journey.

Focus Group: Methods and Recruitment

The focus group for parents of autistic girls was organized in collaboration with ALUT's Family Center,[1] which managed participant recruitment and registration. The group met three times, with each two-hour session being fully recorded and transcribed. The fourth and second authors facilitated the group, while the first author documented the sessions and participated in the third meeting. The sessions were structured progressively:

- First session: An open discussion where parents shared their thoughts and dilemmas about diagnosis disclosure.
- Second session: Featured Ronnie, a 24-year-old autistic woman, who shared her personal experiences. Parents engaged with both Ronnie and author 2, asking questions about their experiences as autistic adults.
- Third session: The first author presented preliminary research findings and recommendations, followed by a final discussion with parents.

The workshop reflected two core principles relevant to the process of diagnosis disclosure. The first is neurodiversity and the understanding that biological diversity is essential to human identity (Baron-Cohen, 2017). The second, "nothing about us without us" or the emancipatory methodology version "no longer researching about us without us" (Johnson, 2009), emphasizes the place of people with disabilities in creating knowledge about them. This principle was implemented in our study in two ways: (1) through the direct involvement of the second and third authors, who themselves are autistic adults and actively shaped the research design, analysis, and interpretation process. The second author facilitated the parent group discussions, while the third author coded the interviews with autistic women, ensuring autistic perspectives were integrated throughout the research process; and (2) through the participation of Ronnie, a 24-year-old autistic woman, in the parent focus group, providing modeling of autistic-parent dialog and offering parents insights into possible futures for their daughters. While the group's primary purpose was research rather than intervention, one mother chose to disclose the diagnosis to her daughter between the second and third meetings. A follow-up survey was conducted one month after the workshop to track any changes in parents' disclosure decisions.

---

[1] ALUT—The Israeli Society for Children and Adults with Autism, one of the first parent NGOs in Israel.

Participants

The group comprised 14 parents of autistic girls: 12 women and two men, consisting of three couples (one of them a couple of moms) and eight mothers. All of the parents described their daughters as high functioning, with an average age of 10. The average age of diagnosis was 5.2 years, which means that the dilemma of disclosing their diagnosis had already been part of their lives for approximately five years. The participants were self-selected parents who attended voluntarily. Their post-workshop feedback emphasized the value of the experience, with recommendations for other parents to attend similar workshops.

Personal Interviews: Methods and Participants

Eighteen semi-structured interviews were conducted with autistic women (age 17–30), all audiotaped and transcribed, lasting 60–120 min. The interviews allowed the participants to express the meanings they ascribed to their disclosure experience. The interview guide and more information are detailed in Almog et al. (2024) (Table 3.1).

Analysis of participants' diagnostic histories revealed two distinct groups: Group 1 (n = 9) experienced significant disclosure delays after early diagnosis (diagnosed at a mean age of 5.7 years), with parents withholding diagnostic information for 2–16 years (M = 8.4, SD = 3.89). Group 2 (n = 9) received immediate disclosure following later diagnoses (mean age 13.38 years). This later age of diagnosis coincided with increased cognitive maturity and self-awareness, making it more challenging for parents to conceal the diagnostic process and associated implications. This natural division provided valuable comparative insights into how disclosure timing impacts identity development and self-understanding."

The study received the approval of Ono College's Ethics Committee, as well as of the Ministry of Welfare and Social Affairs Ethics Committee. All participants' names have been replaced with pseudonyms to protect their privacy.

Table 3.1 Participants of personal interviews

	Group 1 Delayed Disclosure	Group 2 Immediate Disclosure	SUM
Number of participants	9	9	18
Age at Interview	M = 22, SD = 3.27, Range (17–27)	M = 25, SD = 4.06, Range (17–30)	M = 23.5, SD = 3.89
Age at diagnosis	M = 5.27, SD = 4.39	M = 13.38, SD = 4.7	M = 9.3, SD = 6.08
Years between diagnosis to disclosure	M = 8.4, SD = 3.89, Range: 2–16 years	Range: 0–4 weeks	

Findings: Gender-Specific Patterns in Autism Disclosure for Girls

The process of autism diagnosis disclosure to girls presents unique challenges shaped by gender-specific manifestations of autism and societal expectations. Analysis of perspectives from both parents and autistic women reveals how gender influences the diagnostic journey, parental disclosure decisions, and the lived experiences of autistic girls. Building on our previous research with parents of autistic boys (Almog et al., 2023), this chapter examines how parents of girls navigate distinct challenges, particularly around later diagnosis, diagnostic uncertainty, and complex presentation patterns.

This analysis is structured through a unique dual perspective approach: each theme is first examined from the parents' viewpoint and then from the perspective of autistic women who experienced the process during their childhood. This structure enables direct comparison between parental deliberations and the actual experiences of autistic girls, illuminating both the gaps and similarities between parental approaches and the expressed needs of the girls themselves.

Our analysis revealed three themes unique to the experiences of parents of autistic girls and the women themselves:

1. *Delayed Disclosure: Diagnosis Uncertainty and Concealed Identities*
   This theme examines the challenges related to late diagnosis and its impact on disclosure decisions and identity formation.
2. *Knowledge Gaps: Sense of Difference and Partial Information*
   This theme focuses on knowledge gaps between the child, family, and environment, and the ongoing search for self-understanding.
3. *The Masking Paradox: Invisibility and Mental Health Impacts*
   This theme explores the relationship between masking abilities, invisibility, and mental health challenges.

For each theme, we first present the parental perspective—how parents perceive and navigate the issue, followed by the autistic perspective—how autistic women experienced these same issues in their childhood. This parallel analysis provides a deeper understanding of the complex dynamics in the diagnosis disclosure process and offers crucial insights for developing evidence-based support strategies.

Delayed Disclosure: Diagnosis Uncertainty and Concealed Identities

The themes of uncertainty of diagnosis and concealed identities explore the complex interplay between parental doubt regarding autism diagnosis validity and the resulting concealment of autistic identity from the girls themselves. This dynamic creates a significant tension: while parents grapple with diagnostic ambiguity due to the complex presentation of autism in girls, these girls experience a fundamental disconnect from understanding their true selves, as crucial information about their neurodivergent identity remains hidden from them.

Parents' Perspective: Navigating Diagnostic Ambiguity

The focus group participants' daughters predominantly received late autism diagnoses (Average age of diagnosis 5.18, range 1.5–9), following complex diagnostic trajectories. Many girls initially received alternative diagnoses, particularly ADHD, social anxiety, or sensory processing disorder (SPD), before their autism was identified. Sometimes other diagnoses were made early and prevented the possibility of recognizing the autism, as Dorothy describes her daughter, who was diagnosed with autism at age 7:

> There was a very, very clear anxiety component. The anxiety started really, really early (before the age of 3), and actually, when we went for a medical assessment, they told us: 'Well, there are very clear anxiety issues here, first let's do a year of treatment, anxiety medication, and only then can we talk.'

Parents explained their daughters are "difficult to diagnose" and claimed that "girls are more on the edge." This pattern of initial misdiagnosis was also apparent in the autistic women's interviews.

The parents in the focus group frequently questioned the validity of the diagnosis and considered re-evaluation before disclosing it to their daughters, due to their doubts about its validity. These findings were entirely absent from a similar focus group conducted with parents of boys who were deliberating about sharing their child's diagnosis (Almog et al., 2023). Parents' uncertainty about autism diagnosis, particularly in cases of high functioning, was caused by four factors. First, parents observe significant developmental progress, leading them to question initial diagnoses. Some parents noted significant improvements that made them question if autism was still present, as parents of a 14-year-old girl who was diagnosed at age two and a half said: "She made huge progress in many areas, including socially. In elementary school..she was saying 'I don't want friends'… and today she has a group of friends." Second, the parents described symptom mismatch and the fact that most of the girls had previous or parallel psychiatric "labels." In fact, most parents went through a long journey as Theresa described:

> Today she's 7.5 years old. She was diagnosed at the age of 2.9, it was clear ADHD, severe sensory processing issues, and we accepted it, but still had questions… On the first day of first grade, reality hit me. That same day when I saw her at school, I told my partner: 'The child is autistic, I can see it.'

Third, uncertainty was reinforced by educational staff who often don't observe typical autism characteristics in structured school settings. As Victoria said: "'At school they kept saying: We don't see any social problems, she's well-liked, she has friends, there's no reason to accompany her anywhere'." Due to their high cognitive abilities and relatively low support needs in structured settings, these girls' autism characteristics often remained invisible to educational staff, further reinforcing parents' diagnostic uncertainty.

Fourth, the complex nature of these doubts is further complicated by the girls' ability to mask difficulties, as Frances and Audrey, a couple of mothers in the group said "Our daughter's diagnosis came much later (age 9) than our son's, which was identified at a much earlier age (age 3). She masked her difficulties for years until everything exploded during the COVID-19 period." These accounts highlight the dynamic-and context-dependent nature of autism presentation in girls, making diagnostic certainty particularly challenging for parents. Parental certainty in the diagnosis serves as a prerequisite for disclosure to their daughter. Without diagnostic certainty, parental disclosure cannot meaningfully occur.

Autistic Perspective: Uncovering Concealed Identities

The retrospective accounts of autistic women revealed two distinct diagnostic disclosure patterns influencing their identity formation and self-understanding. While one group experienced significant delays between diagnosis and disclosure (averaging 8.4 years), others received immediate disclosure following their later-life diagnoses, when increased cognitive maturity made concealment more challenging for parents, creating fundamentally different pathways to self-discovery. Group 2's later age of diagnosis coincided with increased cognitive maturity and self-awareness, making it more challenging for parents to conceal the diagnostic process and associated implications.

Most participants in the delayed disclosure group didn't have an organized conversation with their parents about the diagnosis. Many of them discovered it through indirect and delayed paths. In some cases, the diagnosis was disclosed by a therapist or educational staff, as Isabella from group 1 described:

> From age 6 to 14, I didn't know I was on the spectrum, and eventually, after a mental breakdown and six months of psychological therapy, my psychologist told me about the diagnosis...My parents initially opposed it, especially my father... It took several meetings between the psychologist and my parents until they gave permission to tell me.

Another participant's story illustrates the common protective approach to diagnosis disclosure. Emma's parents withheld her diagnosis for 14 years, revealing it only at age 16 through an indirect conversation about a social group: "My mom mentioned people with... social difficulties, something along this term, and my dad said that maybe I could find friends there with Asperger's, and before that I didn't know what that word meant." When questioned about this delay, her mother's emotional response—"this isn't something young children need to know about"—reflected a widespread parental belief that withholding the diagnosis serves as protection. However, this approach meant Emma spent her childhood navigating her differences without the framework to understand them. The cases described above illustrate a common parental approach—prioritizing privacy and protection around autism diagnoses, though perspectives on early disclosure have evolved significantly since then. It appears there was a lack of an organized process of sharing the diagnosis by the parents, which sometimes led to delayed or indirect disclosure of the diagnosis. However, when the interviewees discovered their diagnosis, most of them experienced it as something that helped them understand themselves better.

Knowledge Gaps: Sense of Difference and Partial Information

This theme addresses the complex interplay between different forms of knowledge about autism. While parents and professionals hold formal medical knowledge, autistic girls possess experiential knowledge derived from both internal experiences and social comparisons. These different types of knowledge often create gaps in understanding between the child, their family, and their surroundings. Such gaps frequently prompt these girls to question their identity and seek understanding of their perceived differences.

Parents' Perspective: Managing Disclosure Dilemmas

The conflict between partial knowledge about autism and sense of difference was a prominent theme in parental focus group discussions. Parents described how they witnessed their daughters actively seeking information about themselves and their differences, while they struggled with how to respond. As we conceptualized in our earlier work, this process resembles an internal "search engine"—children actively searching for explanations about their experienced otherness through cumulative life experiences (Almog et al., 2024). Parents reported navigating complex questions from their daughters about their perceived differences. As Victoria, a mother of a 15-year-old girl, shared:

> They read *The Curious Incident of the Dog in the Night-Time* at school, and her question was: 'Mom, I feel a bit like in the book.' I choked up because it would have been natural to say yes to her, but it was still something we (both parents) hadn't discussed.

This interaction exemplifies three critical elements in autism disclosure that created conflict for parents: children's intuitive self-recognition through identification with autistic characters in media, parental emotional complexity during potential disclosure moments ("I choked"), and the tension between maintaining parental honesty and managing disclosure implications. Another parent reported their daughter's persistence in seeking clarity: "She knows she's a special child…but it wasn't enough for her. She said to me: 'Yes, but what does that mean? What do they see?'." This illustrates the conflict parents face, where limited disclosure often generates additional questions rather than providing resolution.

Parents in the focus groups expressed multiple fears and ethical dilemmas. One significant fear was that information about the diagnosis would be exposed in an uncontrolled way by various figures in the child's environment. As Grace, one of the mothers in the group stated: "My biggest fear is that she'll hear it from someone... it would be a breach of trust." Other parents mentioned the crisis that might occur due to parental disclosure delay, as Theresa said: "She'll understand on her own and she'll be angry at me, so why shouldn't I tell her." The meanings of damaging the trust when the daughter discovers everyone knew except her, will be presented from the autistic perspective below. Parents also described the ethical dilemma of withholding information from the daughter, as Linda explained:

> I think she needs to give me permission to tell it to the world. I would really love to tell it to the world, I'm waiting for it, but I think I need to respect her and let her be in a place of choice about who knows and how much.

This quote symbolizes how the need to coordinate information with various factors in the daughter's environment is corelated with on the disclosure dilemma.

This analysis captures the multi-dimensional nature of the conflict parents experience, as they grapple with the complexity of knowledge gaps between them, their child and different parties in the child's environment. Both parents and child are aware of something that remains unnamed and undefined. This creates a delicate child-parent dynamic where the truth hovers just below the surface of daily interactions, acknowledged but not directly addressed.

Autistic Perspective: Seeking Explanations for Difference

Curiosity about their autism diagnosis emerged as a central theme in autistic women's interviews. The participants often described an intrinsic awareness of their unique characteristics, even without having the language or framework to define them. This experience of navigating partial and unspoken knowledge manifested in various ways throughout the interviews.

Many participants recounted specific instances that highlighted their sense of difference from neurotypical peers and siblings, spanning from sensory sensitivities to distinct patterns of social interaction and communication. For example, Charlotte shared her experiences of overwhelming classroom noise: "There were several times when I just got up and walked down three flights of stairs and went to sit under a table in the library. Because I couldn't handle being in my class." Similarly, Helen reflected on her heightened sensory experiences, noting "My hearing was always amplified by twenty. Twenty times more than what everyone else actually hears."

These distinctions became particularly salient through direct comparisons in educational and social contexts. As Emma articulated, "It's clear that I knew something about me was a bit different from others." She pointed to concrete examples, such as her brother starting first grade at age six while she remained in kindergarten until age seven, and observed that "he didn't go to many weekly treatments compared to me." The experience of otherness extended even to family dynamics, as evidenced by Olivia's poignant reflection: "I feel this difference especially when I'm with my family. Usually family is the place that embraces you. This is also the family you live with your whole life, and yet with them specifically I feel very strange."

These experiences collectively illuminate a profound conflict. Their accounts reveal a complex interplay of sensory experiences, social interactions, and family dynamics that shaped the women's early awareness of being different. Through everyday moments and interactions, they developed an intricate self-awareness that preceded any formal framework for understanding their autistic identity.

This search for understanding often led to confusing and sometimes traumatic discoveries. Mia described her experience of indirect disclosure in special education:

"Around 7th grade, there was this aunt who asked me why I was in special education. I told her I didn't know, and I got upset. I told my teacher about this aunt, and she answered that we really need to tell each person why they're here. And then indeed, at the end of the year, the tutor and the teacher told me why I was there. But they didn't really tell me; they told me: 'No, it's not because you have PDD, definitely not, you don't have PDD. You have this something… you ask a lot of questions, you say the same thing many times, and it's quite similar to PDD. They didn't want to tell me in words." (Mia).

The impact of discovering one's diagnosis without proper support is further illustrated by Grace's experience. As she describes:

> I was home alone; my parents were abroad... and then there was a knock on the door, and I was given a package of papers that had my name on them and next to it 'National Insurance - Disability' and then I tried to connect between disability and who I am. Because at that time I didn't know that disability was such a complex and broad word. I thought that being disabled meant only physical disability, like being in a wheelchair or something like that. And then I realized something here doesn't make sense. After I checked, I simply threw the papers aside and told myself: 'No, I'm like everyone else and everything is fine.' I went on with my business.

This initial experience was compounded by her mother's attitude, who "doesn't really accept having an autistic daughter." Unsurprisingly, Grace later adopted similar patterns of disclosure: "There was a period when I would say 'Hi, I'm autistic' and then I would run away". The traumatic experience of discovering her diagnosis without support or explanation profoundly shaped her relationship with her autistic identity and her ability to share it with others. This case demonstrates how parental attitudes toward diagnosis disclosure can directly influence a child's future self-disclosure patterns. This represents another type of knowledge gap, where partial information without proper support can be more disruptive than either full disclosure or complete unawareness.

Some participants mentioned their intuitive self-recognition through identification with autistic characters in media, as Isabella said when referring to Sheldon from "The Big Bang Theory":

> They never explicitly say he's diagnosed, but it's a very extreme version of autism… He's not good socially. He's very rigid in the things he does, and usually... usually people laugh about it. But as a child, I sat there, watched it, and said, 'Wow! That's me!' … It was just

> the closest to what I feel, and I could really use him for examples, because like, people saw it on TV. So, if Sheldon needs to sit in a specific spot, I need to sit in a specific spot too!

While partial knowledge itself creates new problems or challenges, getting familiar with an autistic role model leads to better understanding of the self and better self-advocacy due to the use of a familiar example.

The paradox of partial knowledge emerges clearly through these accounts—while some forms of partial knowledge (like media representation) can aid self-understanding, unmediated or incomplete knowledge often creates more confusion than clarity. This partial knowledge frequently results in increased anxiety, confusion about identity, potential misinterpretation of differences, and trust issues when the full information eventually comes to light.

The Masking Paradox: Invisibility and Mental Health Impacts

This theme explores the complex relationship between masking behaviors, invisibility of autism, and mental health challenges. While masking abilities allow autistic girls to blend in socially, this apparent success often comes at a significant psychological cost, creating a paradoxical situation where better social adaptation leads to increased internal distress. Through examining both parental concerns about their daughters' invisible struggles and autistic women's accounts of the psychological toll of maintaining these masks, this theme highlights how gender expectations and autism intersect to create unique challenges.

Parents' Perspective: Confronting the Costs of Invisible Autism

The intersection of invisibility, mental health challenges, and masking behaviors emerged as a distinctive theme that complicated the disclosure process for parents of autistic girls. Unlike the disclosure challenges reported by parents of autistic boys, who primarily worried about stigma and timing (Almog et al., 2023), parents of girls faced additional complexities relating to their daughters' sophisticated masking abilities and the psychological toll these took.

Parents consistently emphasized that their daughters' autism was not immediately apparent or visible to others, often using phrases like "you can't see it on her" or describing them as "very high functioning." However, this invisibility came at a significant psychological cost.

Parents frequently described how their daughters' ability to mask their difficulties was intrinsically linked to mounting mental health challenges. As Frances explained: "The medications sometimes work, sometimes don't work, we switch them, keep switching them—this whole saga is like a movie… Every morning we don't know what we're going to get."

This complexity was particularly evident in cases where daughters were already managing multiple diagnoses, as Theresa, mother of a 7.5-year-old, explained:

> She knows she has ADHD, and she knows she takes Ritalin and Risperdal - she doesn't know the names, but we tell her we need to calm her restless mind and there are all sorts of definitions like that we use. But to introduce the communication (autism) issue? That's like adding fuel to the fire.

This hesitation reflects parents' concerns about overwhelming their daughters with an additional diagnostic label when they were already struggling with anxiety and emotional regulation.

Parents' disclosure considerations were often precipitated by incidents of social difficulties or bullying, particularly when their daughters' masking abilities began to falter. Dorothy, whose 7.5-year-old daughter received her diagnosis just 1.5 months before our group meeting, described how her daughter was experiencing severe bullying at school: "She's already asking questions…she asks me: 'Mom, why is it harder for me to connect and make friends than it is for other children?'" The visibility of social differences in school settings often triggered these considerations, as Beatrice observed:

> She's quite different in class because she avoids many things and finds herself spending half the day, I think, less functional, just observing. And this raises the question of how to mediate this (diagnosis) to her. Because although she's young and maybe it's not the age to talk about it, there's something here that needs to be mediated, for a child who behaves differently.

Parents expressed significant concern about how disclosure might impact their daughters' self-image. Grace, mother of a 15.9-year-old, articulated this dilemma:

> On one hand, knowing can give her inner peace - she has a definition in her head of 'okay, I'm like this and like that, and this is who I am'. On the other hand, what does it give her on the inside, deep inside - self-confidence, how does the world look at me? how do I look at myself?'

This reflection highlights the delicate balance parents sought between providing understanding and potentially burdening their daughters with a stigmatized label.

When approaching disclosure, many parents emphasized the importance of framing autism through a strength-based, empowering lens. One mother described explaining the diagnosis by highlighting her daughter's exceptional abilities: "They saw that your brain works differently… and it works in an amazing way." She specifically emphasized positive attributes such as memory, attention to detail, and perfect pitch, deliberately constructing a narrative that celebrated rather than pathologized these differences. However, parents' efforts to frame autism positively often conflicted with broader societal stigma. As one mother noted, "We're still fighting to this day to establish that 'autistic' isn't a slur." Another parent emphasized this empowerment approach: "I wanted to empower her, I didn't want her to think she was some kind of freak or anything." This ongoing tension between personal empowerment and social stigma significantly influenced both the timing and approach to disclosure, as parents sought to protect their daughters while providing them with the understanding and support they needed.

Autistic Perspective: The Psychological Cost of Camouflaging

The interviews with autistic women revealed complex patterns of masking behaviors and their associated psychological costs. Their accounts highlighted how the intersection of gender expectations and autism created unique challenges around visibility, mental health, diagnosis, and disclosure. Participants described developing sophisticated masking strategies from an early age, often without conscious awareness. As Isabella explained:

> One of the hardest things for me to deal with before I knew I was on the spectrum was that I felt I had a mask, that I was acting. But I didn't understand why I was doing it. I also didn't understand... if I have so many masks and so many protocols for talking to people - who am I really? Who am I? What's the mask, what's acting and what's not?

These masking behaviors manifested across different domains—from consciously modulating voice intonation ("It's very mechanical for me…I fight with myself about when to raise my voice, when to lower it") to adjusting social behavior ("Sometimes I lower my standards and behave at a very low level…I joke around and go with their flow"). The psychological cost of maintaining these masks was significant, leading to exhaustion, anxiety, and profound emotional isolation. As Mary shared: "I was quite lonely, didn't have many close friends and wasn't popular. And I suffered from it... I think people didn't feel my suffering or my difficulty or… like how weak I was…how bad I felt." Mary's story demonstrates how masking behaviors can lead to profound emotional isolation, even when seemingly "successful" at blending in socially. Her reflection on others not perceiving her internal struggles highlights a critical aspect of masking—the disconnect between external presentation and internal experience. This invisibility of suffering compounds the psychological burden, as individuals not only experience distress but feel fundamentally unseen in their struggles.

The effort required to maintain these masks had significant psychological implications. Participants described experiencing exhaustion, anxiety, and identity confusion as a result of constant social performance. The pressure to appear "normal" while internally struggling created what many described as a double life. This was particularly evident in family contexts, as previously exemplified by Olivia's perception of her family's dynamics.

Another recurring theme was how successful masking often delayed diagnosis and support. The better participants were at concealing their challenges, the longer they went without understanding or assistance. This created a paradoxical situation where their coping mechanisms ultimately prevented them from accessing needed support. This was particularly evident in educational settings, where high academic achievement often masked underlying struggles. This pattern is illustrated in Helen's story about her experiences in 11th grade, when her previous coping mechanisms became insufficient: "I had more anxiety attacks, I was more withdrawn, I was always alone, less with others, and this only started in 11th grade." Like many autistic women and as described by parents in the focus group, Helen's struggles became more visible during adolescence, leading to professional intervention and eventual diagnosis. This period marked a shift from successful masking to a point where the emotional and social demands exceeded her ability to maintain her previous compensatory strategies.

For some participants, receiving and understanding their diagnosis provided a framework for developing more authentic self-expression, particularly in supportive environments. This transition from constant masking to selective authenticity often paralleled their journey toward a more positive autism identity. As Evelyn described:

> When I'm with other autistic people or in supportive environments, I can behave how I want, and I feel very liberated. It's somewhat obvious because you're very open and you have friends who supposedly have the same limitation, which is the personality, it's something similar. The traits may be different but there are difficulties that we tell each other about and I feel more secure.

This reflection illustrates how creating safe spaces and positive autism narratives can allow autistic women to move beyond masking toward authentic self-expression, echoing the empowering approach that many parents strive to provide for their daughters.

Finally, after years of integrating their autistic identity, most participants expressed pride in their autistic identity, highlighting unique strengths and abilities. Olivia, who works in a library, articulated how autism-related characteristics enhanced her work performance: "I feel that in the professional domain, autism is an advantage," she explained, detailing specific strengths such as systematic information processing, attention to detail, and strong visual memory. She drew parallels between her work cataloging books and programming, noting how both benefit from autistic traits: "The work requires many repetitive, methodical tasks—you need to go through hundreds of books daily, following a specific system… Each book has an identifying number and designated location, and when you identify that a book has more than one location, you need to consolidate. It's work that has a visual aspect too, remembering many titles and covers."

This recognition of unique autistic strengths was powerfully articulated by Abigail: "I see myself, there are advantages to being autistic. Like, when I focus intensely on something, I'll know it well, the best there is… it's a gift from my perspective. It's something that represents me and I love myself." And as she emphatically stated: "Autism isn't a problem, it's a gift, in my opinion, okay? I'll repeat this a million times because this is what I think."

This theme of finding safe spaces for authentic expression was particularly significant for participants who had spent years masking without understanding why. The diagnosis often provided not just an explanation for their differences, but also a pathway to finding communities and developing a positive autistic identity.

The findings presented above can be synthesized into an integrated model of how gender rules and societal expectations shape the autism disclosure journey for girls (see Fig. 3.1). The model illustrates how gender expectations influence both masking behaviors and diagnostic uncertainty, creating interconnected pathways that affect autistic girls' experiences. Masking and invisibility contribute to mental health impacts, while also connecting to the heightened sense of difference that many autistic girls experience. Simultaneously, diagnostic uncertainty leads to knowledge gaps and partial information, which further contributes to concealed identity. These elements converge in the delayed disclosure of autism, which significantly impacts identity development. However, the model also reveals that when disclosure finally occurs, it often leads to self-understanding and relief, enabling autistic girls to make sense of their experiences and develop a sense of belonging. This framework helps explain why the disclosure process for autistic girls involves unique challenges that differ from those experienced by boys, highlighting the need for gender-sensitive approaches to diagnosis and disclosure.

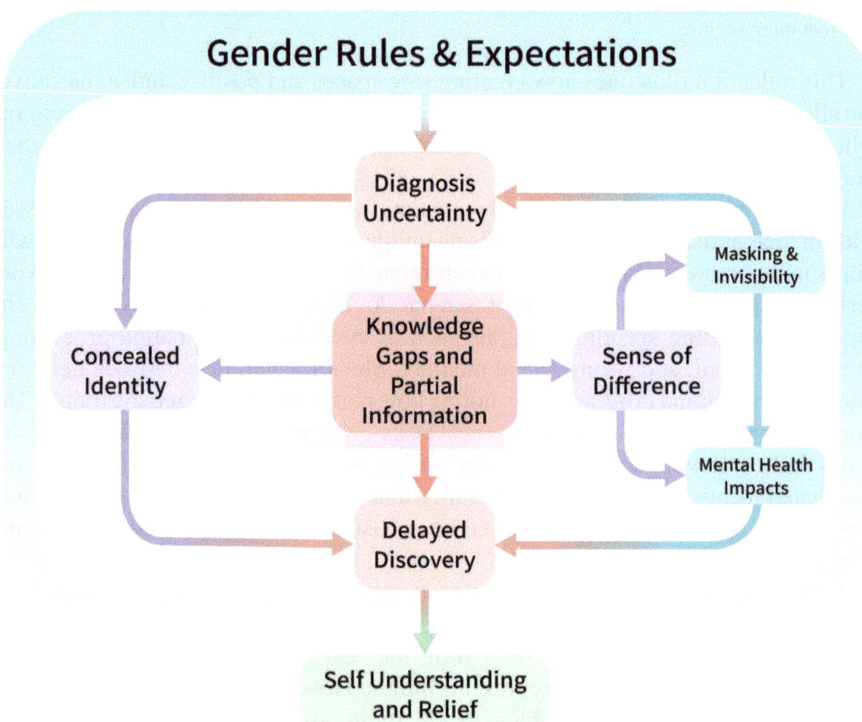

Fig. 3.1 Gender Dynamics Influence on Autism Diagnosis, Disclosure and Disclosure Process in girls

Discussion

This chapter reveals several key insights about the unique challenges and dynamics in autism parental diagnosis disclosure for girls, while contributing to existing theoretical frameworks and practical understanding of this complex process.

Gender-Specific Manifestations and Theoretical Implications

Building on previous research regarding gender differences in autism presentation (Bargiela et al., 2016; Driver & Chester, 2021), our findings highlight distinct patterns that significantly impact both diagnosis and disclosure processes. The prevalent pattern of late diagnosis (average age 5.18 years among parents' daughters and 9.3 years among autistic participants), often following complex diagnostic trajectories, aligns with existing literature on diagnostic challenges for girls (Cammuso & Knapp-Ines, 2024). However, our study reveals additional complexities through what we call the "masking paradox"—where better masking abilities lead to later diagnosis and delayed support, potentially increasing long-term psychological burden.

This paradox extends beyond previous theoretical frameworks by demonstrating how masking not only affects external recognition but actively shapes the internal process of identity formation. While earlier research emphasized masking as a coping mechanism (Bargiela et al., 2016), our dual-perspective analysis shows how masking creates a cyclical pattern affecting both diagnosis and disclosure decisions.

The Complex Knowledge Gap Framework

Our analysis reveals a multi-layered knowledge gap that characterizes the disclosure experience for autistic girls, expanding on Cridland et al. (2014) work on delayed diagnosis impacts. While they primarily focused on the consequences of social isolation, our study reveals a more nuanced pattern of cascading effects through three distinct but interconnected levels:

1. Parent–child knowledge gap;
2. Individual–environmental gap;
3. Professional–family gap.

It is crucial to acknowledge that parental experience encompasses navigating significant knowledge gaps stemming from delayed diagnosis, diagnostic uncertainties, and preliminary labels. This creates a meta-level knowledge gap that lies at the core of multiple information asymmetries and the process of acceptance. This interconnected pattern of information disparities demonstrates how missing information at critical developmental stages leads to increasingly complex challenges in accessing appropriate support, particularly affecting girls' ability to understand and advocate for their needs.

Long-Term Implications for Identity Development

Our findings support and extend Seers and Hogg's (2022) research regarding the relationship between disclosure timing and identity development. While their work emphasized timing as the critical factor, our dual-perspective analysis reveals that the quality and context of disclosure may be equally, if not more, important. This finding aligns with our recent research (Almog et al., 2024), which demonstrated that how and in what context the diagnosis is shared has profound impacts beyond the timing alone. In this chapter, we have identified several significant implications for identity development. First, disclosure experiences directly influence the development of authentic self-expression, as shown through participants' accounts of finding freedom in understanding their differences. Second, this understanding enhances their ability to advocate for personal needs, providing a framework for articulating previously inexplicable challenges. Third, proper disclosure contributes significantly to the formation of autistic identity, allowing girls to recognize strengths alongside challenges. Finally, early disclosure experiences shape patterns of future self-disclosure decisions, creating either positive cycles of openness or reinforcing patterns of concealment. These findings align with and further develop DePape and Lindsay's (2016) emphasis on the importance of recognizing subjective experiences in early development to facilitate healthy identity formation.

Practical Recommendations for Parents and Professionals

- Frame autism through a strength-based, empowering lens while acknowledging sensory experiences, social challenges, and the feeling of otherness.
- Develop and implement gender-sensitive support programs for parents during the disclosure process. Educate parents about how autism intersects with gender roles and social expectations for girls.
- Train parents to recognize and understand the distinct manifestations of autism in girls, particularly regarding masking behaviors. Guide parents in identifying early signs of mental health challenges related to masking and provide specific intervention strategies.
- Equip parents with practical tools to help their daughters navigate social situations while preserving their authentic selves. Coach parents in supporting positive identity development while addressing gender-specific challenges.
- Design stage-specific support strategies that evolve with girls' developmental needs, with particular attention to the intensified social demands of adolescence.

- Establish and maintain safe spaces where autistic girls can freely express themselves. Develop clear protocols for creating environments that celebrate neurodiversity.

This chapter enhances our understanding of autism disclosure in girls while providing a foundation for developing more effective support strategies. Future research should examine the long-term effectiveness of different disclosure approaches and continue to explore the unique needs of autistic girls in this process.

Disclosure:

In this text, we used assistive AI tools to improve the manuscript's word choice, language, grammar, and structure, and for those purposes only.

References

Almog, N., Keren, E. H., Gabai, T., & Kassel, O. (2024). Autistic people's perspectives on parental diagnosis disclosure: A grounded theory study. *Journal of Autism and Developmental Disorders*, 1–15. https://doi.org/10.1007/s10803-024-06468-2

Almog, N., Kassel, O., Levy, N., & Gabai, T. (2023). Mapping the dilemmas parents face with disclosing autism diagnosis to their child. *Journal of Autism and Developmental Disorders, 53*(10), 4060–4075. https://doi.org/10.1007/s10803-022-05711-y

Asperger, H. (1991). Autistic psychopathy in childhood. In U. Frith (Ed.), *Autism and Asperger Syndrome* (pp. 37–92). Cambridge University Press. (Original work published 1944). https://doi.org/10.1017/CBO9780511526770.002

Bargiela, S., Steward, R., & Mandy, W. (2016). The experiences of late-diagnosed women with autism spectrum conditions: An investigation of the female autism phenotype. *Journal of Autism and Developmental Disorders, 46*(10), 3281–3294. https://doi.org/10.1007/s10803-016-2872-8

Barnes, C. (2003). What a difference a decade makes: Reflections on doing 'emancipatory' disability research. *Disability & Society, 18*(1), 3–17. https://doi.org/10.1080/713662197

Baron-Cohen, S. (2017). Editorial perspective: Neurodiversity—a revolutionary concept for autism and psychiatry. *Journal of Child Psychology and Psychiatry, 58*(6), 744–747. https://doi.org/10.1111/jcpp.12703

Browning, J., Osborne, L. A., & Reed, P. (2009). Research section: A qualitative comparison of perceived stress and coping in adolescents with and without autistic spectrum disorders as they approach leaving school. *British Journal of Special Education, 36*(1), 36–43. https://doi.org/10.1111/j.1467-8578.2008.00400.x

Camarena, P. M., & Sarigiani, P. A. (2009). Postsecondary educational aspirations of high-functioning adolescents with autism spectrum disorders and their parents. *Focus on Autism and Other Developmental Disabilities, 24*(2), 115–128. https://doi.org/10.1177/1088357609332675

Cammuso, K., & Knapp-Ines, K. (2024). Autism in girls: Camouflaging, social functioning, and diagnostic dilemmas. *The Brown University Child and Adolescent Behavior Letter, 40*(6), 1–6. https://doi.org/10.1002/cbl.30790

Cassidy, S. A., Robertson, A., Townsend, E., O'Connor, R. C., & Rodgers, J. (2020). Advancing our understanding of self-harm, suicidal thoughts and behaviours in autism. *Journal of Autism and Developmental Disorders, 50*(10), 3445–3449. https://doi.org/10.1007/s10803-020-04643-9

Corden, K., Brewer, R., & Cage, E. (2021). Personal identity after an autism diagnosis: Relationships with self-esteem, mental wellbeing, and diagnostic timing. *Frontiers in Psychology, 12*, Article 699335. https://doi.org/10.3389/fpsyg.2021.699335

Corscadden, P., & Casserly, A. M. (2021). Identification of autism in girls: Role of trait subtleties, social acceptance and masking. *REACH: Journal of Inclusive Education in Ireland, 34*(1). https://reachjournal.ie/index.php/reach/article/view/313

Cridland, E. K., Jones, S. C., Caputi, P., & Magee, C. A. (2014). Being a girl in a boys' world: Investigating the experiences of girls with autism spectrum disorders during adolescence. *Journal of Autism and Developmental Disorders, 44*(6), 1261–1274. https://doi.org/10.1007/s10803-013-1985-6

DePape, A. M., & Lindsay, S. (2016). Lived experiences from the perspective of individuals with autism spectrum disorder: A qualitative meta-synthesis. *Focus on Autism and Other Developmental Disabilities, 31*(1), 60–71. https://doi.org/10.1177/1088357615587504

Dolović, N. (2024). Challenges associated with the identification of autism spectrum condition symptomatology in girls: A grounded theory lite approach. *European Psychiatry, 67*(S1), S467–S467. https://doi.org/10.1192/j.eurpsy.2024.968

Driver, B., & Chester, V. (2021). The presentation, recognition and diagnosis of autism in women and girls. *Advances in Autism, 7*(3), 194–207. https://doi.org/10.1108/AIA-12-2019-0050

Duek-Huri, S. (2014). Gilluy atsmi vesanegor atsmi: Tahalikh shel dialog tippuli, mishpakhti umaarakhti [Self-disclosure and self-advocacy: A process of therapeutic, familial and systemic dialogue]. In S. Lowinger (Ed.), *Meever laqqeshet: Khiddushim beivkhun uvetippul shel yeladim al hassepeqterum haotiseti [Beyond the spectrum: Innovations in the diagnosis and treatment of children on the autism spectrum]* (pp. 235–270). Ach.

Eckerd, M. (2020). Detection and diagnosis of ASD in females. *Journal of Health Service Psychology, 46*(1), 37–47. https://doi.org/10.1007/s42843-020-00006-1

Glaser, B. G., & Strauss, A. L. (1967). *The discovery of grounded theory: Strategies for qualitative research.* Routledge.

Goodall, C., & MacKenzie, A. (2019). What about my voice? Autistic young girls' experiences of mainstream school. *European Journal of Special Needs Education, 34*(4), 499–513. https://doi.org/10.1080/08856257.2018.1553138

Harmens, M., Sedgewick, F., & Hobson, H. (2022). Autistic women's diagnostic experiences: Interactions with identity and impacts on well-being. *Women's Health, 18*, 17455057221137476. https://doi.org/10.1177/17455057221137477

Huws, J. C., & Jones, R. S. P. (2008). Diagnosis, disclosure, and having autism: An interpretative phenomenological analysis of the perceptions of young people with autism. *Journal of Intellectual and Developmental Disability, 33*(2), 99–107. https://doi.org/10.1080/13668250802010394

Johnson, K. (2009). No longer researching about us without us: A researcher's reflection on rights and inclusive research in Ireland. *British Journal of Learning Disabilities, 37*(4), 250–256. https://doi.org/10.1111/j.1468-3156.2009.00579.x

Josefsson, H., & Johansson, S. T. (2024). Adolescent autistic girls navigating their diagnosis in Swedish secondary school. *Frontiers in Education, 9*, 1461054. https://doi.org/10.3389/feduc.2024.1461054

Kanner, L. (1943). Autistic disturbances of affective contact. *Nervous Child, 2*(3), 217–250.

Kiely, B., Adesman, A., Rapoport, E., & Gutman, A. (2020). Patterns and outcomes of diagnosis disclosure to youth with autism spectrum disorder. *Journal of Developmental & Behavioral Pediatrics, 41*(6), 443–451. https://doi.org/10.1097/DBP.0000000000000802

Lockwood-Estrin, G., Milner, V., Spain, D., Happé, F., & Colvert, E. (2021). Barriers to autism spectrum disorder diagnosis for young women and girls: A systematic review. *Review Journal of Autism and Developmental Disorders, 8*(4), 454–470. https://doi.org/10.1007/s40489-020-00225-8

Loubersac, J., Michelon, C., Ferrando, L., Picot, M., & Baghdadli, A. (2021). Predictors of an earlier diagnosis of autism spectrum disorder in children and adolescents: A systematic review (1987–2017). *European Child & Adolescent Psychiatry, 32*, 375–393. https://doi.org/10.1007/s00787-021-01792-9

Mandy, W., Chilvers, R., Chowdhury, U., Salter, G., Seigal, A., & Skuse, D. (2011). Sex differences in autism spectrum disorder: Evidence from a large sample of children and adolescents. *Journal of Autism and Developmental Disorders, 42*(7), 1304–1313. https://doi.org/10.1007/s10803-011-1356-0

Milner, V., McIntosh, H., Colvert, E., & Happé, F. (2019). A qualitative exploration of the female experience of autism spectrum disorder (ASD). *Journal of Autism and Developmental Disorders, 49*(6), 2389–2402. https://doi.org/10.1007/s10803-019-03906-4

Oliver, M. (1992). Changing the social relations of research production? *Disability, Handicap & Society, 7*(2), 101–114. https://doi.org/10.1080/02674649266780141

Riccio, A., Kapp, S. K., Jordan, A., Dorelien, A. M., & Gillespie-Lynch, K. (2020). How is autistic identity in adolescence influenced by parental disclosure decisions and perceptions of autism? *Autism, 25*(2), 374–388. https://doi.org/10.1177/1362361320958214

Sedgewick, F., Hill, V., & Pellicano, E. (2018). 'It's different for girls': Gender differences in the friendships and conflict of autistic and neurotypical adolescents. *Autism, 23*(5), 1119–1132. https://doi.org/10.1177/1362361318794930

Seers, K., & Hogg, R. (2022). "Fake it 'till you make it": Authenticity and wellbeing in late diagnosed autistic women. *Feminism & Psychology, 33*(1), 23–41. https://doi.org/10.1177/09593535221101455

Smith, I. C., Edelstein, J., Cox, B. E., & White, S. (2018). Parental disclosure of ASD diagnosis to the child: A systematic review. *Evidence-Based Practice in Child and Adolescent Mental Health, 3*, 98–105. https://doi.org/10.1080/23794925.2018.1435319

Tierney, S., & Burns, J. (2017). Behind the mask: A qualitative study of autistic women's experiences of 'camouflaging'. In M. J. Legato (Ed.), *Principles of gender-specific medicine* (pp. 203–217). Academic Press. https://doi.org/10.1016/B978-0-12-803506-1.00004-8

Tomlinson, C., Bond, C., & Hebron, J. (2020). The school experiences of autistic girls and adolescents: A systematic review. *European Journal of Special Needs Education, 35*(2), 203–219. https://doi.org/10.1080/08856257.2019.1643154

Tsirgiotis, J. M., Young, R. L., & Weber, N. (2024). A comparison of the presentations of males and females with autism spectrum disorder and those narrowly below the diagnostic threshold. *Autism: The International Journal of Research and Practice, 28*(4), 1029–1044. https://doi.org/10.1177/13623613231190682

Werling, D., & Geschwind, D. (2013). Sex differences in autism spectrum disorders. *Current Opinion in Neurology, 26*(2), 146–153. https://doi.org/10.1097/WCO.0b013e32835ee548

Young, H., Oreve, M. J., & Speranza, M. (2018). Clinical characteristics and problems diagnosing autism spectrum disorder in girls. *Archives De Pediatrie: Organe Officiel De La Societe Francaise De Pediatrie, 25*(6), 399–403. https://doi.org/10.1016/j.arcped.2018.06.008

Culture and Gender

Chapter 4
School Refusal in Autism: Causes, Consequences, and Intervention Strategies

Tal Zacharia and Shiri Pearlman-Avnion

Abstract This paper explores school refusal, a behavioral condition marked by a child's reluctance or avoidance of school attendance, often presenting with physical, emotional, or behavioral symptoms. Although not a formal mental health diagnosis, it is a significant concern affecting an estimated 1–5% of children, particularly those aged 5–10 years. School refusal carries substantial short-term risks like academic decline and long-term consequences such as school dropout, social difficulties, and psychiatric disorders. The sources highlight that school refusal is significantly more prevalent, has an earlier onset, and is more prolonged in autistic children compared to their typically developing peers. Complex factors contribute to this phenomenon in autistic students, including profound difficulties with social functioning and heightened vulnerability to bullying, with victimization rates reaching 46–94%. Other contributing factors include challenges during school transitions (e.g., elementary to high school), sensory sensitivities, and the high comorbidity of psychiatric conditions such as anxiety and depression. The paper emphasizes the critical need for vigilance, early identification, and comprehensive interventions, including managing anxiety, promoting social skills, and preventing bullying, to support autistic students and ensure their educational and socio-emotional well-being.

Keywords School refusal · Absenteeism · Bullying · Anxiety · Depression · Social functioning · Educational challenges · Children's mental health

T. Zacharia (✉)
Educational Psychology Service, Rosh HaAyin, Israel
e-mail: Talzac24@gmail.com

S. Pearlman-Avnion
Tel-Hai College, Kiryat Shmona, Israel

S. Lowinger and S. Pearlman-Avnion (eds.), *Collaborative Care and Partnerships in Autism Diagnosis and Treatment*, Autism and Child Psychopathology Series,
https://doi.org/10.1007/978-3-032-07009-8_4

School Refusal

School refusal is a behavioral condition where children display reluctance or avoidance of attending school, often accompanied by physical, emotional, or behavioral symptoms (Kearney & Albano, 2004; Kearney & Silverman, 1999). It is an important issue among children and adolescents. Education is a fundamental right that prepares children and teenagers for their future lives as active and contributing citizens. Although the right to education is enshrined in legislation in various parts of the world at the national, regional, and local levels, the rate of students who do not attend school regularly is concerning (Nordin et al., 2024; UNESCO, 2020).

School refusal is a phenomenon that involves emotional or behavioral problems, but it is not a formal mental health diagnosis and therefore does not appear in the DSM. This phenomenon has always occurred, but recently there has been an increase in the number of studies on the topic (Ulaş et al., 2024). The prevalence of this phenomenon is difficult to quantify, considering the inconsistency surrounding definitions and the diversity in research methodologies, though the best estimate is between 1–5%, with similar prevalence between genders, and it tends to be more common in children aged 5 to 10 years (Ulaş & Seçer, 2024; Woods & Burns, 2018).

Different studies define the term "school refusal" in various ways. For example, some studies rely on the definition by Kearney (2008), which suggests that this term refers to a child's refusal to attend school or difficulty staying in class for a full day. Another study defined school refusal as failure to attend school due to emotional stress related to being at school, with parents being aware of the absences and making considerable efforts to ensure the child's attendance (Heyne et al., 2019). It can be said that this phenomenon refers to several possible behaviors, such as a child's refusal to learn at school, difficulty staying at school for a full day, missing partial or full school days, skipping classes, or unjustified tardiness. School refusal also refers to a child's inability to continue their studies due to mental health issues like anxiety and depression (Ochi et al., 2020). Additionally, school refusal may be expressed in various ways, including verbal or physical refusal (e.g., pleading, crying, disobedience, clinging to a parent, etc.), verbal and physical aggression, expressions of distress, and somatic complaints. The situation can appear along a continuum, with expressions and timeframes that may vary daily. It is customary to view the phenomenon as a continuum of escalating behaviors. These begin with forced attendance by parents and pleas by children to avoid attending, as well as difficult morning behaviors to avoid school. This is followed by repeated morning tardiness, after which the child attends school. Then, prolonged absences and skipping of classes begins, becoming more urgent, leading to complete absence from school for a certain period, followed by a longer-term absence (Munkhaugen et al., 2017).

School refusal is considered a risk factor in academic, social, and personal domains, with short- and long-term consequences. In the short term, a decline in academic performance, impact on social status, and more negative attitudes toward school can be seen. In the long term, low academic achievements and school dropouts can be observed, as well as difficulties in psychological and social development. Several studies have reported higher rates of language difficulties and learning disabilities. In adulthood, this can lead to difficulties entering the job market, low social status, relationship problems, psychiatric disorders, and more (Munkhaugen et al., 2017; Nordin et al., 2024). Furthermore, it has been found that children and adolescents who refuse school are more likely to experience depression and anxiety, dropout, and suicidal tendencies. School refusal is a major risk factor for violence and substance use (Ochi et al., 2020).

In a study examining the clinical significance of school refusal, its negative impact on the psychological well-being of children and adolescents, and its association with psychopathological conditions during childhood and adolescence, it was found that school refusal is prevalent in neurodevelopmental disorders like autism and ADHD due to behavioral issues and communication skill deficits. Regarding psychiatric disorders, school refusal is particularly common in anxiety disorders, depression, and somatic symptoms (Di Vincenzo et al., 2024). School absenteeism rates are higher in special education schools and among students with special needs regardless of the type of school. This phenomenon may worsen in cases where the special needs are related to social communication difficulties, such as those found in children with autism (Totsika et al., 2020).

School Refusal and Autism

As mentioned, school refusal has significant short- and long-term consequences, making it important to understand how prevalent this issue is among students with autism, what the possible causes are, and what types of support they need (Nordin et al., 2024). Few studies have examined school refusal among children with autism, even though it is considered a serious problem. Even in the existing studies that explore the relationship between the two, there are significant differences in how school refusal is defined, methodological approaches (such as including or excluding children with intellectual disabilities, different sources of reporting by teachers/parents, etc.), and a lack of consideration for the different types of school absences (Totsika et al., 2020).

In a comprehensive review of studies on school absenteeism among autistic children, it was found that autistic children and adolescents were more likely to refuse school than their non-autistic peers (Nordin et al., 2024). Another study found that the average age of onset for school refusal in children with autism was earlier (12.6 years) compared to children without autism (13.8 years) (Ochi et al., 2020). Additionally, it was found that the school refusal rate among children with autism was significantly higher (42.6%) compared to children with typical development (7.1%). Furthermore, this behavior was more prolonged in children with autism. During 20 days of study, 60% of autistic students exhibited school refusal behavior for four or more days, while none of the control group exhibited it for more than three days (Munkhaugen et al., 2017). A similar trend was found in another study that included only autistic students—on average, autistic students missed five school days over a month. Prolonged absenteeism, defined as at least 10% absenteeism, was very common and included 43% of the participants. It is important to note that this study identified various reasons for school absence, with school refusal being the most common cause (Totsika et al., 2020). Another study that supports this found that, on average, autistic children missed six full school days over a four-week period. This is equivalent to almost a third of the school period. The most common reason for a full day's absence was school refusal, while half-day absences were due to medical/therapeutic appointments (Adams, 2022). These findings emphasize the serious situation for autistic students, where the onset is earlier, the prevalence is higher, and the duration is longer compared to non-autistic students.

Factors Contributing to School Refusal in Children with Autism

The reasons for school refusal in children with autism are complex and include social, biological, environmental, and psychological factors. Below, I will briefly outline some of the prominent factors from recent studies in the field.

Social Functioning

Students with autism often experience significant difficulties with reciprocal social interactions and social communication skills, and may sometimes avoid eye contact and display repetitive, atypical patterns of behavior. A study in which all participants were autistic students showed that all exhibited high levels of general social functioning impairments. However, students who also exhibited school refusal were more impaired socially than those who did not show school refusal. Moreover, low social motivation showed the strongest link to school refusal (Munkhaugen et al., 2019). Additionally, students with autism are at a higher risk of being socially excluded in the school environment. They tend to experience daily misunderstandings, feelings of loneliness and differences, and difficulties in forming friendships. They are also more likely to socially withdraw. All these factors can contribute to school refusal (Ochi et al., 2020; Skafle et al., 2020).

Autistic students demonstrate difficulties in adapting to changes in settings, and thus the transition from elementary school to middle school/high school is particularly challenging for them. A significant difference was found in school refusal rates between elementary school and high school. In terms of percentages, about 15% of elementary school students with autism and 65% of high school students with autism exhibited school refusal as partial or total absenteeism (Munkhaugen et al., 2017). Nevertheless, high school is viewed as an important platform for social training and a key place for making new friends. High school can be perceived as a fresh start, especially when the environment is supportive and inclusive (Skafle et al., 2020).

Bullying

Being a victim of bullying is one of the main factors contributing to school refusal. Bullying is defined as aggressive behavior that is repetitive, intentional, and harmful either physically or emotionally (Ochi et al., 2020). Students who experience bullying may be up to six times more likely to refuse school compared to students who are not bullied. School refusal is considered a common coping mechanism among children who experience bullying. Children with autism are at an increased risk of being victims of bullying, with rates of bullying reaching 46–94%. Furthermore, more than a quarter of autistic children who experienced bullying refused to attend school for a period afterward (McClemont et al., 2021). An important outcome of bullying among autistic youth is the desire to avoid returning to the environment where bullying occurred, leading to lower school engagement (Bitsika et al., 2020). A study examining the relationship between bullying and school refusal found that over 80% of autistic adolescents reported being harassed at school, and more than half of those who reported bullying asked their parents if they could avoid going back to school the next day. A significant connection was found between school refusal and the frequency of bullying. Furthermore, bullying explained a larger portion of the variance in school refusal than other factors, such as the child's age, autism-related difficulties, and self-reports of anxiety and depression (Bitsika et al., 2020). Although this study does not allow for causal conclusions, the findings suggest that bullying is a significant predictor of school refusal in autistic adolescents.

One explanation for the bullying described is that children with autism have impaired Theory of Mind (ToM) abilities. ToM is the ability to understand and describe mental states such as beliefs, intentions, and emotions in oneself and others. As a result, children with autism may believe that their peers are bullying them when this is not the case, or they may misinterpret bullying behaviors as non-harmful. Furthermore, repetitive behaviors, rigid routines, and limited areas of interest make children with autism "stand out" socially, making them targets for ridicule. These factors, combined with the social difficulties described above, contribute to social isolation and bullying, which are strongly linked to school refusal (Ochi et al., 2020). A study examining risk and protective factors found that risk factors increasing bullying and school refusal include conflicts with friends, lack of teacher support, and an unsafe school environment. Protective factors that reduce bullying and school refusal include effective classroom management by the teacher, support from teachers, aides, and parents (McClemont et al., 2021).

A recent study examined a concept related to school refusal, called Emerging School Refusal (ESR). ESR refers to signs that school refusal might develop, even before actual absenteeism occurs. The aim of the study was to examine social anxiety and separation anxiety in autistic adolescents at risk for school refusal, based on the ESR sign of asking to stay home after being bullied at school. A little over half of the autistic boys (55%) who reported being bullied asked their parents if they could stay home because of the bullying. In total, it was found that separation anxiety scores were significantly higher in autistic adolescents who exhibited ESR compared to those who did not show ESR. At the same time, there was no significant difference in the overall social anxiety scores (Bitsika et al., 2022a). It is possible that some children and adolescents with autism who report being bullied and request to avoid school lack the knowledge and skills to respond to bullying. In other words, their only coping mechanism is avoidance of school. This finding connects with the factor of impaired social functioning discussed earlier.

Comorbid Conditions

Anxiety and/or depression disorders are diagnosed in about half of the adolescents referred for treatment and assistance for school refusal (Bitsika et al., 2020). Furthermore, compared to adolescents without school refusal, those with moderate school refusal showed a significantly higher likelihood of having generalized anxiety disorder (11 times higher), specific phobia (11 times higher), and social anxiety disorder (7 times higher). These youths also reported specific fears related to school and fear of what will happen at home while they are at school. Additionally, these adolescents were 10 times more likely to meet the diagnostic criteria for depression (Bitsika et al., 2020; Woods & Burns, 2018; Yamada et al., 2020). These findings highlight and clarify the relationship between depression and anxiety and school refusal.

Previous studies have found that autism is associated with other psychiatric disorders, and an increasing number of studies confirm this. Young people with autism often suffer from co-occurring anxiety and depression. It has been found that autistic students with school refusal had significantly higher scores for major depression, generalized anxiety, and separation anxiety, as well as significantly higher levels of somatic symptoms and sleep difficulties (Bitsika et al., 2022b). In another school-related context, children with autism and anxiety have significant difficulties participating in activities that require separation from home and parents (e.g., field trips, tours, camping activities). They often refuse to participate or do not fully engage. This poses a challenge for the school team and requires prior planning and consultation with the child's family for appropriate preparation (Woods & Burns, 2018). Additionally, a study that reviewed studies in the field found that the type of school affects absenteeism in children with autism. When "regular" schools are accompanied by a lack of resources, inadequate teacher knowledge, and a lack of support, the risk for anxiety and depression in autistic children is elevated, as the children's individual needs are not addressed, thereby increasing the phenomenon of school refusal (Sasso & Sansour, 2024). Caamaño et al. (2013) found that children with autism exhibited subclinical psychopathology profiles in areas such as depression, separation anxiety, agoraphobia, specific phobias, OCD, and ADHD. This finding indicates a high risk for co-occurring psychiatric conditions arising from the presence of symptoms that are currently below the clinical threshold. Regarding school refusal, it was found that among items measuring separation anxiety, only school refusal was significantly more common in children with autism. Moreover, depression and anxiety are more prevalent among adolescents with autism, especially those with higher IQs, and during the transition from childhood to adolescence. This finding may be partially explained by the fact that these individuals are able to recognize and communicate their feelings, compared to those with lower-functioning autism. Their heightened awareness of their difficulties may make them more vulnerable due to a limited range of coping mechanisms, thereby exposing them to greater stress, which in turn promotes school refusal. This study highlights the need to be vigilant for the presence of co-occurring disorders in autism, as well as for symptoms that may signal these disorders while still in a subclinical diagnostic phase.

In addition, children with ASD often experience heightened or diminished sensory sensitivities, which can contribute to anxiety in school settings. Sensory sensitivities, such as discomfort from bright lights, loud noises, or certain textures, can make the school environment overwhelming. This sensory overload can trigger school refusal behaviors as children attempt to avoid these distressing stimuli. Similarly, preference for routines and significant distress when faced with changes in their environment or daily schedules (Miller et al., 2007) may be a central discomfort. Changes such as a new teacher, different classroom settings, or disruptions to the daily routine can induce anxiety, contributing to reluctance to attend school. Such transitions may feel unpredictable and overwhelming for children with ASD. Lastly, academic demands can also contribute to school refusal in children with ASD, particularly if the academic content does not align with the child's learning style. For children who struggle with specific academic tasks or who do not receive adequate support, school may become a source of frustration and stress, resulting in avoidance behaviors. Any inclusion process should take into consideration the academic functioning (Pearlman-Avnion, 2018).

Furthermore, research shows that students with ASD and their families encounter significant challenges during school transitions. However, there is limited literature on the specific factors contributing to these difficulties in primary school students with ASD. The study of Sefotho and Onyishi (2021) explored the difficulties that primary school students with ASD face when moving through different grades in South Africa, using a phenomenological approach. The findings highlighted three main challenges. First, academic and skill development struggles—Students with ASD often experience difficulties in their studies and in acquiring essential skills, which hinders their educational progress. Second, social and financial barriers—these learners face challenges in socializing with peers, and financial limitations can add to the difficulty of transitioning smoothly through school levels. Third, behavioral difficulties—various behavioral challenges make learning and social interactions more complicated for students with ASD (Sefotho & Onyishi, 2021). These challenges could all be key contributors to school refusal for students with ASD. These can lead to frustration, anxiety, and fear of failure, making school an overwhelming environment that students may want to avoid. Addressing these challenges through structured transitions, individualized support, and home-school collaboration can help mitigate school refusal behaviors and ensure smoother educational experiences for these students.

Interventions for School Refusal

Typically, interventions for school refusal aim to help children manage anxiety and depression. For example, a case study published recently found that the use of SSRIs (Selective Serotonin Reuptake Inhibitors) in a patient with autism and generalized anxiety disorder improved the social withdrawal and prolonged school refusal that she exhibited (Yamada et al., 2020). At the same time, other interventions suggest adaptations of CBT and DBT therapies for autistic children. Additionally, work is done with parents to help them manage household factors that contribute to maintaining their children's school refusal behavior. For instance, helping parents with their children's sleep issues and creating morning and evening routines have been found to help children wake up on time for school. Furthermore, there is significant importance in interventions aimed at preventing and reducing bullying, as well as improving the sense of security of autistic children at school. These interventions should be implemented at multiple levels: with students, with professional and educational staff, and at the level of the school climate (Bitsika et al., 2020).

Additionally, the study on the ESR concept mentioned earlier highlights the importance of early intervention even before school refusal and absenteeism occur. ESR may reflect the enjoyment and security that children and adolescents with autism gain from staying home with their parents. In this case, parents can help the adolescent cope with separation anxiety, support them, and provide skills to deal with periods of separation. This can help maintain school attendance even after an experience of bullying. In the case of ESR, the negative experience of bullying—whether the bullying is related to the child's autism traits or not—may reduce the motivation to learn at school. In these cases, early intervention to promote school involvement would be crucial, alongside school-wide interventions to prevent bullying (Bitsika et al., 2022a).

Summary and Discussion

School refusal and its connection to autism is a significant issue, and it is important to understand the phenomenon and its causes. Although there are differences in how the phenomenon is defined in various articles and research methodologies, a concerning trend is evident that warrants attention—there is a clear connection between autism and school refusal. School refusal is associated with a reduction in the quality of life for children and adolescents, as well as stress for the family. Frequent absenteeism, which often accompanies the phenomenon, presents a challenge for the school staff.

The reasons for the phenomenon are diverse and complex, and include factors such as impaired social functioning, bullying, and comorbid conditions. Nevertheless, the full picture is still not clear, and environmental factors such as the mode of learning, the classroom environment, school climate, and differences between schools (e.g., between regular and special education, as well as different inclusion and integration approaches) should also be explored.

There is no doubt that autistic children face many challenges in educational settings, and sometimes these challenges are "invisible" to their peers and teachers. Thus, they are not always aware of the daily struggles of these students (Skafle et al., 2020). Additionally, students with autism may have difficulty expressing their feelings regarding situations related to the school setting. They may express their feelings as physical symptoms, such as headaches and nausea. Therefore, it is especially important to pay attention to school refusal, understand the variety of possible behaviors deeply, and interpret them correctly (Munkhaugen et al., 2017). The school staff, particularly the educational psychologist, need to familiarize themselves with the existing literature, theories, and research related to school refusal and autism. Furthermore, it is important that future research in this area focus on the risk and protective factors for the phenomenon and even develop a comprehensive intervention model that includes assistance and support across various domains affecting the phenomenon: social, academic, emotional, and environmental. It is important to remember that school refusal is a red flag for all children, and particularly for autistic children. It is not a phenomenon that passes on its own, and thus prompt action should be taken to prevent it from worsening. Any time a child is not in school represents missed learning opportunities, and when it comes to autistic children and adolescents, school attendance is especially important, as they miss social learning and various treatments that are provided at school. Based on the findings from the studies reviewed above, it is crucial to be vigilant, identify, and detect students who are at risk for this behavior, and conduct interventions, especially in the early stages of the phenomenon.

References

Adams, D. (2022). Child and parental mental health as correlates of school non-attendance and school refusal in children on the autism spectrum. *Journal of Autism and Developmental Disorders, 52*(8), 3353–3365. https://doi.org/10.1007/s10803-021-05211-5

Bitsika, V., Heyne, D. A., & Sharpley, C. F. (2020). Is bullying associated with emerging school refusal in autistic boys? *Journal of Autism and Developmental Disorders, 51*(4), 1081–1092. https://doi.org/10.1007/s10803-020-04610-4

Bitsika, V., Heyne, D. A., & Sharpley, C. F. (2022a). The inverse association between psychological resilience and emerging school refusal among bullied autistic youth. *Research in Developmental Disabilities, 120*, Article 104121. https://doi.org/10.1016/j.ridd.2021.104121

Bitsika, V., Sharpley, C., & Heyne, D. (2022b). Risk for school refusal among autistic boys bullied at school: Investigating associations with social phobia and separation anxiety. *International Journal of Disability, Development and Education, 69*(1), 190–203. https://https://doi.org/10.1080/1034912X.2021.1969544

Caamaño, M., Boada, L., Merchán-Naranjo, J., Moreno, C., Llorente, C., Moreno, D., Arango, C., & Parellada, M. (2013). Psychopathology in children and adolescents with ASD without mental retardation. *Journal of Autism and Developmental Disorders, 43*(10), 2442–2449. https://doi.org/10.1007/s10803-013-1792-0

Di Vincenzo, C., Pontillo, M., Bellantoni, D., Di Luzio, M., Lala, M. R., Villa, M., Demaria, F., & Vicari, S. (2024). School refusal behavior in children and adolescents: A five-year narrative review of clinical significance and psychopathological profiles. *Italian Journal of Pediatrics, 50*(1), 107. https://doi.org/10.1186/s13052-024-01667-0

Heyne, D., Gren-Landell, M., Melvin, G., & Gentle-Genitty, C. (2019). Differentiation between school attendance problems: Why and how? *Cognitive and Behavioral Practice, 26*(1), 8–34. https://doi.org/10.1016/j.cbpra.2018.03.006

Kearney, C. A. (2008). School absenteeism and school refusal behavior in youth: A contemporary review. *Clinical Psychology Review, 28*(3), 451–471. https://doi.org/10.1016/j.cpr.2007.07.012

Kearney, C. A., & Albano, A. M. (2004). The functional profiles of school refusal behavior: Diagnostic aspects. *Behavior Modification, 28*(1), 147–161. https://doi.org/10.1177/0145445503259263

Kearney, C. A., & Silverman, W. K. (1999). Functionally based prescriptive and nonprescriptive treatment for children and adolescents with school refusal behavior. *Behavior Therapy, 30*(4), 673–695. https://doi.org/10.1016/S0005-7894(99)80032-X

McClemont, A. J., Morton, H. E., Gillis, J. M., & Romanczyk, R. G. (2021). Brief report: Predictors of school refusal due to bullying in children with autism spectrum disorder and attention-deficit/hyperactivity disorder. *Journal of Autism and Developmental Disorders, 51*(5), 1781–1788l. https://doi.org/10.1007/s10803-020-04640-y

Miller, L. J., Anzalone, M. E., Lane, S. J., Cermak, S. A., & Osten, E. T. (2007). Concept evolution in sensory processing. *American Journal of Occupational Therapy, 61*(2), 135–140.

Munkhaugen, E. K., Gjevik, E., Pripp, A. H., Sponheim, E., & Diseth, T. H. (2017). School refusal behaviour: Are children and adolescents with autism spectrum disorder at a higher risk? *Research in Autism Spectrum Disorders, 41*, 31–38. https://doi.org/10.1016/j.rasd.2017.07.001

Munkhaugen, E. K., Torske, T., Gjevik, E., Nærland, T., Pripp, A. H., & Diseth, T. H. (2019). Individual characteristics of students with autism spectrum disorders and school refusal behavior. *Autism, 23*(2), 413–423. https://doi.org/10.1177/1362361317748619

Nordin, V., Palmgren, M., Lindbladh, A., Bölte, S., & Jonsson, U. (2024). School absenteeism in autistic children and adolescents: A scoping review. *Autism, 28*(7), 1622–1637. https://doi.org/10.1177/1362361317748619

Ochi, M., Kawabe, K., Ochi, S., Miyama, T., Horiuchi, F., & Ueno, S. I. (2020). School refusal and bullying in children with autism spectrum disorder. *Child and Adolescent Psychiatry and Mental Health, 14*(1), 1–7. https://doi.org/10.1186/s13034-020-00325-7

Pearlman-Avnion, S. (2018). Shitot tippul biyiladim im otizm behityakhes lammisgerot hakhinnukhiyyot [Intervention methods for the treatment of children on the autism spectrum in educational contexts]. In S. Maital & R. Shalhevet-Kaniel (Eds.), Sugyot bifsikhologeyah khinnukhit: Mahalakhah lemaaseh [*Selected issues in educational psychology: From theory to practice*]. Sheffy: Psychological Counseling Service, Ministry of Education.

Sasso, I., & Sansour, T. (2024). Risk and influencing factors for school absenteeism among students on the autism spectrum: A systematic review. *Review Journal of Autism and Developmental Disorders*, 1–14. https://doi.org/10.1007/s40489-024-00474-x

Sefotho, M. M., & Onyishi, C. N. (2021). In-school transition challenges among primary school learners with autism spectrum disorders in South Africa: Parents and teachers' perspectives. *Perspectives in Education, 39*(2), 283–302. https://hdl.handle.net/10520/ejc-persed_v39_n2_a20

Skafle, I., Nordahl-Hansen, A., & Øien, R. A. (2020). Social perception of high school students with ASD in Norway. *Journal of Autism and Developmental Disorders, 50*(2), 670–675. https://doi.org/10.1007/s10803-019-04281-w

Totsika, V., Hastings, R. P., Dutton, Y., Worsley, A., Melvin, G., Gray, K., Tonge, B., & Heyne, D. (2020). Types and correlates of school non-attendance in students with autism spectrum disorders. *Autism, 24*(7), 1639–1649. https://doi.org/10.1177/1362361320916967

Ulaş, S., Gonzálvez, C., & Seçer, İ. (2024). School refusal: Mapping the literature by bibliometric analysis. *Frontiers in Psychology, 15*, 1265781. https://doi.org/10.3389/fpsyg.2024.1265781

Ulaş, S., & Seçer, İ. (2024). A systematic review of school refusal. *Current Psychology: A Journal for Diverse Perspectives on Diverse Psychological Issues, 43*(21), 19407–19422. https://doi.org/10.1007/s12144-024-05742-x

UNESCO. (2020). *Global education monitoring report 2020: Inclusion and education: All means all.* UNESCO.

Woods, M. C., & Burns, J. R. (2018). School camp refusal and reluctance: The role of the school psychologist. *Journal of Psychologists and Counsellors in Schools, 28*(2), 235–247. https://doi.org/10.1017/jgc.2018.11

Yamada, N., Nakadoi, Y., Fukuma, R., & Ohmori, T. (2020). Two children exhibiting social withdrawal, school refusal, and underlying generalized anxiety disorder successfully treated using a selective serotonin reuptake inhibitor. *The Journal of Medical Investigation, 67*(3,4), 355–357. https://doi.org/10.2152/jmi.67.355

Chapter 5
Gender and Age Differences in Eating Patterns Among Children with Autism

Chen Peretz and Shiri Pearlman-Avnion

Abstract Recent studies have documented the connection between eating problems and autism spectrum disorder (ASD) and found that problematic eating behaviors occur in over half of children diagnosed with ASD. However, there is a lack of knowledge regarding differences in eating problems by gender and age. This chapter presents a review of the existing reviews on eating problems and ASD. This is followed by empirical data collected from 31 boys and 28 girls aged 3–18 diagnosed with ASD at varying levels of functioning. The Aut-Eat questionnaire, designed to assess eating problems and habits in children with ASD, was the main research tool. A comparative analysis was conducted on differences in eating problems between boys and girls and between young children and adolescents. The results confirm that eating problems are prevalent among children and adolescents with ASD, but no significant differences were found in overall eating problems by gender or age group, and no interaction was found between age and gender. However, young boys exhibited a significantly higher prevalence of selective eating. These findings indicate that a deeper understanding of the issue is needed to develop effective intervention programs and provide appropriate individualized treatment to help children and youth with ASD address their eating challenges. This comprehensive analysis provides invaluable information for parents, educators, and clinicians, offering a foundation for tailored support and improved quality of life for autistic individuals and their families.

Keywords Eating problems · Selective eating · Gender differences · Age differences · Nutritional challenges · Behavioral interventions · Aut-Eat questionnaire (AEQ)

C. Peretz (✉)
Educational Psychology Service, Acre, Israel
e-mail: Chen-d@akko.muni.il

S. Pearlman-Avnion
Tel-Hai College, Kiryat Shmona, Israel

S. Lowinger and S. Pearlman-Avnion (eds.), *Collaborative Care and Partnerships in Autism Diagnosis and Treatment*, Autism and Child Psychopathology Series,
https://doi.org/10.1007/978-3-032-07009-8_5

Introduction

Eating problems are prevalent among individuals with autism spectrum disorder (ASD), often significantly impacting their nutritional health, development, and quality of life. These can manifest as food selectivity, sensory sensitivities, ritualistic eating behaviors, and aversions to certain food textures, tastes, or smells (Sharp et al., 2013). Food selectivity is particularly common, and many children with ASD prefer a limited variety of foods, often high in carbohydrates and low in fruits and vegetables (Bandini et al., 2010). Sensory processing differences, a hallmark of ASD, are believed to underlie many of these challenges, as individuals may find specific sensory attributes of foods overwhelming or unpleasant (Alibrandi et al., 2023; Cermak et al., 2010).

Furthermore, rigid adherence to routines and repetitive behaviors, both characteristic of ASD, make it difficult for these children to try new foods or accept changes in meal presentation (Schreck et al., 2004). These eating behaviors can lead to nutritional deficiencies, such as inadequate intake of vitamins and minerals, and may also exacerbate gastrointestinal issues, which are more prevalent in individuals with ASD compared to neurotypical populations (Gorrindo et al., 2012). Parents and caregivers often face significant stress and challenges in managing these eating problems, which can strain family dynamics and impact overall well-being (Hubbard et al., 2014). Addressing eating problems associated with ASD requires a multidisciplinary approach, incorporating nutritional, behavioral, and sensory-based interventions tailored to the individual's unique needs. Early intervention and collaboration between healthcare professionals, dietitians, and families are crucial to improving dietary habits and reducing the negative health outcomes associated with these challenges.

Autism Spectrum Disorder (ASD): Present Definition and Characteristics

Autism spectrum disorder (ASD) represents a series of neurodevelopmental impairments characterized by difficulties in social reciprocity, challenges in socially appropriate communication, and restricted and repetitive patterns of behavior and interests. These include repetitive movements, fixed and inflexible interests, sensory processing issues, and heightened environmental sensitivity (American Psychiatric Association [APA], 2022). Individuals on the autism spectrum often manifest behavioral problems and experience other mental and physical health conditions that can impact their lives and the lives of their families (Hurtig et al., 2009). Individuals with ASD may suffer a range of symptoms, including emotional and behavioral issues (such as aggression, tantrums, and self-injurious behaviors), sleep problems, feeding and eating difficulties, intellectual limitations, and learning disabilities. They may also have co-occurring mental health disorders or medical conditions, such as attention-deficit/hyperactivity disorder (ADHD), epilepsy, anxiety, and obsessive–compulsive disorder (Maskey et al., 2013).

Autism Spectrum Disorder and Gender

In the United States, the prevalence of ASD is currently 1:36 (Maenner et al., 2023), but the diagnosis of ASD is 3.8 times more common among boys than girls (Mandy et al., 2012; Maenner et al., 2023; Werling et al., 2016). Some argue that diagnostic tools were developed based on male stereotypes and that differences in the manifestation of symptoms between genders may lead to delays or missed diagnoses in females with ASD (Pearlman-Avnion & Shlain, 2019; Rivet & Matson, 2011). It has also been suggested that genetic factors make ASD harder for clinicians to diagnose in girls than in boys (Zhang et al., 2020).

Few studies have examined symptomatology and gender differences in this population (Christensen et al., 2016). Some research provides evidence of distinct differences in symptoms and clinical presentations between males and females (Holtmann et al., 2007; McLennan et al., 1993; Tsai & Beisler, 1983). However, findings regarding gender differences are ambiguous and inconsistent. For example, one study found that repetitive and stereotyped behaviors are less prevalent in females than males (Bölte et al., 2011), while three other studies reported no gender differences in this domain (Banach et al., 2009; Carter et al., 2007; Holtmann et al., 2007). Further research is needed to better understand the gender-specific characteristics of this disorder.

Autism Spectrum Disorder and Age

Diagnosing children with ASD is possible as early as one year of age, and most evaluations occur between the ages of two and three years. Despite early evaluation, more children are diagnosed with ASD at eight years old than at four years old, because children often exhibit more pronounced symptoms after age four (Christensen et al., 2016). Age may influence potential gender-related differences in autism symptoms. A meta-analysis revealed that among young children with ASD, boys display more restrictive behaviors and interests than girls (Van Wijngaarden-Cremers et al., 2014).

Eating Disorders and Eating Problems

Eating disorders are characterized by an abnormal relationship with body weight and food consumption, leading to atypical eating and behavioral patterns. Eating disorders include anorexia nervosa, bulimia nervosa, binge-eating disorder, avoidant/restrictive food intake disorder, rumination disorder, and pica; definitions of each disorder are given in the *Diagnostic and Statistical Manual of Mental Disorders* (DSM-5-TR, American Psychiatric Association, 2022). Eating disorders are more common among females than males, with a general population ratio of 1:10 (Smink et al., 2014). Anorexia nervosa is one of the most severe psychiatric eating disorders, with a heightened risk of chronic progression and premature death; it affects primarily adolescent girls (Arcelus et al., 2011). The current study uses the general term "eating problems," which is widely used in the literature, to refer to deviations from normative eating or oral patterns that result in health impairments or negative social consequences.

Autism Spectrum Disorder (ASD) and Eating Disorders

Gillberg (1985) first proposed a link between ASD and anorexia nervosa, which is defined in the DSM-5 as being "significantly underweight due to restricted eating driven by fear of weight gain and a distorted body image" (APA, 2022). Recent studies have verified the connection between these two disorders (Westwood et al., 2016). A systematic review of the prevalence of ASD among individuals diagnosed with anorexia nervosa found an average rate of 23% (Huke et al., 2013). However, research demonstrating a potential overlap between ASD and eating disorders has primarily focused on women, with limited knowledge about the eating behaviors of males and females with ASD across age groups. One study found that 23% of women diagnosed with anorexia nervosa also met the criteria for ASD (Wentz et al., 2005). A study among 10 women with eating disorders found that half of them met the criteria for ASD (Mandy & Tchanturia, 2015). A Swedish study found that behaviors characteristic of women diagnosed with ASD also appeared among women diagnosed with anorexia nervosa (Karjalainen et al., 2024). The shared traits between ASD and eating disorders are concerning, as they can significantly affect behavior management, learning acquisition, and the development of social relationships in individuals with ASD, all of which greatly impact their functioning.

Although some types of eating problems (e.g., food refusal) are common in the general pediatric population, studies have found that the prevalence of eating problems is significantly higher among children with ASD, with estimated rates ranging from 46 to 89% of children with ASD. A meta-analysis revealed that children with ASD are four times more likely to develop eating problems compared to their typically developing peers (Sharp et al., 2010). These eating problems include frequent food refusal, food selectivity limiting consumption to a limited repertoire of specific food categories, and excessive consumption of a few foods (Ledford & Gast, 2006; Margari et al., 2020; Maskey et al., 2013).

Other eating problems identified among children with ASD include difficulties chewing and swallowing, repetitive behaviors, overeating, pica (repeated ingestion of non-food items), and problematic behaviors during meals, such as aggression and tantrums (Beecroft et al., 1998; Matson & Fodstad, 2009; Matson et al., 2013; Provost et al., 2010). Children with ASD may insist on specific food preparation methods or mealtime rituals, such as presenting food in a particular order (Ahearn et al., 2001). These eating problems pose significant health risks and impact family routines, creating a primary source of concern and considerable difficulty in daily life for these children and their families (Cermak et al., 2010; Schreck et al., 2004).

Selective eating is the most common eating problem throughout life among children with ASD and is 15–20% more prevalent in this population compared to children with typical development (Bandini et al., 2010; Cermak et al., 2010; Kuschner et al., 2015; Mascola et al., 2010; Schreck et al., 2004; Sharp et al., 2013; Williams et al., 2005; Zimmer et al., 2012; Zucker et al., 2015). Studies comparing types of eating problems, such as food selectivity by type and texture or food refusal, verify the high prevalence of eating problems in individuals on the autism spectrum (Ahearn et al., 2001; Dominick et al., 2007; Schreck & Williams, 2006). Selective eating among children with ASD has been linked to extreme sensory problems linked to features of foods such as smell, smell, texture, color, and temperature (Alibrandi et al., 2023).

Age plays a role in the manifestation of eating problems among children diagnosed with ASD. A positive correlation was found between eating problems and age in children with ASD, showing that as age increased, there was a rise in food selectivity, monotony, and ritualistic eating behaviors (Vissoker et al., 2019). A study of 18 children with ASD at two points in time (average age 6.3 and 13.2 years) observed a decrease in food repertoire during the study period, with 65% of the children having reduced the number of foods they consumed (Bandini et al., 2017).

Methods for Assessing Eating Disorders Among Children with ASD

While many studies have identified and described eating problems in this population, few have examined the development of these problems throughout childhood and adolescence or compared differences between boys and girls regarding eating problems.

Issues surrounding eating and the nutritional implications for children and adolescents with ASD pose significant concerns for parents and for people working in educational frameworks who are trying to incorporate healthy nutrition into curricula and provide intervention programs. Among children with ASD who are integrated into mainstream schools, 55% suffer from frequent eating problems (Maskey et al., 2013). Identifying and addressing medical issues among children with ASD can improve their performance in school (Bellando & Lopez, 2009). This underscores the importance of raising school nurses' awareness of problems and treatment options and providing individualized guidance to these students to help them achieve academic success (Bellando & Lopez, 2009).

Research Goals, Hypotheses, and Data Collection

This research aimed to characterize the eating problems of young and adolescent boys and girls with ASD. The findings can be used to form the basis for developing intervention programs that would benefit parents and professionals in providing guidance, adapting environments, and managing problematic behaviors related to eating. Assessing whether there are gender- and age-dependent differences in eating problems in this population could help provide appropriate individualized care that would significantly reduce the distress experienced by them and their families.

Hypotheses

A recent study by one of this chapter's authors (Peretz, 2024) examined whether there are differences in eating problems between boys and girls and between young children and adolescents diagnosed with ASD. The following hypotheses were proposed for the current study.

Hypothesis 1: Differences in eating problems will be found between boys and girls diagnosed with ASD, with girls exhibiting eating problems more frequently than boys, regardless of age.

Hypothesis 2: Differences in eating problems will be found between children and adolescents diagnosed with ASD, with adolescents exhibiting eating problems more frequently than children, regardless of gender.

Hypothesis 3: An interaction between gender and age will be observed, according to which the difference between girls and boys will increase as the participants' age increases.

Hypothesis 4: Differences in eating problems will be found according to gender, with young boys exhibiting eating problems on the food selectivity scale more frequently than young girls.

Hypothesis 5: Differences in eating problems will be found between adolescents and young children, with adolescents exhibiting eating problems on the food selectivity scale and the rigidity and ritualistic eating scale more frequently than young children.

Study Design

To assess gender- and age-based differences in eating problems among children and adolescents with ASD, a cross-sectional correlational design was employed. The independent variables were the gender and age of participants (categorical variables). The dependent variable was eating problems (a quantitative variable). A pilot study was conducted in Israel among a sample of boys aged 3–8 diagnosed with ASD. Some of the children were enrolled in special educational settings, and others were integrated into regular educational settings.

Study Population

The current study population included 59 children and youth aged 3–18. There were 31 boys and 28 girls. The participants were divided into four groups based on gender and age: boys aged 3–8 ($n = 21$), adolescent boys aged 12–18 ($n = 10$), girls aged 3–8 ($n = 19$), and adolescent girls aged 12–18 ($n = 9$).

All had been diagnosed with ASD according to the DSM-5 criteria for autism (American Psychiatric Association, 2022) by a neurologist, child psychiatrist, or certified psychologist recognized by the Israeli National Insurance Institute. Participants were recruited using a convenience sampling method. Recruitment was conducted via direct contact with parents of children and adolescents with ASD and through online forums. Participation was voluntary.

Aut-Eat Questionnaire (AEQ)

The Aut-Eat Questionnaire (AEQ) was designed to assess the specific eating problem profiles and eating habits of children with ASD and to serve as a basis for clinical intervention. There is a version for parent reporting (for children and adolescents with lower functioning) and a self-report version (for high-functioning adolescents). The questionnaire comprises three sections. The first collects demographic data, including age and gender. It also has open-ended questions regarding the child's development with open-ended questions such as "Does your child sit at the table during meals?" and "Does your child eat regular meals?" The second section includes 44 statements related to eating-related behaviors, such as "Eats foods only when they are at a specific temperature" and "Ensures that foods do not touch each other on the plate." Respondents rank each on a Likert scale from 0 (never) to 5 (very frequent behavior). These items can be categorized into six subscales of eating problems: (a) chewing and swallowing difficulties, b) food avoidance, (c) selective eating, (d) rigidity/uniformity and eating rituals, (e) overeating; and (f) mealtime behavioral difficulties. The third section has a list of 137 specific foods categorized into food groups. The respondents ranked each on a Likert scale from 1 (avoids) to 5 (frequently eats) (Gal et al., 2022).

In the current study, the parent report version was used. Participating parents of children with ASD were asked to complete the AEQ. The questionnaire was administered in Hebrew; for details on the translation process, see Gal et al. (2022).

The questionnaire has internal reliability within the acceptable range, with Cronbach's alpha ranging from 0.74 (for the food avoidance category) to 0.93, and high discriminant validity among populations (Gal et al., 2022). This study only used the first two sections of the questionnaire, with a focus on demographic data and eating problems. The open-ended questions about eating habits were not included.

The study was approved by the ethics committee of Tel-Hai College, Israel. Parents were provided with an explanation of the study and signed an informed consent form to participate. Children in the adolescent group also provided their consent. Parents completed the AEQ independently and at their convenience via an online link. To ensure anonymity, each participant was assigned a serial number, and identifying details were removed from the participants' forms.

Data Analysis

Data processing was conducted using SPSS software, with a significance level of $p < 0.05$ for all tests. Before testing the hypotheses, descriptive statistics of the research variables were calculated to examine the characteristics of the study population. To examine the relationship between gender and age, a preliminary chi-squared test was conducted.

To test the hypotheses, one-way ANOVA, two-way ANOVA, and one-way multivariate ANOVA (MANOVA) tests were used. The two-way ANOVA was designed to examine differences between groups with two categorical independent variables and one quantitative dependent variable.

Two-way ANOVA tests were conducted to test the first, second, and third hypotheses regarding differences in eating problems between boys and girls with ASD, differences in eating problems between young children and adolescents with ASD (main effect), and the interaction effect between gender and age, respectively. This allowed for an examination of the combined effect of the two independent variables on the dependent variable.

A one-way ANOVA was performed to test the fourth hypothesis predicting selective eating based on gender among younger participants. Finally, a one-way multivariate ANOVA (MANOVA) was performed to test the fifth hypothesis regarding differences specifically related to the selective eating and rigidity/rituals subscales based on age (between adolescents and young children) using Hotelling's trace criterion.

Results

The results indicated that selective eating is the most prevalent eating problem in this study population. Examination of minimum and maximum values suggests the presence of a "floor effect" in several scales, particularly in the swallowing difficulties and behavioral difficulties scales. The preliminary chi-squared test showed no significant relationship between gender and age [$\chi 2$ (1, $N = 59$) = 0.001, ns].

The two-way ANOVA showed no significant difference in eating problems between boys and girls diagnosed with ASD [F (1,55) = 2.53, ns]. The mean eating problem level for girls ($M = 1.18$, SD = 1.08) was not significantly different from that of boys ($M = 1.63$, SD = 0.81). This finding refutes Hypothesis 1.

The two-way ANOVA results indicated no significant difference in eating problems between younger children and adolescents with ASD [F (1,55) = 0.24, ns]. The mean eating problem score for younger children ($M = 1.40$, SD = 0.99) was not significantly different from that of adolescents ($M = 1.54$, SD = 0.94). This finding refutes Hypothesis 2.

The two-way ANOVA results showed no significant interaction between gender and age regarding eating problems [F(1,55) = 0.01, ns]. The difference between girls and boys did not vary significantly by age, refuting Hypothesis 3.

A one-way ANOVA revealed a significant difference in selective eating between boys and girls [F (1,38) = 6.99, $p < 0.05$]. The mean level of selective eating among boys ($M = 2.70$, SD = 1.56) was significantly higher than that of girls ($M = 1.86$, SD = 1.42). This supports Hypothesis 4.

A one-way multivariate ANOVA (MANOVA) assessed selective eating and rigidity/ritual eating problems based on age using Hotelling's trace. The analysis revealed no significant differences in the levels of selective eating and rigidity/ritual eating problems between younger children and adolescents [F (1,57) = 0.19, ns]. Separate one-way ANOVA tests also showed no significant effect of age on selective eating [F (1,57) = 0.23, ns] or on rigidity and rituals in eating [F (1,57) = 0.39, ns]. These findings refute Hypothesis 5.

The findings confirm prior research showing a high prevalence of eating problems in children diagnosed with ASD (e.g., Ahearn et al., 2001; Dominick et al., 2007; Ledford & Gast, 2006; Margari et al., 2020; Maskey et al., 2013; Schreck & Williams, 2006; Sharp et al., 2010). The data showed no significant differences in overall eating problems between boys and girls with ASD. However, a non-significant trend indicated higher eating problem scores among young boys, which aligns with meta-analytic findings indicating that boys with ASD exhibit more restrictive behaviors and interests than girls (Van Wijngaarden-Cremers et al., 2014). These restrictive behaviors may manifest in eating, which helps explain the higher prevalence of selective eating problems among boys.

Contrary to previous findings that eating problems, such as selective eating, intensify with age (e.g., Bandini et al., 2017; Vissoker et al., 2019), analysis of the data collected in this study did not find significant differences in eating problems between young children and adolescents. Importantly, Alibrandi et al. (2023) found that significant challenges in eating behavior and food selectivity among children with ASD strongly correlated with sensory sensitivities—particularly to smell, taste, texture, color, and temperature—and with impaired motor skills. Nevertheless, early diagnosis of ASD and interventions among the study participants in the present study may have mitigated eating problems in early childhood. Additionally, the small sample size of adolescents ($N = 19$), approximately half of whom were boys ($N = 10$), may have contributed to the lack of significant findings, as prior studies on eating problems in adolescents primarily included male participants.

Limitations

Several limitations should be noted. The small sample of 59 participants, with varying subgroup sizes, limits the generalizability of the findings. A larger sample might yield different results. Participants were recruited through convenience sampling, making the demographic characteristics of the sample unrepresentative of the general Israeli population. The reliance on parent-reported data for assessing eating problems may introduce reporting bias.

Future research should consider conducting larger and more representative study populations to enhance the understanding of eating problems in this population and explore the influence of functioning levels (low, medium, high) on eating problems in children and adolescents with autism.

Implications and Recommendations

This study of children and adolescents aged 3–18 with ASD yielded multiple insights that can directly inform clinical and educational practices.

Awareness and Intervention in Educational Settings

The findings confirm the prevalence of eating problems among children and adolescents with ASD in both regular and special education settings. Increased awareness among educators could foster the development of targeted intervention programs to address eating difficulties in schools.

Selective Eating by Young Boys

Intervention programs should account for the higher prevalence of selective eating among young boys. Appropriate mediation and guidance in therapeutic and educational settings may help children and adolescents manage persistent eating difficulties, improving their quality of life and that of their families. The study and analysis contribute to the growing body of knowledge on eating problems in children and adolescents with ASD, offering a foundation for tailored interventions to reduce distress in this population and their families.

Such knowledge could serve as a foundation for developing age- and gender-appropriate treatments for children and adolescents with ASD. Therefore, it is crucial to further examine whether differences exist between genders and age groups to facilitate the development of new treatment approaches and effective intervention strategies to minimize the distress experienced by these children and their families. Since persistent eating difficulties may pose nutritional and health risks and impair the young people's quality of life and that of their families, the ability to assess differences in eating behaviors among children with ASD can be highly valuable for providing appropriate individualized care.

References

Ahearn, W. H., Castine, T., Nault, K., & Green, G. (2001). An assessment of food acceptance in children with autism or pervasive developmental disorder-not otherwise specified. *Journal of Autism and Developmental Disorders, 31*(5), 505–511. https://doi.org/10.1023/a:1012221026124

American Psychiatric Association [APA]. (2022). *Diagnostic and statistical manual of mental disorders, text revision* (5th ed.) [DSM-5-TR]. American Psychiatric Association. https://www.mredscircleoftrust.com/storage/app/media/DSM%205%20TR.pdf

Alibrandi, A., Zirilli, A., Loschiavo, F., Gangemi, M. C., Sindoni, A., Tribulato, G., Lo Giudice, R., & Famà, F. (2023). Food selectivity in children with autism spectrum disorder: A statistical analysis in southern Italy. *Children, 10*(9), 1553. https://doi.org/10.3390/children10091553

Arcelus, J., Mitchell, A. J., Wales, J., & Nielsen, S. (2011). Mortality rates in patients with anorexia nervosa and other eating disorders: A meta-analysis of 36 studies. *Archives of General Psychiatry, 68*(7), 724–731. https://doi.org/10.1001/archgenpsychiatry.2011.74

Banach, R., Thompson, A., Szatmari, P., Goldberg, J., Tuff, L., Zwaigenbaum, L., & Mahoney, W. (2009). Brief report: Relationship between non-verbal IQ and gender in autism. *Journal of Autism and Developmental Disorders, 39*(1), 188–193. https://doi.org/10.1007/s10803-008-0612-4

Bandini, L. G., Anderson, S. E., Curtin, C., Cermak, S., Evans, E. W., Scampini, R., Maslin, M., & Must, A. (2010). Food selectivity in children with autism spectrum disorders and typically developing children. *The Journal of Pediatrics, 157*(2), 259–264. https://doi.org/10.1016/j.jpeds.2010.02.013

Bandini, L. G., Curtin, C., Phillips, S., Anderson, S. E., Maslin, M., & Must, A. (2017). Changes in food selectivity in children with autism spectrum disorder. *Journal of Autism and Developmental Disorders, 47*(2), 439–446. https://doi.org/10.1007/s10803-016-2963-6

Beecroft, N., Bach, L., Tunstall, N., & Howard, R. (1998). An unusual case of pica. *International Journal of Geriatric Psychiatry, 13*(9), 638–641. https://doi.org/10.1002/(SICI)1099-1166(199809)13:9%3c638::AID-GPS837%3e3.0.CO;2-N
Bellando, J., & Lopez, M. (2009). The school nurse's role in treatment of the student with autism spectrum disorders. *Journal for Specialists in Pediatric Nursing, 14*(3), 173–182. https://doi.org/10.1111/j.1744-6155.2009.00195.x
Bölte, S., Duketis, E., Poustka, F., & Holtmann, M. (2011). Sex differences in cognitive domains and their clinical correlates in higher-functioning autism spectrum disorders. *Autism: The International Journal of Research and Practice, 15*(4), 497–511. https://doi.org/10.1177/1362361310391116
Carter, A. S., Black, D. O., Tewani, S., Connolly, C. E., Kadlec, M. B., & Tager-Flusberg, H. (2007). Sex differences in toddlers with autism spectrum disorders. *Journal of Autism and Developmental Disorders, 37*(1), 86–97. https://doi.org/10.1007/s10803-006-0331-7
Cermak, S. A., Curtin, C., & Bandini, L. G. (2010). Food selectivity and sensory sensitivity in children with autism spectrum disorders. *Journal of the American Dietetic Association, 110*(2), 238–246. https://doi.org/10.1016/j.jada.2009.10.032
Christensen, D., Bilder, D., Zahorodny, W., Pettygrove, S., Durkin, M., Fitzgerald, R., Rice, C., Kurzius-Spencer, M., Baio, J., & Yeargin-Allsopp, M. (2016). Prevalence and characteristics of autism spectrum disorder among 4-year-old children in the autism and developmental disabilities monitoring network. *Journal of Developmental and Behavioral Pediatrics, 37*(1), 1–8. https://doi.org/10.1097/DBP.0000000000000235
Dominick, K. C., Davis, N. O., Lainhart, J., Tager-Flusberg, H., & Folstein, S. (2007). Atypical behaviors in children with autism and children with a history of language impairment. *Research in Developmental Disabilities, 28*(2), 145–162. https://doi.org/10.1016/j.ridd.2006.02.003
Gal, E., Gal-Mishael, R., Vissoker, R. E., Hedley, D., Bury, S. M., & Stolar, O. (2022). Eating challenges in children with autism spectrum disorder: Development and validation of the "Aut-Eat" questionnaire (AEQ). *Journal of Autism and Developmental Disorders, 52*(2), 811–822. https://doi.org/10.1007/s10803-021-04978-x
Gillberg, C. (1985). Autism and anorexia nervosa: Related conditions? *Nordisk Psykiatrisk Tidsskrift, 39*(4), 307–312. https://doi.org/10.3109/08039488509101911
Gorrindo, P., Williams, K. C., Lee, E. B., Walker, L. S., McGrew, S. G., & Levitt, P. (2012). Gastrointestinal dysfunction in autism: Parental report, clinical evaluation, and associated factors. *Autism Research, 5*(2), 101–108. https://doi.org/10.1002/aur.237
Holtmann, M., Bölte, S., & Poustka, F. (2007). Autism spectrum disorders: Sex differences in autistic behaviour domains and coexisting psychopathology. *Developmental Medicine & Child Neurology, 49*(5), 361–366. https://doi.org/10.1111/j.1469-8749.2007.00361.x
Hubbard, K. L., Anderson, S. E., Curtin, C., Must, A., & Bandini, L. G. (2014). A comparison of food refusal related to characteristics of food in children with autism spectrum disorder and typically developing children. *Journal of the Academy of Nutrition and Dietetics, 114*(12), 1981–1987. https://doi.org/10.1016/j.jand.2014.04.017
Huke, V., Turk, J., Saeidi, S., Kent, A., & Morgan, J. F. (2013). Autism spectrum disorders in eating disorder populations: A systematic review. *European Eating Disorders Review, 21*(5), 345–351. https://doi.org/10.1002/erv.2244
Hurtig, T., Kuusikko, S., Mattila, M. L., Haapsamo, H., Ebeling, H., Jussila, K., Joskitt, L., Pauls, D., & Moilanen, I. (2009). Multi-informant reports of psychiatric symptoms among high-functioning adolescents with Asperger syndrome or autism. *Autism, 13*(6), 583–598. https://doi.org/10.1177/1362361309335719
Karjalainen, S., Aro, T., & Parviainen, T. (2024). Coactivation of autonomic and central nervous systems during processing of socially relevant information in autism spectrum disorder: A systematic review. *Neuropsychology Review, 34*(1), 214–231. https://doi.org/10.1007/s11065-023-09579-2
Kuschner, E. S., Eisenberg, I. W., Orionzi, B., Simmons, W. K., Kenworthy, L., Martin, A., & Wallace, G. L. (2015). A preliminary study of self-reported food selectivity in adolescents and

young adults with autism spectrum disorder. *Research in Autism Spectrum Disorders, 15*, 53–59. https://doi.org/10.1016/j.rasd.2015.04.005
Ledford, J. R., & Gast, D. L. (2006). Feeding problems in children with autism spectrum disorders: A review. *Focus on Autism and Other Developmental Disabilities, 21*(3), 153–166. https://doi.org/10.1177/10883576060210030401
Maenner, M. J., Warren, Z., Williams, A. R., Amoakohene, E., Bakian, A. V., Bilder, D. A., Durkin, M. S., Fitzgerald, R. T., Furnier, S. M., Hughes, M. M., Ladd-Acosta, C. M., McArthur, D., Pas, E. T., Salinas, A., Vehorn, A., Williams, S., Esler, A., Grzybowski, A., Hall-Lande, J., … Shaw, K. A. (2023). Prevalence and characteristics of autism spectrum disorder among children aged 8 years: Autism and developmental disabilities monitoring network, 11 sites, United States, 2020. *MMWR. Surveillance Summaries, 72*(2), 1–14. https://doi.org/10.15585/mmwr.ss7202a1
Mandy, W., Chilvers, R., Chowdhury, U., Salter, G., Seigal, A., & Skuse, D. (2012). Sex differences in autism spectrum disorder: Evidence from a large sample of children and adolescents. *Journal of Autism and Developmental Disorders, 42*(7), 1304–1313. https://doi.org/10.1007/s10803-011-1356-0
Mandy, W., & Tchanturia, K. (2015). Do women with eating disorders who have social and flexibility difficulties really have autism? *A Case Series. Molecular Autism, 6*(1), 1–10. https://doi.org/10.1186/2040-2392-6-6
Margari, L., Marzulli, L., Gabellone, A., & de Giambattista, C. (2020). Eating and mealtime behaviors in patients with autism spectrum disorder: Current perspectives. *Neuropsychiatric Disease and Treatment*, 2083–2102. https://doi.org/10.2147/NDT.S224779
Mascola, A. J., Bryson, S. W., & Agras, W. S. (2010). Picky eating during childhood: A longitudinal study to age 11 years. *Eating Behaviors, 11*(4), 253–257. https://doi.org/10.1016/j.eatbeh.2010.05.006
Maskey, M., Warnell, F., Parr, J. R., Le Couteur, A., & McConachie, H. (2013). Emotional and behavioural problems in children with autism spectrum disorder. *Journal of Autism and Developmental Disorders, 43*(4), 851–859. https://doi.org/10.1007/s10803-012-1622-9
Matson, J. L., & Fodstad, J. C. (2009). The treatment of food selectivity and other feeding problems in children with autism spectrum disorders. *Research in Autism Spectrum Disorders, 3*(2), 455–461. https://doi.org/10.1016/j.rasd.2008.09.005
Matson, J. L., Rieske, R. D., & Williams, L. W. (2013). The relationship between autism spectrum disorders and attention-deficit/hyperactivity disorder: An overview. *Research in Developmental Disabilities, 34*(9), 2475–2484. https://doi.org/10.1016/j.ridd.2013.05.021
McLennan, J. D., Lord, C., & Schopler, E. (1993). Sex differences in higher functioning people with autism. *Journal of Autism and Developmental Disorders, 23*(2), 217–227. https://doi.org/10.1007/BF01046216
Pearlman-Avnion, S., & Shlain, R. (2019). Adult women on the high-functioning autism spectrum. In Lowinger, S., & Pearlman-Avnion, S. (Eds.), *Autism in Adulthood* (pp. 89–112). Springer. https://doi.org/10.1007/978-3-030-28833-4_5
Peretz, C. (2024). *Differences in eating problems between boys and girls and between young children and adolescents diagnosed with autism.* (Unpublished Master's Dissertation), Tel-Hai College, Israel.
Provost, B., Crowe, T. K., Osbourn, P. L., McClain, C., & Skipper, B. J. (2010). Mealtime behaviors of preschool children: Comparison of children with autism spectrum disorder and children with typical development. *Physical & Occupational Therapy in Pediatrics, 30*(3), 220–233. https://doi.org/10.3109/01942631003757669
Rivet, T. T., & Matson, J. L. (2011). Review of gender differences in core symptomatology in autism spectrum disorders. *Research in Autism Spectrum Disorders, 5*(3), 957–976. https://doi.org/10.1016/j.rasd.2010.12.003
Schreck, K. A., & Williams, K. (2006). Food preferences and factors influencing food selectivity for children with autism spectrum disorders. *Research in Developmental Disabilities, 27*(4), 353–363. https://doi.org/10.1016/j.ridd.2005.03.005

Schreck, K. A., Williams, K., & Smith, A. F. (2004). A comparison of eating behaviors between children with and without autism. *Journal of Autism and Developmental Disorders, 34*(4), 433–438. https://doi.org/10.1023/B:JADD.0000037419.78531.86

Sharp, W. G., Berry, R. C., McCracken, C., Nuhu, N. N., Marvel, E., Saulnier, C. A., Klin, A., Jones, W., & Jaquess, D. L. (2013). Feeding problems and nutrient intake in children with autism spectrum disorders: A meta-analysis and comprehensive review of the literature. *Journal of Autism and Developmental Disorders, 43*(9), 2159–2173. https://doi.org/10.1007/s10803-013-1771-5

Sharp, W. G., Jaquess, D. L., Morton, J. F., & Herzinger, C. V. (2010). Pediatric feeding disorders: A quantitative synthesis of treatment outcomes. *Clinical Child and Family Psychology Review, 13*(4), 348–365. https://doi.org/10.1007/s10567-010-0079-7

Smink, F. R., van Hoeken, D., Oldehinkel, A. J., & Hoek, H. W. (2014). Prevalence and severity of DSM-5 eating disorders in a community cohort of adolescents. *International Journal of Eating Disorders, 47*(6), 610–619. https://doi.org/10.1002/eat.22316

Tsai, L. Y., & Beisler, J. M. (1983). The development of sex differences in infantile autism. *The British Journal of Psychiatry, 142*(4), 373–378. https://doi.org/10.1192/bjp.142.4.373

Van Wijngaarden-Cremers, P. J., van Eeten, E., Groen, W. B., Van Deurzen, P. A., Oosterling, I. J., & Van der Gaag, R. J. (2014). Gender and age differences in the core triad of impairments in autism spectrum disorders: A systematic review and meta-analysis. *Journal of Autism and Developmental Disorders, 44*(3), 627–635. https://doi.org/10.1007/s10803-013-1913-9

Vissoker, R. E., Latzer, Y., Stolar, O., Rabenbach, A., & Gal, E. (2019). Eating problems and patterns among toddlers and young boys with and without autism spectrum disorders. *Research in Autism Spectrum Disorders, 59*, 1–9. https://doi.org/10.1016/j.rasd.2018.12.001

Wentz, E., Lacey, J. H., Waller, G., Råstam, M., Turk, J., & Gillberg, C. (2005). Childhood onset neuropsychiatric disorders in adult eating disorder patients: A pilot study. *European Child & Adolescent Psychiatry, 14*(8), 431–437. https://doi.org/10.1007/s00787-005-0494-3

Werling, D. M., Parikshak, N. N., & Geschwind, D. H. (2016). Gene expression in human brain implicates sexually dimorphic pathways in autism spectrum disorders. *Nature Communications, 7*(1), 10717. https://doi.org/10.1186/s13293-016-0112-8

Westwood, H., Stahl, D., Mandy, W., & Tchanturia, K. (2016). The set-shifting profiles of anorexia nervosa and autism spectrum disorder using the Wisconsin Card Sorting Test: A systematic review and meta-analysis. *Psychological Medicine, 46*(9), 1809–1827. https://doi.org/10.1017/S0033291716000581

Williams, K. E., Gibbons, B. G., & Schreck, K. A. (2005). Comparing selective eaters with and without developmental disabilities. *Journal of Developmental and Physical Disabilities, 17*(3), 299–309. https://doi.org/10.1007/s10882-005-4387-7

Zhang, L., Huang, C. C., Dai, Y., Luo, Q., Ji, Y., Wang, K., Deng, S., Yu, J., Xu, M., Du, X., Tang, Y., Shen, C., Feng, J., Sahakian, B., Lin, C.-P., & Li, F. (2020). Symptom improvement in children with autism spectrum disorder following bumetanide administration is associated with decreased GABA/glutamate ratios. *Translational Psychiatry, 10*(1), 9. https://doi.org/10.1038/s41398-020-0692-2

Zimmer, M. H., Hart, L. C., Manning-Courtney, P., Murray, D. S., Bing, N. M., & Summer, S. (2012). Food variety as a predictor of nutritional status among children with autism. *Journal of Autism and Developmental Disorders, 42*(4), 549–556. https://doi.org/10.1007/s10803-011-1268-z

Zucker, N., Copeland, W., Franz, L., Carpenter, K., Keeling, L., Angold, A., & Egger, H. (2015). Psychological and psychosocial impairment in preschoolers with selective eating. *Pediatrics, 136*(3), e582–e590. https://doi.org/10.1542/peds.2014-2386

Chapter 6
Educational Choices for Autistic Children in Religious Communities

Liat Maia Schvarzman Sinai and Shiri Pearlman-Avnion

Abstract This study investigates the nuanced educational choices made by Jewish national-religious (JNR) families in Israel for their children diagnosed with Autism Spectrum Disorder (ASD). It examines how parental worldviews, knowledge of ASD, and the severity of the child's symptoms influence decisions between regular and special education settings. Through a mixed-methods approach, collecting both quantitative and qualitative data from 20 mothers, the research reveals a trend: parents with greater ASD knowledge and children exhibiting higher cognitive functioning, particularly in language development, were more likely to opt for inclusive educational environments. A core finding highlights the significant emotional and social complexities parents face, including profound fear of social stigma, guilt, and isolation related to their child's diagnosis. The study emphasizes the dilemma of seeking specialized education versus maintaining community integration within their religious society, often leading to a choice of regular settings despite challenges. This research underscores the critical need for professional support and guidance for these families, advocating for informed parental choice that respects their unique cultural and communal values when determining educational placement for children with autism in Israel.

Keywords Parental decision-making · Jewish national-religious · Inclusive education · Special education · Social stigma · Community integration

---

L. M. S. Sinai (✉)
School Psychology Service, Elkana, Israel
e-mail: liat@elkana.org.il

S. Pearlman-Avnion
Tel-Hai College, Qiryat Shmona, Israel

S. Lowinger and S. Pearlman-Avnion (eds.), *Collaborative Care and Partnerships in Autism Diagnosis and Treatment*, Autism and Child Psychopathology Series,
https://doi.org/10.1007/978-3-032-07009-8_6

Introduction

The current chapter explores the choice of educational framework among parents with children who have been diagnosed with autism spectrum disorder (ASD). It looks at how the connections between the parents' worldviews, knowledge of ASD, and the severity of their child's disability affect this choice. The population under consideration is the Jewish national-religious (JNR) community in Israel. The Jewish population of Israel is divided into various sectors, reflecting differences in religious beliefs. These beliefs influence attitudes toward disabilities and educational choices.

The chapter offers a review of the relevant literature and then presents an analysis of data collected from parents in the Jewish national-religious community in Israel regarding their decision of whether to enroll their child diagnosed with ASD into regular or special education settings. Qualitative and quantitative data were collected from twenty mothers in the target population. Questionnaires examined the parents' knowledge of ASD and the severity of their children's symptoms. The interviews provided in-depth and nuanced insights into the considerations that led to their choice of educational setting.

The data analysis revealed a trend whereby parents of children with a great deal of knowledge about ASD and whose children exhibit a high level of functioning were more likely to choose to integrate their children into a regular educational setting while parents with less knowledge about ASD and whose children exhibited a low level of functioning were more likely to choose to integrate their children into a special educational setting. However, there were cases in which the parents' choice of educational setting was arbitrary and not based on either the severity of the child's symptoms or the parents' level of knowledge.

The analysis emphasizes the emotional and social complexity that parents face when making this decision. Many of the surveyed parents said they feared disclosing their child's diagnosis of ASD due to social stigma in their social environment and feelings of guilt and/or isolation. Despite this fear of exposure, due to lack of suitable solutions within the religious settings, many parents from the Jewish national-religious community choose to enroll their children in regular educational settings out of a desire to provide them with a religious education and to integrate them into religious society. The conclusions pertain to parents' great need for professional support and guidance when making choices regarding their children's education, especially among this population in which multiple community-related complexities affect the decision.

The uniqueness and importance of the research lie in two focal points. First, the combination of quantitative and qualitative methods provides an in-depth structure for the considerations underlying the decision in a way that is not possible in purely quantitative research, as the qualitative examination offers a critique and tells an accurate story that explains the quantitative data. The second arises from how this combination of methods deepens the understanding of the dilemma between the fear of stigma versus the fear of exclusion from the special community to which children on the autism spectrum belong. This is the dilemma faced by a small community within a broader context, in that transitioning to special education represents the child's removal from the community and its values, while keeping the child within the community at all costs means dealing with the stigma of the diagnosis, and perhaps, with appropriate professional help, an opportunity to change and maybe remove the stigma.

Autism Spectrum Disorder in Israeli Society

Autism spectrum disorder is a developmental neurobiological disability that manifests in two main symptoms: a persistent deficit in interpersonal communication with the environment and preoccupation with a narrow field of interest and repetitive behavior. To be diagnosed with ASD, a person must exhibit symptoms that meet the five criteria listed in the *DSM-5-TR* (American Psychiatric Association, 2022, pp. 56–57). Cognitive abilities are not among the criteria.

In recent years, there has been a significant increase in the prevalence of ASD in Israel; the rate of diagnosis is currently approximately 15%, similar to that in other Western countries. This trend has been documented in multiple studies. For example, the number of applications for disability benefits in Israel due to a diagnosis of ASD increased between 2003 and 2007 (Segev et al., 2019). The prevalence of ASD diagnoses in Israel rose between 2017 and 2021, with a 4.4-fold increase among children between the ages of two and three years old and a 2.3-fold increase among children between the ages of four and six (Ilan et al., 2023). These increases occurred among the general population, with smaller increases observed among minority populations.

The Jewish population in Israel is divided into three main sectors according to degree of religiosity: secular, traditional, and religious. Religious Jews can be further divided into two subgroups: the *Haredi* (ultra-Orthodox) community and the national-religious community. Members of the Haredi community strictly observe traditional Jewish religious laws and precepts, maintain gender segregation, and largely isolate themselves from secular life (Shaked & Bilu, 2006). In contrast, members of the national-religious community are more fully integrated into the secular community, although they maintain Orthodox religious practice and strive toward the realization of a religious Jewish state in Israel (Schwartz, 2018).

Orthodox Jewish tradition is based on obedience to its laws and scriptures, in which a person diagnosed with ASD may be classified as a "simpleton" and thus exempt from observing the religious commandments. At the same time, parents in religious Jewish communities want their children to uphold a religious lifestyle, which makes it difficult for them to accept this disability (Shaked, 2005).

Models of Perceptions Regarding Disability

Gershoni (2018) described models that explain people's perceptions of disability, which may be divided into two categories. The first category encompasses models with a paternalistic approach, according to which people with disabilities are viewed as being dependent on the goodwill of others in their social environment. The second category includes models with an empowering approach according to which people with disabilities are active agents who can utilize their environment to realize their potential. Gershoni's study on perceptions of people with disabilities in Jewish religious society in Israel found that the two main models expressed among this population are the charitable model and the religious model, both of which fall under the paternalistic approach.

According to the charitable model, people with disabilities are experiencing a terrible lifelong tragedy, and the community is responsible for supporting them in order for them to survive. This approach of charity and compassion toward people with disabilities can also be recognized in Islamic and Christian communities (McMahon-Panther & Bornman, 2025; Mehmood & Parveen, 2024).

According to the religious model, disability can be viewed negatively, as a curse, or positively, as something holy. Negative societal attitudes cause a sense of guilt on the part of families of people with disabilities. In such cases, people with disabilities are hidden from the community lest they damage the family's image and other family members' eligibility in marital matchmaking. In contrast, a positive attitude views a person with disabilities as a sacred being who was brought to this world to redeem society and should be treated with gentleness and tolerance. The attitude toward people with disabilities is determined by religious leaders. Each case is examined individually, based on biblical (Torah) sources and interpretations, and the religious leaders' perspectives and decisions are considered indisputable (Gershoni, 2018).

Rights for People with Disabilities in Israel

Special Education

Integrating children with ASD into society in general and a religious community specifically reflects the ways in which the world at large is learning to accommodate, assist, and support such integration. In 2006, the United Nations Convention on the Rights of Persons with Disabilities was drafted, and Israel became a signatory in 2007 (United Nations, 2006). Israel's Special Education Law of 1988 provides for educational frameworks appropriate for children with special needs (Special Education Law, 1988).

Israel's Rehabilitative Daycare Law (2000) and the Special Education Law enable parents of children diagnosed with ASD to choose between three educational frameworks: a special education setting, a special education setting integrated into a regular education setting, or a regular educational setting accompanied by a personal assistant (for details, see the Special Education Law of 1988 with Amendments No. 7, 2002 and No. 11 and the Rehabilitation Day Care Law, 2000).

State Religious Education

According to Israel's State Education Law of 1953, religious State education is "State education, with the distinction that its institutions are religious as to their way of life, curriculum, teachers and inspectors," and "an official education institution in which State religious education is being provided and which educates to a life of Torah and mitzvoth [religious commandments] according to the religious tradition and in the spirit of religious Zionism." Special education settings within the religious State education system have been adapted for this community and are under the supervision of the Ministry of Education (Maoz, 2005; State Education Law, 1953). Although the number of children in the non-religious state education system diagnosed with ASD is larger, a higher percentage of parents from the nation-religious community choose to integrate their child into regular religious State educational frameworks.

Parental Choice of Educational Setting

A study that examined why parents choose to place their children in a regular or special educational setting found that in over 85% of cases, the choice is arbitrary and not based on the severity of the autistic symptoms (Jeong et al., 2023). Ilan et al. (2021) examined differences between children between the ages of two and five with ASD who were in special education settings and those who were integrated into regular education. They found no significant differences between settings in the children's overall scores on the well-established Autism Diagnostic Observation Schedule (ADOS). In some cases, the choice of setting was based on the child's linguistic abilities; children with normative language development were enrolled in regular educational settings while those exhibiting linguistic delay were placed in special education. Further, the parents' level of education was found to affect the decision. Parents with a high level of education and high incomes were more likely to place their children in regular educational settings and finance paramedical treatments privately, while parents with a low level of education and low incomes were more likely to place their children in special education settings where they could receive state-funded paramedical treatments as part of the services provided in the school (Ilan et al., 2021).

When parents choose to integrate their child with ASD into regular education, they are effectively disclosing their child's difficulties to others in their social environment. Due to a desire to appear "normative," many families keep the diagnosis of ASD to themselves and avoid revealing the complexities associated with this diagnosis. Parents of children with disabilities may experience feelings of guilt, stress, isolation, and social exclusion. Many fear the stigma and social labeling associated with their child's disability (Isham, 2020).

A qualitative study found that some parents hide the ASD diagnosis from the child in question because this enables the parents to remain in denial and avoid explaining the challenges and behaviors associated with ASD to the child and others in the social environment (Almog et al., 2022). Parents who disclose the diagnosis to their child and community must first acknowledge and accept the diagnosis. In addition, they must find an appropriate way to explain to the child and others how the syndrome is expressed in their child. Parents must help their children find ways to cope with their difficulties and support them along the way. In other words, while the concealment process is passive and the disclosure process is active, both require emotional stamina to deal with the consequences of their choice daily.

An interesting comparison can be made to the little research that has been done on the same question within the Amish communities. Research on special education for children in Amish communities, particularly those with autism or other developmental disabilities, is relatively limited due to the Amish commitment to maintaining their traditional lifestyle, which often includes resistance to modern educational practices and external interventions. However, some studies have explored how special education needs are addressed within these communities, showing that parents often prefer to address educational challenges, including special education needs, within the family or community rather than seeking formal, outside interventions. The small, tight-knit nature of Amish communities means that children with disabilities might receive more individualized attention from peers and teachers, but specialized resources and formal diagnoses (such as for autism) are generally avoided or are less emphasized. In some cases, Amish communities may seek assistance from professionals outside the community but prefer to do so discreetly, without exposing children to the broader societal structure (Kraybill, 2001). Other studies focused on barriers to formal special education for Amish children, showing that Amish children are often excluded from state-funded special education programs, as the Amish typically do not participate in the public education system beyond eighth grade. Because of religious beliefs, Amish parents tend to be skeptical about modern medical or psychological diagnoses, including those related to autism spectrum disorder. This resistance to formal intervention often leads to a reliance on informal support systems within the community. There are instances where Amish children with disabilities are enrolled in special needs programs outside their community, but these interventions may not always align with Amish values, creating tensions between their cultural beliefs and educational needs. Lastly, some studies have focused on the need for culturally sensitive approaches to special education when working with Amish children. Professionals who provide services to Amish families need to be aware of Amish values, particularly their preference for privacy and their wariness of medical or psychological labels. Findings show that culturally sensitive educational practices that respect the Amish way of life can help in creating more effective interventions for children with autism and other special needs. Approaches that emphasize family and community involvement, rather than formal diagnoses or external therapies, are more likely to be accepted by Amish families. There is a growing recognition among educational professionals of the need to work with Amish communities in a manner that respects their religious beliefs, which can involve providing support that aligns with their cultural and community-based values. The following study will present an interesting way and findings regarding the parental choice of educational setting in the national-religious Jewish community in Israel.

Data Collection, Aims of the Current Study, and Research Questions

The current study examined the factors that influence parental choice of educational setting for children with ASD in the national-religious Jewish community in Israel. It looks at why parents in this community choose regular or special educational settings for their children. Data are presented and analyzed that examine the influence that parental perceptions and the severity of the child's disability have on the choice of educational setting among the study population. Analysis of the interviews enriches the results of the quantitative survey and sheds light on how parents from this population choose an educational setting and how this relates to their perceptions of ASD.

The study focused on four main research questions. Two are *quantitative research questions.* Among children diagnosed with ASD from the Jewish national-religious population in Israel, how do their levels of functioning differ between those who are in special education settings and those who are integrated into regular education settings? Among parents of children diagnosed with ASD in this population, how does their level of knowledge about ASD differ between those who chose to enroll their child in special education and those who chose to integrate their child into regular education? Two are *qualitative research questions***.** How do the symptoms of ASD exhibited by the child relate to the parents' choice of educational setting? How do the meanings that parents from the Jewish national-religious community in Israel attribute to ASD explain their choice of educational setting for their child?

Hypotheses

Children diagnosed with ASD who exhibit more severe symptoms will be enrolled in special education settings.

Among parents from the Jewish national-religious population in Israel, those who exhibit a great deal of knowledge about ASD are more likely to enroll their child in special education settings, while those exhibiting little knowledge about ASD are more likely to integrate their child into regular religious State schools.

The child's level of symptoms of ASD and the parents' level of knowledge about ASD will positively correlate with the child's placement in a given educational setting.

Collection and Analysis of Quantitative Data

The study population included 20 mothers who are affiliated with the Jewish national-religious community in Israel and who have a child between the ages of 3 and 10 diagnosed with ASD. Fourteen of the children were in kindergarten, and the other six were in elementary school. Only mothers, not fathers, were surveyed, which avoided the potential for differences based on gender.

To recruit participants, announcements were posted in special education settings and in online groups for parents in this community who have children with ASD. Twenty mothers who responded to the messages and agreed to participate were included in the study.

This mixed-method study used quantitative and qualitative research tools. First, the participating mothers completed two questionnaires. This was followed by an in-depth interview. The interviewer was blind to the questionnaire results, so there was no connection between the answers in the questionnaires and the interview.

The first quantitative research tool was the Autism Knowledge Survey-Revised (AKS-R). The questionnaire, taken from Ables et al. (2011), is a revised and updated version of the original AKS (Stone, 1987). The version used for the current study was translated into Hebrew through a back-translation process. The questionnaire assesses knowledge about ASD, including etiology, diagnosis, intervention, treatment, and outcomes of the syndrome. The questionnaire includes 20 statements. Participants were asked to rate their level of agreement with each item on a scale from 1 (strongly agree) to 6 (strongly disagree). Ratings from 1 to 3 reflect agreement, while ratings from 4 to 6 reflect disagreement. Sample items from the questionnaire include: "Children with ASD can grow up to live independent lives" and "There are now treatments that can cure ASD."

The second quantitative tool used was the Australian Scale for Asperger's Syndrome (ASAS). The questionnaire was taken from Attwood (1997) and translated into Hebrew by Yael Lehman. The questionnaire examines whether there is a reasonable chance of diagnosing high-functioning autism based on social, emotional, cognitive, and motor skills. The questionnaire includes 24 statements. Participants rate the frequency of occurrence of each within the previous two weeks on a scale from 0 to 6. Ratings from 0 to 2 indicate the events never or rarely occur, and ratings from 4 to 6 indicate they occur frequently. The questionnaire also includes 10 statements to which participants are asked to indicate whether the characteristics described are met (yes/no). Sample items from the questionnaire are: "Does the child have an odd gait when running?" and "When in a conversation, does the child tend to use less eye contact than you would expect?".

The qualitative research tool was an in-depth interview, a well-documented and valuable way to understand how people perceive experiences and what meanings they attribute to them (Shkedi, 2003). In the interviews conducted in the current study, the mothers were asked to address the following areas: family and environmental background; feelings that arose during the diagnostic process; feelings, emotions, and experiences after receiving the diagnosis; the child's daily functioning; attitudes toward the child in their social environment; considerations that led to the choice of an educational setting; and feelings and emotions regarding the educational setting.

Combining quantitative and qualitative research methods, known as mixed methods research, has gained prominence for its ability to provide comprehensive insights into complex phenomena. This approach leverages the strengths of both methodologies, allowing for a more nuanced understanding than either method could offer independently (Fetters et al., 2013; Plano Clark & Ivankova, 2016). This combination is unique to the present study and adds to its validity and reliability.

The researcher and each mother decided where and when the interviews would be conducted. At the researcher's request and with the mothers' consent, all interviews were recorded. After being transcribed, the interviews were deleted in a controlled manner. The interviews lasted between 30 min and one hour. There was no need for additional meetings. Analysis of the interview results was carried out using the qualitative-constructivist method (Shkedi, 2003). The data analysis process began simultaneously with conducting the interviews. As categories emerged in the analysis of the interviews, new questions were formulated and asked in subsequent interviews. These focused questions enabled the researchers to delve deeper and obtain broad and detailed information regarding those categories. After all the interviews were completed, a focused mapping of the data obtained was carried out, and the basis of the results was built according to the existing theoretical knowledge.

Summary of the Quantitative and Qualitative Research Findings

Quantitative Results

Data on the level of functioning of children diagnosed with ASD who were in special educational settings and those in regular educational settings were compared, based on the ASAS questionnaire that the mothers completed at the beginning of the meeting with the researcher. The results were used to test the hypothesis that children diagnosed with ASD who exhibit fewer symptoms would be integrated into regular schools in the national-religious State education system and that those exhibiting more severe symptoms would be enrolled in special education settings.

Two-tailed independent t-tests were conducted to assess differences in the level of functioning of children diagnosed with ASD according to the type of educational setting chosen by the parents. The level of functioning of children with ASD in regular education settings (M = 3.94, SD = 0.88) was slightly higher than that of children with ASD in special education (M = 3.74, SD = 0.79), but the difference was not significant ($T(2,18) = 0.534$, $P = 0.600$).

Next, differences in the parents' level of knowledge were examined using the mothers' responses to the AKS-R questionnaire, which tests knowledge about ASD. It was hypothesized that parents with a great deal of knowledge about ASD would choose special education settings where their child could be provided with a wide range of treatments, while parents who exhibited little knowledge about ASD would integrate their child into regular schools of the national-religious State school system. The two-tailed independent T-test found that the level of knowledge of parents of children with ASD who are integrated into regular education (M = 3.78, SD = 0.38) was slightly higher than that of parents of children with ASD who are in special education (M = 3.68, SD = 0.34), but this difference was also not significant ($T(2,18) = 0.585$, $P = 0.566$). Thus, the hypothesis was not confirmed. Instead, parents with a great deal of knowledge were found to prefer regular education, while parents with less knowledge preferred special education, although the difference was not significant.

In summary, no significant differences were found in the variables examined between the types of educational frameworks chosen. However, a trend was noted that children with a higher level of functioning and whose parents have greater knowledge about ASD were more likely to be integrated into regular education, while children with a lower level of functioning and whose parents have less knowledge about ASD were more likely to be enrolled in special education.

Qualitative Results

The qualitative findings are presented according to the order of the qualitative research questions and analyzed in the context of the quantitative research findings. The themes that emerged from the analysis of the interviews supported the results of the quantitative analysis as described above. No significant differences were found in the mothers' reports of the manifestations of the characteristics of ASD that explained the parents' choice of educational placement. Nevertheless, a trend emerged in the interviews regarding several core symptoms expressed in the children's behaviors. One is cognitive flexibility, and the second pertains to interpersonal communication and language development.

Cognitive Flexibility

The mothers' responses indicated that they deal with a variety of challenges regarding their children's behavior in situations that require cognitive flexibility, such as changes in the daily routine, hosting friends, going to the playground, etc. The findings found no consistent trend linking the needs of children with ASD outside of school or kindergarten and the type of educational setting in which they are integrated.

Children's ability to cope with change reflects their cognitive flexibility. Van Eylen et al. (2011) found that cognitive flexibility in children with ASD is individual and inconsistent. Therefore, the differences in the mothers' reports may reflect variations in their children's cognitive flexibility. Mothers of children in special education kindergartens or schools spoke about issues they had to cope with, as shown in the following quotes.

"He [my son] needs a very clear routine, and this makes it very difficult for us. I can't decide to go to my mother's spontaneously because I know it would be too difficult for him, and he wouldn't agree to go." (Interview 3).

"I can't go to the playground with her [my daughter] alone after kindergarten or on Saturdays. I must have someone else with me who can chase her in case she decides to run away. Even though she really loves playing outside, I rarely take her out because I am afraid that she will run into the road, and I won't be able to catch her in time." (Interview 4).

"The kindergarten teacher tells me how calm he [my son] is and how he listens to instructions, but at home, I just ask him for something small, and he immediately starts screaming." (Interview 19).

The sentiments expressed in interviews with mothers of children integrated into regular learning settings were similar.

"If something happens and his daily routine changes, he gets into a loop with himself and he will only go to bed at ten after barely touching dinner, not showering, and with incessant screaming." (Interview 11).

Interpersonal Communication and Language Development

Another theme that characterizes ASD is interpersonal communication and language development. Although delayed language development is not a mandatory symptom for the diagnosis of ASD, it is often an early sign that motivates parents to assess their child's development. Interpersonal communication and language development are among the most prominent symptoms of ASD and are recognizable by late infancy.

Language development is based on joint attention and the development of brain mechanisms for language acquisition (Adamson et al., 2019; Keen et al., 2016). Although language development is individual, by the age of two, children are expected to acquire their first words and initiate and respond with joint attention to children and adults. Many children who are later diagnosed with ASD initially showed delays in language acquisition and joint attention. Although delayed language development is not a criterion for diagnosing ASD, it is an early sign.

Many of the mothers who had enrolled their children in special education settings said that one of the reasons for this choice was their child's delayed language development, although some said that the child's early language development was normative.

One mother of a child in a special education kindergarten said:

"The teacher at the kindergarten called us in for a meeting. At the meeting, she told us that a child of her [my daughter's] age is expected to already use a variety of words. Our T. didn't really have any words. She's our oldest daughter, and at the time, we didn't know what was expected at each age." (Interview 14).

"The mother of another child in special education said, "I don't remember when he [my son] started talking. There probably wasn't anything unusual, because if there was, I would remember." (Interview 3).

Another mother whose child was in a special education class reported,

"We saw that something was wrong with his development. He is not our first child, so we had something to compare it to. True, we always say not to compare children, but his older brother said his first words at the age of one, and at that age, he barely made sounds." (Interview 7).

In contrast, the mothers of children integrated into regular educational settings were more likely to say their child exhibited normative language development. "His first words were 'auto' and 'water'. We did expect him to say 'dada' or 'Bamba' [an Israeli snack food] first, as is common in all sorts of places, but that's not what bothered us." (Interview 16) "Thank God, motor and language development were normal, nothing unusual." (Interview 18). However, some children in regular education exhibited significant delays in language development. "Our communication with him is through an iPad and his hand movements." (Interview 9).

In conclusion, the mothers' reports indicate a trend that when interpersonal communication and language development are normal, mothers prefer to include their children in regular education rather than in special education settings.

Perceptions of ASD and Perceptions of Revealing or Concealing the Diagnosis

There are two main themes that are important to distinguish between: one theme is attitudes toward the diagnosis, and the second theme is attitudes toward its disclosure, both to the child and to the environment. The first theme, regarding attitudes toward the diagnosis, shows that parents' perceptions of autism spectrum disorder range along two main axes. The first axis is a negative attitude toward the diagnosis, expressed through concealment and a desire to "fix" the individual from autism. The second axis is a positive attitude toward the diagnosis, expressed through acceptance of autism as part of the person. According to reports from mothers, these two axes overlap and change over time, regardless of the children's ability levels or the type of placement chosen.

The second theme, regarding disclosure or concealment, ranges from reports of complete concealment of the diagnosis to full disclosure to the child, even meaningfully influencing the child's behavior following the exposure. Similar perceptions can be seen in how parents share the diagnosis with extended family. In some cases, parents avoided telling the family about the diagnosis, while in other cases, a family member was involved throughout the process and served as a supportive anchor for the mothers. The dilemma regarding whether to disclose the child's diagnosis to the family and environment is a challenge faced by many parents of children on the autism spectrum. The gap between the "invisibility" of the disability and the child's high cognitive abilities, as well as the gap between these abilities and the behavior that does not always align with the child's age and the accompanying social difficulties, sharpens the question of the need to share with society (Almog et al., 2022). In both groups, the dilemma of disclosing to the environment arose, particularly when the child was described as having age-appropriate cognitive and language abilities. Mothers who chose to share with the environment reported understanding and acceptance from society, even in unpleasant situations. These mothers were often those who chose to integrate their child into mainstream educational settings. In contrast, mothers who chose not to share, particularly when their child was in special education, expressed that it was a private matter and that others did not need to know.

As stated by one mother who chose not to share the diagnosis with her community and extended family: "We didn't tell anyone for a long time. To this day, many don't know that he was diagnosed. They hardly ever see him, so they don't ask us." (Interview 8).

Other mothers initially chose not to publicly share the diagnosis, but due to unpleasant reactions from the community, decided to reveal it.

"At first, we were very afraid to tell. We didn't know what people would say or how they would say it, what label he would receive, so we chose not to tell. But then we started to hear rumors that other parents labeled him a problem child who was always hitting. That was our signal to step out of the box and start talking. We realized that it was important for people to know that he wasn't acting like that because he was a bad kid or something, but because it was hard for him. Thank God, after we started telling people, the incidents of aggression also decreased significantly, and he had more friends." (Interview 19).

Some mothers chose to reveal the diagnosis from the very beginning, especially among those whose children were integrated into regular education throughout their years of schooling.

"We didn't hide the diagnosis for a moment. Everyone sees that he is different, so why hide it? They accepted him somehow." (Interview 13).

"We live in a small community, so I can't hide it. Besides, there is the fact that he goes to kindergarten with everyone else and has a personal assistant, so it's clear to everyone that something is wrong. The fact that the parents know doesn't make them keep their children away from him. On the contrary, he has lots of friends." (Interview 17).

"We shared it with our immediate family, especially his [my husband's] parents and mine. Thank God we have quite a few children, and we need help. We had to tell them so they could help us." (Interview 10).

"My mother was with me when I received the diagnosis. She was with me throughout the entire process. I don't know how I would have gotten through the diagnosis process without her." (Interview 12).

Discussion: Significance of Parents' Choice of Educational Setting

The recent significant increase in the number of children diagnosed with ASD requires adjustments in the education system to respond to the needs of children along the entire autism spectrum. The general State and religious State education systems in Israel offer a variety of educational frameworks for these children. As noted, according to Israeli law, parents decide which type of framework their child diagnosed with ASD will attend (Amendment No. 11 to the Special Education Law, 2018). However, some of the interviewed parents said that they did not feel they had an appropriate option for their child with ASD within their community. This may be the case for many parents of children with ASD in this population and may explain why some choose regular educational settings.

The data analyzed in this study show that it is not possible to clearly predict which setting parents will choose for their child based on the child's level of functioning and parental knowledge about ASD. However, a trend was noted in that parents with greater knowledge of ASD and whose children exhibit normative linguistic development are more likely to integrate their children into regular education settings. These results confirm those of Ilan et al.'s (2021), finding of similar ADOS scores of children in special and regular educational settings in Israel. However, significant differences were found in parental level of knowledge about ASD and their children's language abilities. For many parents, the choice of educational setting is one point in a long process they have undergone and continue going through in raising a child with ASD.

Some of the surveyed mothers said that taking their children out of the small special education setting and integrating them into a regular education setting was like rebirthing the child into the big world. The intimate settings in which the interviews were conducted enabled the mothers to recount the story of their child's life and reflect on the long process they had gone through, like creating a historical documentary. We asked them to talk about their child from infancy and about their journey, which one described as "a journey between mountains and hills with almost no plain" (Interview 13). The journeys included naiveté, disappointment, hope, and anticipation for a better future.

It emerged that the child's level of ASD symptoms does not have a significant impact on the parents' choice of educational setting. Societal perceptions of disability do affect this choice and a core finding of the study is that the parents' fear of stigma against their family impacts their willingness to reveal or hide the disability, and this, in turn, affects the choice of educational setting.

The dilemma regarding revealing or concealing the diagnosis can be explained by Gershoni's (2018) religious model, according to which the parents' fear of societal stigma imposed on their family and its consequences causes parents to choose a small educational framework that will suit the children's needs and prepare them to participate in society, alongside reinforcing concealment and dealing with feelings of shame. However, parents who integrate their children into regular education also operate according to the religious model, but with the positive perception that society should adapt itself to the needs of the child. The parents want to maintain their child's place in their community. They realize that despite the physical invisibility of this disability, their child exhibits behaviors that put them in situations that may require them to reveal and explain the diagnosis. These parents move from being passive to taking an active role in protecting and standing up for their child by explaining ASD and its implications to others in their community (Almog et al., 2022).

Combining quantitative and qualitative research strengthened the findings, as the same participants completed the questionnaires and opened up during the in-depth interviews. The study participants were ready to share their feelings about the processes they had gone through, both those who said they continued to conceal their child's diagnosis and those who were not afraid of disclosing it.

Based on the findings of the current study and previous research, it is recommended that parents continue to be given the choice of what type of educational setting they prefer for their children with ASD. Parents know better than others what is right for their children, and their choices are made against the background of the attitudes and worldviews according to which the family lives. It is important that children with ASD are raised with the same values and way of life. Additionally, it is essential to give parents professional support and guidance throughout the process of choosing the educational setting for their children so that their choice is informed and focused on the child's best interests.

The fear of stigma and the dilemma between receiving specialized education in special education versus the possibility of being excluded from the community also intersect with the fear of the future. What will happen to my child? Will the community be able to accept his autism, or will it reject him? What will serve him better? Belonging to a community at any cost, including attaching stigma to him and his family, or exclusion and more precise care tailored to his needs, including learning acceptance of others and recognition of them, focused social work, self-advocacy training, and the development of personalized learning methods?

Future research in these domains might benefit from combining quantitative and qualitative methods, since this offers a deep understanding of decision-making, where qualitative analysis critiques and explains the quantitative data. This combination enhances the understanding of the dilemma faced by children on the autism spectrum, torn between the fear of stigma and the risk of exclusion from their special community. This dilemma revolves around the choice between removing the child from the community for special education or keeping them in the community despite the stigma, with the potential for change through professional intervention.

References

Ables, E., Ashby, I., & Swiezy, N. (2011). Autism knowledge survey-revised: Comparison of knowledge across role and experience. *Paper presented at the Applied Behavior Analysis International*, Denver, CO, 27–30 May 2011.

Adamson, L. B., Bakeman, R., Suma, K., & Robins, D. L. (2019). An expanded view of joint attention: Skill, engagement, and language in typical development and autism. *Child Development, 90*(1), e1–e18. https://doi.org/10.1111/cdev.12973

Almog, N., Kessel, A., Gabbay, T., & Levy, N. (2022). "Even if you don't tell, everybody knows": Dilemmas of parents of autistic children regarding diagnosis disclosure. *Mifgash: Journal of Social Educational Work, 30*(54).

American Psychiatric Association. (2022). *Diagnostic and statistical manual of mental disorders, text revision* (5th ed.) [DSM-5-TR]. American Psychiatric Association. https://www.mredscircleoftrust.com/storage/app/media/DSM%205%20TR.pdf

Attwood, A. (1997). *Asperger's syndrome: A guide for parents and professionals.* Jessica Kingsley Publishers.

Fetters, M. D., Curry, L. A., & Creswell, J. W. (2013). Achieving integration in mixed methods designs: Principles and practices. *Health Services Research, 48*(6 pt2), 2134–2156. https://doi.org/10.1111/1475-6773.12117

Gershoni, H. (2018). Siakh shivyon hazzekhuyot shel anashim im mugbaluyot baqqehillah hakharedit [The discourse of equal rights for people with disabilities in the Haredi community]. *Mishpat Khevrah Vetarbut [law, Society and Culture], 1*, 323–359.

Ilan, M., Faroy, M., Zachor, D., Manelis, L., Waissengreen, D., Michaelovski, A., Avni, I., Menashe, I., Koller, J., Dinstein, I., & Meiri, G. (2023). Children with autism exhibit similar longitudinal changes in core symptoms when placed in special or mainstream education settings. *Autism, 27*(6), 1628–1640. https://doi.org/10.1177/13623613221142394

Ilan, M., Meiri, G., Manelis-Baram, L., Faroy, M., Michaelovski, A., Flusser, H., Binoun-Chaki, H., Segev-Cojocaru, R., Dotan, D., Schtaierman, H., Menashe, I., & Dinstein, I. (2021). Young autism spectrum disorder children in special and mainstream education settings have similar behavioral characteristics. *Autism Research, 14*(4), 699–708. https://doi.org/10.1002/aur.2400

Isham, M. (2020). "Shakhor taltallim venavon": Al hammerots hayyisreeli lattinoq hammushlam uzekhuyotehem shel horim leatid liyiladot veyililadim im mugbalut "Black curls and wise": On the Israeli quest for the perfect infant and the rights of parents to plan for the future of newborns and children with disabilities. *Mishpat Refui Uviyyoetiqah [medical Law and Bioethics], 8*, 44–78.

Jeong, H. I., Kim, S. G., Youn, H., Lee, J., & Lee, S. I. (2023). A pilot study on the validity and reliability of Korean school readiness inventory on children with autism spectrum disorder. *Psychiatry Investigation, 20*(10), 940–945. https://doi.org/10.30773/pi.2023.0137

Kraybill, D. B. (2001). The Amish and the educational system. *Mennonite Quarterly Review, 75*(3), 337–357.

Keen, D., Meadan, H., Brady, N. C., & Halle, J. W. (2016). *Prelinguistic and minimally verbal communicators on the autism spectrum.* Springer.

Mehmood, M. U., & Parveen, Z. (2024). Exploring the Islamic perspective on special persons: A study of the Quran and Hadith. *AL-Īmān Research Journal, 2*(03), 114–128.

McMahon-Panther, G., & Bornman, J. (2025). Persons with disabilities in the Christian church: A scoping review on the impact of expressions of compassion and justice on their inclusion and participation. *Journal of Disability & Religion, 29*(1), 81–108. https://doi.org/10.1080/23312521.2024.2331461

Maoz, A. (2005). Religious education in Israel. *University of Detroit Mercy Law Review, 83*, 679.

Plano Clark, V., & Ivankova, N. (2016). Mixed methods research: A guide to the field. *Sage Publications.* https://doi.org/10.4135/9781483398341

Rehabilitative Day Care Law, Israel. (2000). *Khoq meonot yom*. shiqqumiyyim, https://he.wikisource.org/wiki/%d7%97%d7%95%d7%a7_%d7%9e%d7%a2%d7%95%d7%a0%d7%95%d7%aa_%d7%99%d7%95%d7%9d_%d7%a9%d7%99%d7%a7%d7%95%d7%9e%d7%99%d7%99%d7%9d

Schwartz, D. (2018). Meakhdut leribbuy: Sippurah shel hattodaah hatsiyyonit-datit [*From unity to multiplicity: The story of religious Zionist consciousness*]. Bialik Institute.

Segev, A., Weisskopf, M. G., Levine, H., Pinto, O., & Raz, R. (2019). Incidence time trends and socioeconomic factors in the observed incidence of autism spectrum disorder in Israel: A nationwide nested case–control study. *Autism Research, 12*(12), 1870–1879.

Shaked, M. (2005). The social trajectory of illness: Autism in the ultraorthodox community in Israel. *Social Science & Medicine, 61*(10), 2190–2200. https://doi.org/10.1016/j.socscimed.2005.04.022

Shaked, M., & Bilu, Y. (2006). Grappling with affliction: Autism in the Jewish ultraorthodox community in Israel. *Culture, Medicine and Psychiatry, 30*(1), 1–27. https://doi.org/10.1007/s11013-006-9006-2

Shkedi, A. (2003). Mimmillim hammenassot lagaat: Mekhqar ekhutani—teoreyah veyissum [*Words that try to touch: Qualitative research—theory and application*]. Ramot.

Special Education Law, Israel. (1988). *Khoq khinnukh meyukhad*, 1988 https://he.wikisource.org/wiki/%D7%97%D7%95%D7%A7_%D7%97%D7%99%D7%A0%D7%95%D7%9A_%D7%9E%D7%99%D7%95%D7%97%D7%93

Special Education Law, Amendment No. 7. (2000). *Khoq khinnukh meyukhad*. https://fs.knesset.gov.il/15/law/15_lsr_300594.pdf

Special Education Law, Amendment No. 11. (2018). https://fs.knesset.gov.il/20/law/20_lsr_504077.pdf

State Education Law, Israel. (1953). https://www.adalah.org/uploads/oldfiles/Public/files/Discriminatory-Laws-Database/English/24-State-Education-Law-1953.pdf

Stone, W. L. (1987). Cross-disciplinary perspectives on autism. *Journal of Paediatric Psychology, 12*, 615–630. https://doi.org/10.1093/jpepsy/12.4.615

United Nations. (2006). *Convention on the rights of persons with disabilities (CRPD)*. United Nations. https://www.un.org/disabilities/documents/convention/convoptprot-e.pdf

Van Eylen, L., Boets, B., Steyaert, J., Evers, K., Wagemans, J., & Noens, I. (2011). Cognitive flexibility in autism spectrum disorder: Explaining the inconsistencies? *Research in Autism Spectrum Disorders, 5*(4), 1390–1401. https://doi.org/10.1016/j.rasd.2011.01.025

Chapter 7
Sexual Education for Autistic Children: Insights from Parents

Anastasia Frid Juliusberger and Shiri Pearlman-Avnion

Abstract This study addresses the critical, yet often neglected, area of parental sexual education for children with autism spectrum disorder (ASD), recognizing its vital role in healthy development and safety. An empirical study conducted in Israel investigated the characteristics of 42 mothers and 31 fathers of children with ASD and their communication about sexuality. It is hypothesized that mothers provide more comprehensive sexual education than fathers, particularly for daughters, and that higher parental knowledge of sexuality and ASD would predict broader education. Results indicate that mothers provide significantly more comprehensive sexual education across most topics, including privacy, sexual abuse prevention, and sexual maturation, compared to fathers. Mothers also discussed more sexual maturation topics with daughters than with sons. Crucially, mothers' knowledge about sexuality significantly predicted the extent of their sexual education on topics like privacy, relationships, and general sexuality. However, fathers' knowledge, whether of sexuality or ASD, did not predict their sexual education efforts. Knowledge about ASD did not predict sex education for either parent. These findings highlight the central and distinct role of mothers in sexual education for children with ASD and emphasize the need for tailored interventions to promote the sexual health and safety of this vulnerable population.

Keywords Autism spectrum disorder (ASD) · Sexual education · Parental role · Sexuality knowledge · Children's sexual health

---

A. F. Juliusberger (✉)
Educational Psychology Service, Qiryat Bialik, Israel
e-mail: Anastasia.frid@qbialik.org.il

S. Pearlman-Avnion
Tel-Hai College, Kiryat Shmona, Israel

S. Lowinger and S. Pearlman-Avnion (eds.), *Collaborative Care and Partnerships in Autism Diagnosis and Treatment*, Autism and Child Psychopathology Series,
https://doi.org/10.1007/978-3-032-07009-8_7

Introduction

Sexual education for children with Autism Spectrum Disorder (ASD) is a critical yet often overlooked area of parenting and caregiving. Parents play a vital role in addressing their children's sexual development and providing them with essential knowledge to navigate relationships and self-care. Sexual education provided by parents has positive effects on children's health, particularly among those on the autism spectrum. Research suggests differences in the roles that mothers and fathers play and the challenges they face in educating their children about sexuality. This chapter will examine the relationship between the characteristics of parents of children on the autism spectrum and their communication with their children about topics related to sexuality.

In addition to an up-to-date literature review on the topic, the chapter is followed by results of an empirical study carried out in Israel among parents of children with ASD. The study had two hypotheses. The first was that mothers provide more comprehensive sexual education compared to fathers and that the gap is larger in the sexual education of daughters. The second hypothesis proposed that higher knowledge about sexuality and ASD would predict broader sexual education. The extent of sexual education was measured by the number of sexuality-related topics that parents discussed with their children. Forty-two mothers and thirty-one fathers completed online self-report questionnaires regarding sexual education, knowledge of sexuality, and knowledge of ASD. The study found that mothers provide more comprehensive sexual education to their children compared to fathers in most topics. Among the fathers, no correlation was found between knowledge of sexuality and ASD and the extent of sexual education. Among mothers, knowledge of sexuality alone significantly predicted the extent of sexual education on topics of privacy, relationships, and sexuality. The study indicates that mothers of children on the autism spectrum play a central role in sexual education, like mothers of children with typical development. The factors predicting the extent of parental sexual education are not fully clear, but these findings shed light on the different influences on mothers and fathers of children with ASD. The chapter discusses important topics of sexuality that parents talk about with their children, as ultimately, it aims to expand sexual education to contribute to the sexual health and safety of children on the autism spectrum and their later lives as adults.

Literature Review

Recent research reviews highlight the variation in rates of diagnoses of ASD worldwide. Globally, the prevalence ranges from 0.10% to 4.36% with a median of 1%. In the United States, as of 2020, the rate of children with ASD was 2.7%, equivalent to one in 36 children (Sacco et al., 2022). In Europe, the rate of ASD diagnoses for those aged 5–18 ranges between 0.8% and 1.4% (Sacco et al., 2022).

Studies show a significant gender difference, with a rate of ASD diagnosis among boys 3.8 times higher compared to girls. Similarly, a study in Europe found a ratio of 3.5:1 boys to girls diagnosed with ASD (Sacco et al., 2022).

Sexual Development and Sexual Expressions Among Children With ASD

Until the 1990s, the prevailing view was that people on the autism spectrum were not interested in intimacy and sexuality, and therefore, the topic did not receive in-depth research attention (Fernandes et al., 2016; Hartmann et al., 2019; Sala et al., 2020). However, today it is known that for children with ASD, like their peers with typical development, healthy sexual development is an important developmental milestone during adolescence. Adolescents with ASD experience physiological changes, express desire and interest in sexual interactions and activities, and participate in romantic relationships (Brown-Lavoie et al., 2014; Duarte et al., 2022; Hartmann et al., 2019; Kellaher, 2015; Sala et al., 2020; Stanojević et al., 2021). However, people in their social environment, especially parents, often struggle to accept this reality (Shier, 2015).

Sexual development includes three primary areas: sexual socialization, sexual behavior, and developing the psycho-sexual self. Sexual socialization is a process that begins in childhood and continues throughout life, as individuals acquire skills, knowledge, attitudes, values, motivations, norms, arts, and language according to the culture in which they live. Sexual socialization plays an important role in learning acceptable and healthy ways to fulfill sexual needs. The most significant socialization agents for adolescents are family members. Sexual behavior includes actions undertaken alone or with one or more other people. The psycho-sexual self refers to the aspects that compose the individual's positive sexual well-being, such as sexual interests, sexual orientation, gender identity, and recognition of oneself as a sexual being (Stanojević et al., 2021). Sexual development and the ability to participate in intimate relationships are important parts of the transition from childhood to adulthood and have a positive impact on the individual's physical and mental health (Holmes et al., 2019).

The characteristic difficulties of people on the autism spectrum affect sexual development and sexual health. In the realm of sexual socialization, children and adolescents with ASD struggle to acquire knowledge about sexually appropriate behaviors for their environment and culture, and they have difficulty regulating themselves during social interactions. Additionally, they have fewer opportunities to develop the necessary skills to understand complex social dynamics, and they struggle to acquire these skills through observation and modeling from their peer group and family (Duarte et al., 2022; Stanojević et al., 2021).

In the psycho-sexual self-domain, higher percentages of non-heterosexual sexual orientation, gender diversity, and gender dysphoria have been found among people on the autism spectrum, compared to the general population (Sala et al., 2020). Some studies have found a connection between non-heterosexual orientation and comorbidity with developmental intellectual disability and language difficulties (Fernandes et al., 2016).

In the sexual behavior domain, people on the autism spectrum engage in sexual behaviors like all people: hugs, caresses, kisses, self and mutual masturbation, oral sex, anal sex, and vaginal intercourse. However, their sexual behavior is often categorized as concerning, problematic, and inappropriate. It appears that due to difficulty distinguishing between private and public spaces, and difficulty understanding others' perspectives, people on the autism spectrum may adopt socially unacceptable behaviors such as compulsive masturbation, sexual fears and obsessions (Stanojević et al., 2021), and inappropriate sexual behavior (Sala et al., 2020). Moreover, despite wanting to participate in romantic relationships, they rarely date because they struggle to understand how to do so (Duarte et al., 2022).

It is important to note that most research on the sexual behavior of people on the autism spectrum is based on parental reports and it has been found that parents tend to underestimate their children's sexual experiences (Dewinter et al., 2016). A study that examined both parental reports and self-reports of young people on the autism spectrum found that young people reported more sexual behaviors, desire for private time, and sexual vulnerabilities than their parents reported. Conversely, there was alignment between parents' and children's answers regarding interest in romantic relationships (or lack thereof), sexual orientation, and whether sexual contact occurred. Additionally, the study's results indicated that the sexual activity of young people on the autism spectrum with partners does not differ from young people not on the autism spectrum (Hartmann et al., 2019).

Parents of children with ASD often report inappropriate sexual manifestations by their children and difficulty controlling their sexual impulses, such as public masturbation or seeking physical contact through hugs and kisses unexpectedly and without the other person's consent, and they seem to be unaware of social boundaries (Sullivan & Caterino, 2008).

These parents are concerned about their children's inappropriate sexual behavior, such as sexual behavior in public places and inappropriate touching of other people. Additionally, they fear misinterpretation of their children's behavior, unwanted pregnancies, and sexual abuse (Corona et al., 2016). A study conducted among adolescents and young adults on the autism spectrum and their parents found that nearly one-third of the youth with ASD engaged in inappropriate sexual behavior. The most common behavior was masturbation in a public place, followed by undressing (Fernandes et al., 2016).

Shier (2015) examined reports from parents and caregivers of children and adults aged 8–25 and found connections between autism severity, stage of puberty, and language skills with inappropriate sexual behaviors of touching intimate body parts and undressing in public places. However, no connection was found between these variables and masturbation or inappropriate touching of others. The direction of the relationship between variables could not be tested as the analysis of findings was through chi-square tests. Surveyed parents expressed concern that their children might be sexually abused or that their inappropriate behavior might be interpreted as assault, but the study did not examine factors related to parents' reactions and concerns. Furthermore, differences in perceptions between mothers and fathers and differences in perceptions between people of different ethnic and religious origins were not examined.

Sexual Education for Children on the Autism Spectrum

The understanding of issues related to sexuality and romance develops through formal and informal sexual education throughout life (Duarte et al., 2022). Informal learning begins in the family context, where knowledge, attitudes, and norms are passed on, influencing individual behavior in later life (Stanojević et al., 2021). Adolescents' level of knowledge about sexuality is related to the sex education provided by their parents (Flores & Barroso, 2017). Improving parents' knowledge helps them to engage in sex education with their children (Wight & Fullerton, 2013). However, these studies did not examine gender differences or differences between mothers and fathers. Many parents of children on the autism spectrum are not well-versed in their children's sexuality and sexual needs (for example, Corona et al., 2016), which may make them less likely to discuss these topics.

Sexual education focuses on two main aspects: promoting healthy sexuality and reducing sexual coercion and violence. Formal sexual education programs typically address the negative consequences of sexuality and do not adequately focus on the positive aspects, such as emotional and physical pleasure from sex, self-efficacy in sexual contexts, and positive self-image related to sexuality and pleasure (Kaye-Tzadok, 2019).

According to the recently developed holistic sexual education approach, sexual education should address the cognitive, emotional, social, and physical aspects of sexuality. This approach is based on a positive view of sexuality, seeing it as a potential source of joy and happiness. The desired outcomes are knowledge of the human body, the development of personal and behavioral skills, such as the ability to be in an intimate relationship, and the development of values, such as respectful attitudes toward sexual diversity and gender differences (Ketting et al., 2016).

Sexual education is especially important for individuals on the autism spectrum, as they are at higher risk for sexual exploitation, abuse, sexually transmitted diseases, pre-cancerous cervical conditions, unintended pregnancy, excessive pornography use, inappropriate sexual behavior, abuse of others, and difficulties in forming meaningful relationships (Ballan, 2012; Mackin et al., 2016; Sala et al., 2020). Furthermore, it has been found that people on the autism spectrum have less knowledge about sexually transmitted diseases, contraception, and reproduction compared to the general population. They are twice as likely to receive relevant knowledge from unreliable sources such as the internet and television, and four times less likely to receive it from parents, teachers, or peers (Kellaher, 2015; Sala et al., 2020).

A study comparing young individuals on the autism spectrum with a control group from the general population found that participants from the first group relied more on non-social sources of knowledge, such as media, magazines, informational pamphlets, and pornography, compared to the control group. They used fewer social knowledge sources, such as parents, teachers, peers, partners, religious figures, and counselors. The group with ASD had less accurate and perceived knowledge about sexual matters compared to the control group. Additionally, ASD was found to increase the likelihood of experiencing unwanted sexual contact by 3 times, sexual coercion by 2.7 times, and rape by 2.4 times. Finally, researchers found a link between actual knowledge of sexuality and victimization, with lower knowledge levels increasing the likelihood of becoming a victim in the sexual domain (Brown-Lavoie et al., 2014).

Parents play an important role in their children's sexual education (Corona et al., 2016; Flores & Barroso, 2017; Kaye-Tzadok, 2019; Wisnieski et al., 2015). The American Academy of Pediatrics recommends that all parents talk to their children about sexual health, reproduction, dating, sexual orientation, sexually transmitted diseases, and contraception. The values that parents instill in their children regarding these issues are expected to stay with them into adulthood (Kenny et al., 2020). Communication between parents and adolescents about sexuality reduces risky behaviors, teenage pregnancy, and sexually transmitted diseases. However, many parents avoid discussing sexuality due to feelings of shame, insecurity about their knowledge, and uncertainty about when and how to talk about sexuality (Kaye-Tzadok, 2019), and which topics should be discussed at each age (De Looze et al., 2015; Wisnieski et al., 2015).

Most parents of children and adolescents on the autism spectrum believe they are the primary educators regarding sexuality, in collaboration with professionals (Ballan, 2012; Mackin et al., 2016). However, studies show that parents of children on the autism spectrum communicate less with their children about sexuality compared to parents of typically developing children. In a study of young people on the autism spectrum and their parents, the parents reported that their children received most of their sexual education from school, while the children themselves reported that most of their knowledge came from the internet, watching images, videos, and reading. Most of the young participants (95%) and their parents (98%) reported that additional sexual education would have helped them (Hartmann et al., 2019). Moreover, many parents are unsure whether sexuality is relevant to children on the autism spectrum, what healthy sexuality looks like for these individuals, and how to teach them appropriate sexual behavior (Corona et al., 2016).

Among parents of typically developing adolescents, the most frequently discussed topics in sexual education are romantic relationships, respecting personal and partner boundaries, and contraception (De Looze et al., 2015). In contrast, parents of adolescents with ASD most often discuss hygiene, types of physical contact, privacy, private body parts, and puberty (André et al., 2020).

Holmes and Himle (2014) examined what sexual topics parents discuss with their children on the autism spectrum and what child characteristics (functional level, autism symptoms, and age) predict parental communication about sexuality. Autism symptoms were measured using the Social Responsiveness Scale, which assessed social motivation, social cognition, social awareness, social communication, and repetitive behaviors, based on parent reports. Communication was assessed using a parent sexual education questionnaire in which parents indicated (in yes/no questions) whether they had discussed each topic with their child. The results were analyzed separately for parents of children with high functioning (IQ average or above) and low functioning (IQ below average). It was found that parents of high-functioning children covered a wider range of topics. The study showed that parents of high-functioning children covered topics such as privacy, sexual abuse prevention, puberty, hygiene, types of families, and gender roles. However, they did not discuss romantic relationships, healthy sexuality, prevention, and sexuality in general, such as sexual activities. Parents of low-functioning children covered topics like privacy, sexual abuse prevention, puberty, and reproduction but did not discuss romantic relationships, healthy sexuality, prevention, inappropriate behaviors, and sexuality in general. Additionally, among the high-functioning group, children's social motivation and social cognition predicted the extent of parental communication about sexuality, with parents of children with higher social motivation and cognition discussing sexuality more with their children.

In another study of parents of adolescent girls on the autism spectrum aged 12–18, it was found that almost all parents covered basic topics like puberty, privacy, and reproduction, but few addressed issues related to sexual activities, intercourse, protection, and sexual abuse prevention. One of the primary concerns of the parents was sexual abuse of their daughters (Holmes et al., 2019). Another qualitative study examined parent–child communication about sexuality among parents (16 mothers and 3 fathers) of children on the autism spectrum aged 6–13 and found that most parents had difficulty imagining a future in which their child might be sexually active in an appropriate way. As a result, these parents did not address their children's reproductive and healthy sexual needs. Additionally, they expressed reluctance to discuss sexual matters and focused their conversations on safety and social norms. The parents in this study expressed concerns that people in their environment might misinterpret their children's sexual and non-sexual behaviors, and they viewed normative sexual behaviors, such as masturbation, as stigmatizing and frightening (Ballan, 2012).

In a study examining parents' perceptions of the sexual education needs of children aged 14–20 on the autism spectrum, it was found that all parents discussed sexual topics with their children to some extent. However, most focused on their own concerns and fears rather than positive aspects and sexual health. For example, parents talked about boundaries and fears of exploitation, fearing that their children might misinterpret their behaviors. The primary goal of the parents' sexual education was to avoid negative stereotypes. Parents in the study also expressed concern that they were not speaking to their children correctly and noted that they lacked the knowledge, resources, and support to provide their children with the sexual education they desired (Mackin et al., 2016).

Gender Differences: Parental Roles in Sexual Education for Children with ASD

Mothers often assume a more active role in addressing the sexual education of children with ASD compared to fathers. Cultural expectations frequently position mothers as primary caregivers responsible for guiding children through sensitive topics, including sexuality (Elsabbagh et al., 2024). Mothers are also more likely to engage in discussions about personal boundaries, puberty, and safeguarding against potential sexual abuse (Holmes & Himle, 2014).

Fathers tend to take a less active role, often due to discomfort or uncertainty about how to approach the subject. This discrepancy may leave children with limited exposure to a diverse range of perspectives on sexual education (Van Nieuwenhuizen et al., 2015). Research indicates that the limited involvement of fathers could also stem from traditional gender norms, which assign emotional and educational caregiving responsibilities primarily to mothers (Elsabbagh et al., 2024).

Both mothers and fathers encounter significant challenges in providing sexual education to children with ASD. These include a lack of accessible resources, fear of exposing their children to inappropriate material, and uncertainties about the timing and content of discussions. Holmes and Himle (2014) noted that parents often delay or avoid sexual education entirely, fearing that their children might not understand or that the information could be misinterpreted. Additionally, parents of children with ASD express concerns about the social vulnerabilities of their children, such as difficulties in understanding social cues and potential risks of exploitation (Van Nieuwenhuizen et al., 2015). These concerns often heighten the emotional weight of sexual education, making it a stressful endeavor for parents.

A key issue in parental roles is the gap in knowledge about their children's sexual development and experiences. Van Nieuwenhuizen et al. (2015) found that parents, particularly fathers, often underestimate the extent of their children's sexual curiosity and activities. This lack of awareness may hinder effective communication about sexuality, leaving children without the necessary guidance to make informed decisions.

In the general population, mothers play a more prominent role than fathers in educating their children. The research literature suggests that mothers take a more significant role in educating their children about sexual matters (Flores & Barroso, 2017), and that communication on sexuality between parents and children is influenced by the gender of the child. A study conducted in the Netherlands among parents of teenagers found that mothers discussed sexual topics more with their children compared to fathers and that both parents talked about sexual matters more with sons than with daughters. Topics explored in this study included physiological differences between boys and girls, physical changes during adolescence, romantic relationships, physical touch, consent and refusal, homosexuality, pregnancy, reproduction, and contraception (De Looze et al., 2015).

In a study examining gender differences in sexual communication between parents and their children in the general population, it was found that mothers covered more topics than fathers. Additionally, mothers spoke with their daughters about abstinence until marriage more than with their sons, and they discussed condom use more with sons than with daughters. No significant differences were found on other topics. Among fathers, it was found that they spoke with their daughters more about engaging or not engaging in various sexual activities and abstinence until marriage, while fathers spoke more with their sons on other topics (Sneed et al., 2013).

A qualitative study conducted among young women in the general population revealed that mothers were their primary source of information on reproductive matters, even when the relationship with their mothers was not particularly close. While fathers were not the primary source of information, they were available for consultations on romantic relationships (Wisnieski et al., 2015).

A study conducted among young African American men regarding the sexual education they received from their parents between the ages of 10 and 18 found that they talked more with their mothers than with their fathers about topics like contraception, protection against sexually transmitted diseases, abstinence, peer pressure to have sex, and coping with it (Harris et al., 2013).

Many parents in the general population find it difficult to communicate about sexuality with children of the opposite gender because they feel embarrassed and uncomfortable and assume their children will have similar feelings. Additionally, it has been found that boys receive less sexual education because they deal with fewer reproductive topics (Kamangu et al., 2017). In some cultures, discussions between fathers and daughters about sexuality are considered taboo (Mullis et al., 2021). This research also shows that mothers are more comfortable talking about sexuality than fathers, especially with their daughters, and the most productive conversations about sexuality occur between mothers and daughters. One hypothesis is that mothers feel comfortable being naked around their daughters but not their sons and that nudity provides an opportunity to communicate about the human body and sexuality. Additionally, it was found that mothers' sexual education tends to be future-oriented, with a focus on protecting their daughters and ensuring their future, which is why they talk to them more about sexuality (Flores & Barroso, 2017).

One study among British families found that mothers talk with their children about sexual matters more than fathers, and fathers struggle to discuss sexuality with their children because they themselves received limited sexual education as children. Furthermore, the study found differences in how mothers provide sexual education to sons compared to daughters. Mothers spoke more coldly and impersonally with sons and more warmly with daughters, covering a wider range of topics (Turnbull et al., 2008).

In a qualitative study among the general population (Walker, 2001) among 50 parents, it was found that in most families, mothers rather than fathers were responsible for the sexual education their children received at home. Many fathers reported leaving the topic of sexual education to the mothers, believing that women have better interpersonal skills than men. Some fathers even said they were embarrassed to discuss sexuality, so they avoided the subject. The mothers in the study indicated that they felt more comfortable discussing sexuality with their daughters than with their sons because they could share more of their life experiences with their daughters. Additionally, mothers stated that there were topics they did not discuss with their sons, and one of their difficulties was not knowing what it feels like to be a boy. In families without a father, or where the father did not participate in the sexual education of the sons, participants reported that the sexual education of the sons suffered.

Although gender differences in sexual education among the general population have been studied extensively, the subject has not yet been researched in the autistic spectrum population. Girls and boys on the autism spectrum may have distinctive needs, as girls are more likely to have a homosexual sexual orientation and gender diversity and are more vulnerable to emotional abuse and sexual coercion (Holmes et al., 2019).

Knowledge About Sexuality

The Research literature indicates that many parents lack sufficient knowledge about topics related to sexuality, which may negatively affect their ability to provide comprehensive sexual education to their children. Some barriers preventing parents from discussing sexual matters with their children include gaps in knowledge about protective measures, the sexuality of the opposite gender, and non-heterosexual orientations (Flores & Barroso, 2017).

In a study that examined various factors affecting parental communication with children on sexuality, including knowledge of HIV, it was found that the higher the level of knowledge, the more mothers (but not fathers) covered a wide range of sexual topics (Harris et al., 2013).

In a study examining the intentions of parents of children on the autism spectrum to discuss sexuality and sexual abuse with their children, it was found that parents were well aware of their children's vulnerability to sexual harm and were concerned about it, so many parents indeed spoke to their children about the topic. When asked for reasons why they shouldn't talk to their children about sexuality and sexual abuse, the most common responses were that they believed their children would not understand the topic or that the topic did not interest them. Additionally, many parents said they did not know how to explain the subject to their children and could not find information that would help them (Kenny et al., 2020).

In various populations studied, it was found that higher knowledge about sexuality is associated with a greater perceived ability to engage in sexual education. For example, in a study conducted among Israeli teacher education students, a comparison was made between students who took a course on human sexuality and those who did not. It was found that the students who took the course had improved their knowledge about sexual education topics and reported higher self-efficacy to engage in sexual education with children and adolescents after completing the course.

In a study that examined the effectiveness of various intervention programs aimed at improving communication between parents and children about sexuality in the general population (Wight & Fullerton, 2013), two effective intervention programs that focused on increasing parents' knowledge were identified. In the first program, parents of children in preschool were given a two-hour workshop to improve their ability to answer their children's questions. Parents who participated in the program were more prepared and skilled in discussing sexuality with their children compared to the control group that did not receive the training. In the second program, parents of children aged five and above received 42 h of training on human sexuality. After participating in the program, there was an improvement in parent–child communication on sexuality among the participants.

More recently, Alhassan and Gharaibeh (2024) pointed out that mothers provide timely sexual education and safety orientation. However, since parents and caregivers do not understand their children's sexual requirements, children with autism and other impairments generally get less comprehensive education. Training and assistance lessen the risk of sexual exploitation or abuse. Their study aimed to discover how much mothers in Jordan know about the sexual abuse of their children with autism, and how a training program has helped them learn more. In addition, the training program was used to see how Jordanian mothers' education level affected their children's knowledge and development. Among the research sample ($n = 91$), 12 mothers were trained to understand sexual assault, and an awareness scale examined before and after the impact of the training program. The training boosted mothers' comprehension of sexual abuse, yet the educational qualification of the mother was a central predictor of the significance of the results: Mothers with bachelor's or postgraduate degrees learned more than those with secondary education. This study suggested that children with autism may benefit from sex education to lessen sexual assault risks, as well as an opportunity to understand healthy sexuality.

Knowledge About Autism

The relationship between parental knowledge of autism spectrum disorder and communication about sexuality between parents and children has not been explored in the research literature. In the current study, it is hypothesized that there is a relationship between these variables for two reasons. First, because the recognition of the sexual needs of people on the spectrum is relatively new. Some 30 years ago, professionals and parents believed that people on the autism spectrum were not interested in sexuality (Fernandes et al., 2016; Hartmann et al., 2019; Sala et al., 2020). Even today, most sexual education provided to children on the autism spectrum focuses on hygiene, privacy, and the human body, rather than sexuality and relationships (André et al., 2020). Many parents report having insufficient knowledge about the sexual aspects of autism (Ballan, 2012; Corona et al., 2016; Hartmann et al., 2019; Mackin et al., 2016). Therefore, parents may not talk to their children about certain aspects of sexuality due to a lack of knowledge about autism or its sexual aspects.

Second, because parental coping with their child's diagnosis is complex, and a lack of knowledge about the diagnosis may influence their willingness to engage in sexual education. Parents of children on the autism spectrum are characterized by higher levels of stress and anxiety, which are partly influenced by the parents' level of knowledge about autism. One study found that family resources and social support can reduce parents' stress and that high levels of perceived parental efficacy and knowledge about autism can reduce parental distress when children exhibit multiple behavioral problems (Lindsey & Barry, 2018). Parental stress levels for parents of children on the autism spectrum are higher compared to parents of typically developing children, especially among parents of daughters (Zamora et al., 2014).

Studies on knowledge about ASD have found that there is not always a match between perceived knowledge about autism and actual knowledge (Williams et al., 2011), and that familial closeness to someone on the autism spectrum does not necessarily increase knowledge about autism (Gillespie-Lynch et al., 2015). Additionally, it has been found that parents with limited knowledge about autism rely less on extended family and neighbors for support (Johnson & Simpson, 2013).

There is no doubt that communication about sexuality between parents and children is important and has an impact on children's health. Communication about sexuality is especially important between parents and children on the autism spectrum, who are at increased risk for negative sexual outcomes, but have fewer opportunities to receive reliable information from other sources. Therefore, it is crucial to understand the factors that may influence the sexual education provided by parents to their children. Most research in the academic literature has focused on sexual education for typically developing children, and studies concerning children on the autism spectrum have primarily concentrated on the characteristics of the children and the topics discussed by parents, but not on the characteristics of the parents themselves.

A recent study (Juliusberger, 2023) examined the characteristics of parents of children on the autism spectrum that relate to the extent of sexual communication they engage in with their children. Specifically, the study investigates whether there is an interaction between the gender of the parent and the gender of the child regarding the extent of sexual education and whether parents' levels of knowledge about sexuality and autism predict the scope of sexual education they provide to their children.

Understanding the characteristics of parents that may influence their attitudes toward their children's sexuality and the extent of sexual education they provide has implications for the work of school psychologists. These characteristics can help psychologists design interventions aimed at promoting discussions among parents about their children's sexuality and improving the sexual education they provide, for example, in parent groups or parent training sessions. Such understanding can also help identify a more accurate and tailored way to assist parents who require these interventions. Research has shown that the effectiveness of educational programs in sexual education is higher when the program is part of a broader universal initiative, including training for both teachers and parents (Kaye-Tzadok, 2019).

It was hypothesized that mothers generally provide more comprehensive sexual education to their children compared to fathers, with greater gaps observed in the education of daughters. Additionally, it was hypothesized that among both mothers and fathers, higher levels of knowledge about sexuality and autism predict more comprehensive sexual education.

Methods

Participant Recruitment

Participants were sampled using non-probabilistic sampling methods of volunteers and snowball sampling. Recruitment was conducted through social networks, with the criteria for participation being parents of a child on the autism spectrum aged 5–21. A demographic questionnaire was administered including questions about gender, age, religion, religiosity level, family status, education, income, residential area, number of children, child's gender, child's age, child's functioning level, and child's communication level (verbal/non-verbal).

Research Tools

The study used several previously published questionnaires, translated from English into Hebrew using a back-translation process. The Parent Sex Education Inventory assesses the number of sexuality topics parents cover in communication with their children (Holmes & Himle, 2014). The 50-item survey included general questions about parent and child demographics and 39 items specifically on parent–child communication about sexuality. This section was divided into six subtopics: privacy (e.g., private body parts); consent and sexual abuse prevention (e.g., the importance of not pressuring people to have sex); puberty and reproduction (e.g., physical development of males and females; how women get pregnant and give birth); relationships (e.g., how to ask someone on a date); sexual health and contraception (e.g., preventing sexually transmitted diseases, using contraceptives); and sexuality (e.g., what sexual intercourse feels like; sexual decision-making). Participants were asked to mark each item as "yes" if they discussed the topic with their child or "no" if they did not. The final score was calculated by summing the number of positive responses, with a higher score reflecting more comprehensive sexual education. Strong internal reliability was found in the original questionnaire ($\alpha = 0.98$) and in the current study ($\alpha = 0.93$). Items for the survey were chosen based on previous research on this topic (Beckett et al., 2009; Koller, 2000; Nichols & Blakeley-Smith, 2010; Travers & Tincani, 2010; Wolfe et al., 2009).

The Autism Knowledge Survey-Revised (AKS-R) was taken from Ables et al. (2011); it is an updated version of Stone's (1987) Autism Knowledge Survey. The questionnaire examines knowledge about ASD, including etiology, diagnosis, intervention, treatment, and outcomes. Participants rate their level of agreement with each of 20 statements on a scale from one (completely agree) to six (completely disagree). Ratings between one and three reflect agreement, while ratings between four and six reflect disagreement. Example items from the questionnaire include "Children with autism do not show emotion" and "Autism can be diagnosed at 18 months". For the current study, an additional statement was added: "People with autism have sexual needs like all people", so the final questionnaire included 21 items. In this study, participants received 1 point for agreeing with a correct statement and 0 points for disagreeing with a correct statement or agreeing with an incorrect statement, with the final score calculated by summing the points. The original questionnaire was found valid in Tukey's honest significance test, with strong internal reliability ($\alpha = 0.74$) and strong test–retest reliability, but weak internal reliability in the current study ($\alpha = 0.61$).

The Sexual Knowledge Questionnaire, from a comprehensive questionnaire on sexual education and family life education (Brosh, 2007), examines knowledge, attitudes, and willingness to engage in sexual education in schools. For the current study, only the last section was used, with 17 questions testing knowledge about anatomy, physiology of sexual organs, contraception, and sexual orientations. The questionnaire contains true/false questions (e.g., "A girl can receive a prescription for birth control pills without her parents' knowledge") and multiple-choice questions (e.g., "The man's testicles produce the hormone: 1. Progesterone, 2. Estrogen, 3. Testosterone"). Each question included a "don't know" option, and participants were asked to avoid guessing and select this option if they did not know the answer. Each correct answer earns a point, with the final score being the sum of correct answers (ranging from 0 to 17). The internal reliability of the questionnaire in this study was found to be weak ($\alpha = 0.63$).

The research was approved by the ethics committee of Tel Hai College in Israel. Participation in the study involved online responses to questionnaires using Google Forms. After an explanation of the research purpose and consent to participate, participants answered a demographic questionnaire, sexual education questionnaire, autism knowledge questionnaire, and sexual knowledge questionnaire. Participant recruitment was carried out using snowball sampling and publication on Facebook groups related to parenting, sexual education, autism, and parenting children on the autism spectrum.

Study Participants

The research sample included 73 participants with an average age of 45.33 years (standard deviation 10.28). The average number of children per participant was 2.82 (standard deviation 2.82). Most participants were parents of boys (54.8% of the fathers and 69% of the mothers). The majority were women (57.5%). Most belonged to the Jewish religion (87.8%), with the remainder being Druze (12.3%), which largely reflects the demographic makeup of the targeted audience of Israeli families with children in general public schools (Israel Central Bureau of Statistics, 2024). Most defined themselves as secular (57.5%), with the remainder relatively equally divided between traditional (20.5%) and religious (21.9%). Most participants were married or in a common-law partnership (82.8%), 12.3% were divorced, and small percentages were single (2.7%) or widowed (2.7%).

Educational levels were as follows: 41.1% held a bachelor's degree, 24.7% held a master's degree or higher, 20.5% had professional education, and 13.7% had high school education. Regarding income, 47.9% had average income, 32.9% earned above average, and 19.2% earned below average.

The average age of participants' children was 12.37 years, ranging from 5 to 21 years. The majority of the participants' children were boys (63%), had a high functioning level (71.2%), and could communicate verbally (89%).

Results

Differences Between Mothers and Fathers in Sexual Education Provided to Their Children

Results of two-way between-subjects ANOVA tests found a significant main effect for parent gender on the overall number of sexual education topics covered beyond child gender [$F(1,69) = 9.81$, $p < 0.01$]. The average number of topics covered by mothers ($M = 13.92$, SD = 8.00) was significantly higher than the average number of topics covered by fathers ($M = 8.87$, SD = 7.34). No significant interaction effect was found between parent gender and child gender [$F(1,69) = 9.81$, n.s.].

Each education sub-topic was examined separately. For privacy, a significant main effect was found for parent gender [$F(1,69) = 5.51$, $p < 0.05$] showing that mothers covered more privacy topics on average ($M = 2.67$, SD = 0.69) compared to fathers ($M = 2.16$, SD = 1.16). Regarding sexual abuse prevention and consent, a significant main effect was found for parent gender [$F(1,69) = 6.66$, $p < 0.05$], and mothers covered more topics on this subject on average ($M = 2.11$, SD = 1.38) compared to fathers ($M = 1.26$, SD = 1.53). A significant main effect for parent gender [$F(1,69) = 15.91$, $p < 0.001$] was also found for topics related to sexual maturation/reproduction, with significant interaction between parent and child gender [$F(1,69) = 5.03$, $p < 0.05$]. Simple effects analysis revealed no significant differences between mothers and fathers for the sexual education of sons, but significant differences were found for daughters, with whom mothers covered more topics on average ($M = 3.54$, SD = 1.33) compared to fathers ($M = 1.29$, SD = 1.38).

Additional analysis of the interaction by child gender showed no significant differences among fathers in the topics covered with their children. Significant differences were found among mothers. They covered more topics with daughters ($M = 3.54$, SD = 1.33) compared to their sons ($M = 2.69$, SD = 1.50). Regarding sexuality, there was a significant main effect for parent gender [$F(1,69) = 7.64$, $p < 0.01$]. Mothers covered more sexuality topics on average (M = 2.10, SD = 2.01) compared to fathers ($M = 1.00$, SD = 1.44). No significant effects were found for relationship topics and sexual health/contraception. In summary, the first research hypothesis was partially confirmed.

Prediction of the Extent of Sex Education by Parental Knowledge Levels of Sexuality and Autism

In order to examine whether the level of knowledge of mothers and fathers about sexuality and autism predicts the extent of sex education they provide to their children, a series of multiple regression models were constructed. Among fathers, none of the multiple regression models examined were found to be significant. However, among mothers, the prediction model for the number of general sexuality topics based on knowledge about autism and knowledge about sexuality was found to be significant [$F(2,39) = 3.87, p < 0.05$], explaining 12% of the variance in the number of sexuality topics mothers discuss with their children. The standardized regression coefficients (β) indicate that the contribution of knowledge about sexuality is significant, while the contribution of knowledge about autism is not significant.

When fragmented into subtopics of sexuality, the model predicting the number of topics related to privacy was found to be significant [$F(2,39) = 3.89$, $p < 0.05$], explaining 12% of the variance. The standardized regression coefficients (β) indicate a significant contribution from knowledge about sexuality, while the contribution of knowledge about autism was found to be non-significant. Additionally, the model predicting the number of topics related to relationships was found to be significant [$F(2,39) = 3.44$, $p < 0.05$], explaining 11% of the variance. Finally, the model predicting the number of topics related to sexuality was found to be significant [$F(2,39) = 3.68$, $p < 0.05$], explaining 12% of the variance. In this model as well, the standardized regression coefficients (β) indicate a significant contribution from knowledge about sexuality, while the contribution of knowledge about autism was found to be non-significant.

In other words, the higher the level of knowledge mothers have about sexuality, the more comprehensive the sex education they provide their children, covering topics related to privacy, relationships, and sexuality. The models predicting the number of topics related to sexual abuse/consent, sexual maturation and reproduction, and sexual health and contraception were not found to be significant. In conclusion, the second research hypothesis was only partially confirmed.

In summary, the models for fathers did not show any significant relationship between their knowledge of sexuality and ASD and the amount of sex education they provided. Research indicates that the limited involvement of fathers could stem from traditional gender norms, which assign emotional and educational caregiving responsibilities primarily to mothers (Elsabbagh et al., 2024). Among mothers, knowledge of sexuality significantly predicted the number of general sexuality topics discussed with their children. This model explained 12% of the variance in the number of topics covered. However, knowledge of autism did not have a significant effect. Specific topics such as privacy, relationships, and sexuality were significantly influenced by the mother's knowledge of sexuality, but knowledge of autism was not significant.

Regarding subtopics of sexual education, knowledge of sexuality significantly influenced the number of privacy topics covered. Similarly, knowledge of sexuality was significant for relationship-related topics. Knowledge of sexuality predicted the number of topics covered under general sexuality, yet no significant effects were found for these production and sexual health/contraception. Regarding differences in education scope according to parent gender, mothers provided more comprehensive sex education than fathers, covering more topics related to privacy, sexual abuse prevention, sexual maturation, and sexuality. Also, there was a significant interaction between parent gender and child gender. Mothers discussed more sexual maturation topics with daughters than with sons and covered more topics with daughters compared to sons in several areas, particularly sexual maturation.

Discussion and Long-Term Conclusions

The presented study examined which characteristics of parents of children on the autism spectrum are associated with the extent of their communication with their children regarding sexuality. The topics of sexuality examined included privacy, consent and sexual abuse prevention, puberty and reproduction, relationships, sexual health and contraception, and sexuality.

The first hypothesis of the study posited that mothers provide more comprehensive sex education compared to fathers, meaning they discuss a broader range of sexuality topics with their children, and that the gap is larger in the education of daughters. This hypothesis was partially supported. Although it was found that mothers discuss more topics with their children compared to fathers, the differences between boys and girls—i.e., the interaction between a parent's gender and the child's gender—were not found to be statistically significant. Out of 39 topics in total, for the boys, mothers discussed an average of 13 topics, and fathers discussed an average of 10, while for the girls, mothers discussed an average of 17 topics, and fathers discussed an average of 7 topics. It is possible that the differences did not reach statistical significance due to the relatively small sample size, particularly since the number of mothers with daughters in this sample was limited.

The gaps between mothers and fathers were statistically significant in communication on topics of privacy, sexual abuse prevention, consent, and sexuality. An interesting finding was that in topics related to sexual maturation and reproduction, fathers discussed the same number of topics with both genders, while mothers discussed more topics with daughters compared to sons. A possible explanation for this is that girls deal with more reproductive-related topics, such as menstruation, pregnancy, and childbirth, and mothers believe they need to provide guidance on these issues. Additionally, mothers may feel more comfortable talking about these topics with their daughters. In one study conducted on the general population, it was found that boys receive less comprehensive sex education because they deal less with reproductive issues, and parents feel more comfortable discussing these topics with children of the same gender (Kamangu et al., 2017). Further support for this hypothesis can be found in another study (Flores & Barroso, 2017), which found that mothers discuss sexuality topics with their daughters more than with their sons, both because they see each other as having a natural connection that encourages conversations about the human body and sexuality, and because they want to prepare them for the future. That is, part of the preparation for the future for girls may involve communication on topics unique to females, related to sexual maturation and reproduction, and the mother's ability to be nude around her daughters facilitates discussions on bodily changes during maturation.

No statistically significant differences were found between parents' communication with their children on topics of relationships, sexual health, and contraception. A plausible explanation is that communication on these topics was generally limited, and the sample size was relatively small, thus small differences did not reach statistical significance. For example, out of eight topics related to relationships, mothers discussed an average of only three topics, while fathers discussed an average of only two. Another example is the topic of sexual health and contraception, which included ten possible topics, and mothers discussed an average of only one topic, while fathers discussed an average of less than one. These findings align with those of a meta-analysis, which found that relationships and contraception use were among the least discussed topics between parents and their children on the autism spectrum, in contrast to parents of typically developing children who tend to discuss these topics more frequently (André et al., 2020).

These findings are especially concerning because children on the autism spectrum are at higher risk for sexual behaviors, sexual abuse, exploitation in relationships, sexually transmitted diseases, and unwanted pregnancies (Ballan, 2012; Mackin et al., 2016; Sala et al., 2020). One significant factor that can reduce the level of risk is communication with parents about sexuality (Kaye-Tzadok, 2019).

The second hypothesis of the study proposed that higher levels of knowledge about sexuality and autism predict more comprehensive sex education, meaning communication about a broader range of sexuality topics. This hypothesis was tested separately for fathers and mothers and was only partially supported. The level of knowledge about autism did not predict communication on any sexuality topics for either gender. This is the first study to examine the level of knowledge about autism in the context of sex education, so this finding cannot be compared to previous studies, and further research is needed to determine whether and how parental knowledge about autism may influence communication on sexuality.

An interesting finding was that the level of knowledge about sexuality was a significant predictor for mothers, but not for fathers. That is, for fathers, neither the level of knowledge about autism nor sexuality significantly predicted the number of sexuality topics discussed with their children. However, for mothers, a higher level of knowledge about sexuality alone predicted communication about a greater number of sexuality topics in general, as well as specific topics like privacy, relationships, and sexuality. This confirms the findings of Harris et al. (2013), who found that as the level of knowledge about sexuality increased, mothers—but not fathers—discussed a greater number of sexuality topics with their children, though the researchers did not provide an explanation for this. It is possible that men and women face different barriers that hinder their ability to talk to their children about sexuality, and it would be interesting to ask them about this in future studies. Qualitative studies examining the differences between mothers and fathers in the sex education they provide to their children have found that fathers reported difficulties discussing sexuality topics because they did not receive comprehensive sex education in childhood (Turnbull et al., 2008), they believe that mothers have better interpersonal skills for the task and that the subject embarrasses them (Walker, 2001).

In conclusion, it seems that mothers of children on the autism spectrum play a more prominent role in their children's sex education compared to fathers. This is consistent with many studies conducted with parents of typically developing children, which found that mothers discuss more sexuality topics with their children than fathers (De Looze et al., 2015; Elsabbagh et al., 2024; Flores & Barroso, 2017; Harris et al., 2013; Sneed et al., 2013; Wisnieski et al., 2015). Furthermore, it appears that the factors predicting the extent of sex education provided to children on the spectrum differ between mothers and fathers, and further exploration of potential factors is needed. This issue is of great importance because, as noted, parent–child communication on sexuality may reduce risky sexual behaviors, and children on the autism spectrum are at an increased risk. Understanding the factors influencing parent–child communication on sexuality can help improve communication and promote child safety.

Implications for Practice

The present data and the literature review have some practical implications for the work of educational psychologists in schools, as well as other professional staff working with parents of children with ASD. The research literature shows that in order to increase the success rate of sex education programs, interventions should also target teachers and parents of children (Kaye-Tzadok, 2019). This study provides important insights into the sexuality topics that Israeli parents of children on the autism spectrum discuss with their children. This information allows for a more tailored approach to sex education programs, where more attention can be given to topics that are often not discussed at home with parents. In addition, interventions with parents can be conducted to expand the range of sex education they provide to their children and to support them in this process, through lectures for parents at the school, parent support groups, and parent workshops. Improving the extent of sex education provided to students on the autism spectrum can help promote their sexual health and safety.

To address these challenges, researchers have emphasized the importance of providing parents with training and resources tailored to the unique needs of children with ASD. Programs that enhance parents' understanding of sexual development and equip them with strategies for discussing sexuality have proven effective (Elsabbagh et al., 2024). Such programs also help parents recognize and address their own biases and discomforts, fostering a more open and supportive environment for sexual education.

Given the critical role of parents in sexual education, healthcare providers and educators should actively involve both mothers and fathers in training programs. Encouraging fathers to participate more actively and providing them with tools to overcome discomfort could balance parental involvement and ensure children receive well-rounded guidance. Furthermore, resources must address the specific challenges faced by children with ASD, such as difficulties with social interactions and sensory sensitivities.

References

Ables, E., Ashby, I., & Swiezy, N. (2011). Autism knowledge survey-revised: Comparison of knowledge across role and experience. *Applied Behavior Analysis International*. Paper presented at the Applied Behavior Analysis International, Denver, CO, 27–30 May 2011.

Alhassan, A. A. H., & Gharaibeh, M. (2024). Mothers' awareness of sex education and training programs for children with autism. *Sexuality and Disability, 42*(4), 905–921. https://doi.org/10.1007/s11195-024-09859-6

André, T. G., Valdez-Montero, C., Márquez-Vega, M. A., Ahumada-Cortez, J. G., & Gámez-Medina, M. E. (2020). Communication on sexuality between parents and adolescents with autism spectrum disorder: A systematic review. *Sexuality and Disability, 38*(2), 217–229. https://doi.org/10.1007/s11195-020-09628-1

Ballan, M. S. (2012). Parental perspectives of communication about sexuality in families of children with autism spectrum disorders. *Journal of Autism and Developmental Disorders, 42*(5), 676–684. https://doi.org/10.1007/s10803-011-1293-y

Beckett, M. K., Elliott, M. N., Martino, S., Kanouse, D. E., Corona, R., Klein, D. J., & Schuster, M. A. (2009). Timing of parent and child communication about sexuality relative to children's sexual behaviors. *Pediatrics, 125*, 34–42. https://doi.org/10.1542/peds.2009-0806

Brosh, E. (2007). *Mudaut, teda unechonut lehitmoded im hachinuch hamini bebeit hasefer, bekerev studentim lehora'a [Awareness, knowledge, and willingness to address sexual education in schools among teaching students.]* Mofet Institute.

Brown-Lavoie, S. M., Viecili, M. A., & Weiss, J. (2014). Sexual knowledge and victimization in adults with autism spectrum disorders. *Journal of Autism and Developmental Disorders, 44*, 2185–2196. https://doi.org/10.1007/s10803-014-2093-y

Corona, L. L., Fox, S. A., Christodulu, K. V., & Worlock, J. A. (2016). Providing education on sexuality and relationships to adolescents with autism spectrum disorder and their parents. *Sexuality and Disability, 34*, 199–214. https://doi.org/10.1007/s11195-015-9424-6

De Looze, M., Constantine, N. A., Jerman, P., Vermeulen-Smit, E., & Ter Bogt, T. (2015). Parent–adolescent sexual communication and its association with adolescent sexual behaviors: A nationally representative analysis in the Netherlands. *The Journal of Sex Research, 52*(3), 257–268. https://doi.org/10.1080/00224499.2013.858307

Dewinter, J., Vermeiren, R. R. J. M., Vanwesenbeeck, I., & Elsabbagh, C. (2016). Parental awareness of sexual experience in adolescent boys with autism spectrum disorder. *Journal of Autism and Developmental Disorders, 46*, 713–719. https://doi.org/10.1007/s10803-015-2622-3

Duarte, L., Figueiredo, R., & Alves, J. C. (2022). Psychosexual education and training for adolescents with autism spectrum disorder: A systematic review. *Nascer E Crescer-Birth And Growth Medical Journal, 31*(2), 123–129. https://doi.org/10.25753/BirthGrowthMJ.v31.i2.24777

Elsabbagh, M., Divan, G., & Koh, Y. J. (2024). Challenges and strategies for parents in addressing sexual education in children with Autism Spectrum Disorders. *Sexuality Research and Social Policy, 21*(3), 456–470. https://doi.org/10.1007/s11195-024-09859-6

Fernandes, L. C., Gillberg, C. I., Cederlund, M., Hagberg, B., Gillberg, C., & Billstedt, E. (2016). Aspects of sexuality in adolescents and adults diagnosed with autism spectrum disorders in childhood. *Journal of Autism and Developmental Disorders, 46*, 3155–3165. https://doi.org/10.1007/s10803-016-2855-9

Flores, D., & Barroso, J. (2017). 21st century parent–child sex communication in the United States: A process review. *The Journal of Sex Research, 54*(4–5), 532–548. https://doi.org/10.1080/00224499.2016.1267693

Gillespie-Lynch, K., Brooks, P. J., Someki, F., Obeid, R., Shane-Simpson, C., Kapp, S. K., Daou, N., & Smith, D. S. (2015). Changing college students' conceptions of autism: An online training to increase knowledge and decrease stigma. *Journal of Autism and Developmental Disorders, 45*(8), 2553–2566. https://doi.org/10.1007/s10803-015-2422-9

Harris, A. L., Sutherland, M. A., & Hutchinson, M. K. (2013). Parental influences of sexual risk among urban African American adolescent males. *Journal of Nursing Scholarship, 45*(2), 141–150. https://doi.org/10.1111/jnu.12016

Hartmann, K., Urbano, M. R., Raffaele, C. T., Qualls, L. R., Williams, T. V., Warren, C., Kreiser, N. L., Elkins, D. E., & Deutsch, S. I. (2019). Sexuality in the Autism Spectrum Study (SASS): Reports from young adults and parents. *Journal of Autism and Developmental Disorders, 49*, 3638–3655. https://doi.org/10.1007/s10803-019-04077-y

Holmes, L. G., & Himle, M. B. (2014). Brief report: Parent–child sexuality communication and autism spectrum disorders. *Journal of Autism and Developmental Disorders, 44*(11), 2964–2970. https://doi.org/10.1007/s10803-014-2146-2

Holmes, L. G., Strassberg, D. S., & Himle, M. B. (2019). Family sexuality communication for adolescent girls on the autism spectrum. *Journal of Autism and Developmental Disorders, 49*, 2403–2416. https://doi.org/10.1007/s10803-019-03904-6

Israel Central Bureau of Statistics. (2024). *The Druze population of Israel*. Israel Central Bureau of Statistics. https://www.cbs.gov.il/he/mediarelease/DocLib/2024/124/11_24_124b.pdf

Johnson, N. L., & Simpson, P. M. (2013). Lack of father involvement in research on children with autism spectrum disorder: Maternal parenting stress and family functioning. *Issues in Mental Health Nursing, 34*(4), 220–228. https://doi.org/10.3109/01612840.2012.745177

Juliusberger, A. F. (2023). *The relationship between the characteristics of parents of children on the autistic spectrum and the extent of their communication with their children about sexuality*. [Unpublished Master's Dissertation, Tel-Hai College, Israel].

Kamangu, A. A., John, M. R., & Nyakoki, S. J. (2017). Barriers to parent-child communication on sexual and reproductive health issues in East Africa: A review of qualitative research in four countries. *Journal of African Studies and Development, 9*(4), 45–50. https://doi.org/10.5897/JASD2016.0410

Kaye-Tzadok, A. (2019). *Qiddum beriut minit umeniat pegiot miniyyut baqqerav mitbaggerimo/t utseirimo/t*]*Promoting healthy sexuality and preventing sexual violence among adolescents: A literature review*[. Israel Ministry of Labor, Social Affairs, & Social Services.

Kellaher, D. C. (2015). Sexual behavior and autism spectrum disorders: An update and discussion. *Current Psychiatry Reports, 17*, 1–8. https://doi.org/10.1007/s11920-015-0562-4

Kenny, M. C., Crocco, C., & Long, H. (2020). Parents' plans to communicate about sexuality and child sexual abuse with their children with autism spectrum disorder. *Sexuality and Disability, 39*, 357–375. https://doi.org/10.1007/s11195-020-09636-1

Ketting, E., Friele, M., Michielsen, K., & European Expert Group on Sexuality Education. (2016). Evaluation of holistic sexuality education: A European expert group consensus agreement. *The European Journal of Contraception & Reproductive Health Care, 21*(1), 68–80.https://doi.org/10.3109/13625187.2015.1050715

Koller, R. (2000). Sexuality and adolescents with autism. *Sexuality and Disability, 18*, 125–135. https://doi.org/10.1023/A:1005567030442

Lindsey, R. A., & Barry, T. D. (2018). Protective factors against distress for caregivers of a child with autism spectrum disorder. *Journal of Autism and Developmental Disorders, 48*(4), 1092–1107. https://doi.org/10.1007/s10803-017-3372-1

Mackin, M. L., Loew, N., Gonzalez, A., Tykol, H., & Christensen, T. (2016). Parent perceptions of sexual education needs for their children with autism. *Journal of Pediatric Nursing, 31*(6), 608–618. https://doi.org/10.1016/j.pedn.2016.07.003

Mullis, M. D., Kastrinos, A., Wollney, E., Taylor, G., & Bylund, C. L. (2021). International barriers to parent-child communication about sexual and reproductive health topics: A qualitative systematic review. *Sex Education, 21*(4), 387–403. https://doi.org/10.1080/14681811.2020.1807316

Nichols, S., & Blakeley-Smith, A. (2010). "I'm not sure we're ready for this ...": Working with families toward facilitating healthy sexuality for individuals with autism spectrum disorders. *Social Work in Mental Health, 8*(1), 72–91. https://doi.org/10.1080/15332980902932383

Sacco, R., Camilleri, N., Eberhardt, J., Umla-Runge, K., & Newbury-Birch, D. (2022). The prevalence of autism spectrum disorder in Europe. In M. Carotenuto (Ed.), *Autism spectrum disorders: Recent advances and new perspectives*. InTech Open. https://doi.org/10.5772/intechopen.108123

Sala, G., Pecora, L., Hooley, M., & Stokes, M. A. (2020). As diverse as the spectrum itself: Trends in sexuality, gender and autism. *Current Developmental Disorders Reports, 7*, 59–68. https://doi.org/10.1007/s40474-020-00190-1

Shier, K. L. (2015). *Sexual behavior in children, adolescents, and young adults with autism spectrum disorder.* [Doctoral Dissertation, Azusa Pacific University]. ProQuest Dissertations & Theses, no. 10002618.

Sneed, C. D., Somoza, C. G., Jones, T., & Alfaro, S. (2013). Topics discussed with mothers and fathers for parent–child sex communication among African-American adolescents. *Sex Education, 13*(4), 450–458. https://doi.org/10.1080/14681811.2012.757548

Stanojević, Č, Neimeyer, T., & Piatt, J. (2021). The complexities of sexual health among adolescents living with autism spectrum disorder. *Sexuality and Disability, 39*(2), 345–356. https://doi.org/10.1007/s11195-020-09651-2

Stone, W. L. (1987). Cross-disciplinary perspectives on autism. *Journal of Paediatric Psychology, 12*(4), 615–630. https://doi.org/10.1093/jpepsy/12.4.615

Sullivan, A., & Caterino, L. C. (2008). Addressing the sexuality and sex education of individuals with autism spectrum disorders. *Journal of Education and Treatment of Children, 31*, 381–394. https://www.jstor.org/stable/42899984

Travers, J., & Tincani, M. (2010). Sexuality education for individuals with autism spectrum disorders: Critical issues and decision-making guidelines. *Education and Training in Autism and Developmental Disabilities*, 284–293. https://www.jstor.org/stable/23879812

Turnbull, T., Van Wersch, A., & Van Schaik, P. (2008). A review of parental involvement in sex education: The role for effective communication in British families. *Health Education Journal, 67*(3), 182–195. https://doi.org/10.1177/0017896908094636

Van Nieuwenhuizen, C., Nijman, H., & Van Daalen, E. (2015). Parental awareness of their adolescent children's sexual experiences: Parents of children with Autism Spectrum Disorders versus typically developing adolescents. *Journal of Autism and Developmental Disorders, 45*(11), 3326–3336. https://doi.org/10.1007/s10803-015-2497-5

Walker, J. L. (2001). A qualitative study of parents' experiences of providing sex education for their children: The implications for health education. *Health Education Journal, 60*(2), 132–146. https://doi.org/10.1177/001789690106000205

Wight, D., & Fullerton, D. (2013). A review of interventions with parents to promote the sexual health of their children. *Journal of Adolescent Health, 52*(1), 4–27. https://doi.org/10.1016/j.jadohealth.2012.04.014

Williams, K. L., Schroeder, J. L., Carvalho, C., & Cervantes, A. (2011). School personnel knowledge of autism: A pilot survey. *The School Psychologist, 65*(2), 7–9. https://digitalcommons.tamuc.edu/educ-faculty-publications/7

Wisnieski, D., Sieving, R., & Garwick, A. (2015). Parent and family influences on young women's romantic and sexual decisions. *Sex Education, 15*(2), 144–157. https://doi.org/10.1080/14681811.2014.986798

Wolfe, P. S., Condo, B., & Hardaway, E. (2009). Sociosexuality education for persons with autism spectrum disorders using principles of applied behavior analysis. *Teaching Exceptional Children, 42*(1), 50–61. https://doi.org/10.1177/004005990904200105

Zamora, I., Harley, E. K., Green, S. A., Smith, K., & Kipke, M. D. (2014). How sex of children with autism spectrum disorders and access to treatment services relates to parental stress. *Autism Research and Treatment*. https://doi.org/10.1155/2014/721418

Parents and Children: Identity Development

Chapter 8
Self-Disclosure and Self-Advocacy: A Process for Family and Systemic Therapeutic Dialogue

Sigal Dwek and Susan Lowinger

Abstract This chapter details the crucial processes of self-disclosure and self-advocacy for individuals diagnosed with Autism Spectrum Disorder (ASD), particularly children and adolescents, to facilitate their successful integration into various community settings. Self-advocacy involves individuals speaking for themselves to ensure their needs are met and rights respected, thereby maximizing their potential. However, effective self-advocacy necessitates prior self-disclosure, where individuals learn to articulate their unique characteristics, including strengths, abilities, difficulties, and challenges. This is particularly complex for people with ASD due to impaired self-awareness and communication difficulties, which are core aspects of the disorder. The chapter emphasizes that self-disclosure should ideally begin in early childhood, fostering self-awareness and familiarization with one's traits through an integrative process with therapists and parents. This long-term process involves multiple stages, including defining abilities and difficulties across various environments and eventually conceptualizing them under a diagnostic term. Self-advocacy requires both child readiness—built on a developed emotional, cognitive, and communicative infrastructure—and crucially, environmental readiness, which involves preparing the community, including peers, teachers, and authority figures, to be accepting and understanding of autistic traits. A multi-axis, integrative dialogue, involving therapeutic, family, professional, educational and community interactions, is essential for building this supportive infrastructure and enabling individuals with ASD to effectively explain their needs and behaviors. The success of these processes relies on collaboration and a common language among all involved parties.

Keywords Self-disclosure · Self advocacy · Diagnostic disclosure · Dialogue process · Environmental readiness · Child developmental readiness

---

S. Dwek (✉)
Speech and Language Pathologist, Kfar Yona, Israel
e-mail: Sigal329@bezeqint.net

S. Lowinger
Developmental Psychology, Kishurim Clinic, Jerusalem, Israel

S. Lowinger and S. Pearlman-Avnion (eds.), *Collaborative Care and Partnerships in Autism Diagnosis and Treatment*, Autism and Child Psychopathology Series,
https://doi.org/10.1007/978-3-032-07009-8_8

Introduction

In recent years, an increasing number of children, youth, and adults diagnosed with autism spectrum disorder (ASD) are being integrated into community, educational, academic, cultural, recreational, and workplace settings. This has created a growing need for these individuals to be able to explain their situation, the characteristics and components of ASD in general, and how they pertain to the specific individual; this includes strengths and abilities as well as difficulties and challenges (Townson et al., 2007; Wehmeyer & Smith, 2012). Parallel to this, the communities into which individuals with ASD are being integrated need information about the traits and components of the disorder in general and how they pertain to the individuals being integrated (Abernathy & Taylor, 2009).

Meeting the needs of people with ASD who are being integrated, as well as those of the receiving community, requires a dialogue that promotes a beneficial integration process for both. Therefore, individuals with ASD must understand the disorder's characteristics and components and how these manifest in their case in specific. There is growing recognition that individuals must acquire the skills and tools to understand and communicate about their situation and take part in an ongoing dialogue. This means creating a process of self-advocacy that is suited to their evolving needs (Barnard-Brak & Fearon, 2012). The skills and tools for self-advocacy may be acquired in therapeutic, educational, and family settings. The educational and therapeutic team, in collaboration with the family, faces the challenge of helping the person with ASD develop an emotional, cognitive, and communicative infrastructure to enable the acquisition and application of self-advocacy skills. Self-advocacy has become accepted around the world as appropriate in a discourse in which one party is claiming their rights to advance their own interests, while other parties are required to provide those rights.

The topic of this chapter pertains to how people with ASD learn to describe themselves to others and explain their difficulties and abilities, so that members of the community to which they belong will treat them with tolerance and consideration regarding their behavior. Such discourse is based on self-disclosure of their personal, neurological, and developmental identity. Further, the discourse should emphasize the shared responsibility of all partners to understand the needs of the person with ASD and implement the necessary adjustments.

This chapter describes processes of self-disclosure, self-advocacy, and dialogic discourse among children and adolescents with ASD, both within the therapeutic framework and outside it. Differences between these processes and how they complement each other will be explained.

The chapter discusses in detail dialogue with the nuclear and extended family of children and adults with ASD, relevant professionals in the educational, support, therapeutic, paramedical, and medical teams, and clinical dilemmas. Additionally, the chapter presents a comprehensive plan for an inclusive intervention plan for collaboration among families and the therapeutic and educational systems to enable children and adolescents with ASD to stand before their communities and explain their disabilities, challenges, unique characteristics, and needs. The plan includes a protocol and steps for developing a process of self-disclosure and self-advocacy.

The process is presented in its entirety, including the difficulties, clinical dilemmas, and thoughts about the future. At the end of the chapter, points for discussion and topics for further developing self-advocacy among people with ASD will be raised.

Definitions of Self-Advocacy and Self-Disclosure

Self-Advocacy

The concept of self-advocacy is familiar from the fields of law, psychology, social work, and education. Previously, the recognition that students can and should talk about their special needs has been largely limited to the realm of learning disabilities (Pocock et al., 2002). Recently, there has been increased exposure to and awareness of the existence of a large population of students with ASD among professionals in healthcare, education, and welfare systems around the world. As a result, there is growing recognition that children, adolescents, and adults diagnosed with ASD must learn to communicate their needs and advocate for themselves (Wehmeyer & Smith, 2012).

Self-advocacy involves individuals speaking for themselves, taking actions, and representing and promoting their personal interests. The aims are to create change in their lives, to ensure that their needs are met, their rights are respected, and that they receive the services and conditions they need and to which they are entitled, so that they can function to their full potential (Wehmeyer & Schalock, 2001).

Through self-advocacy, individuals take responsibility for their lives and for coping with their disability, thus improving their chances of influencing people in their environment so they can have their needs met. The individual plays a central role in shaping the functional environment (home, classroom, school) and in making decisions regarding the course of his functioning in the environment.

Kozminsky's (2005) guide to self-advocacy for children with learning disabilities defines prerequisites for effective self-advocacy, including awareness of one's own strengths, abilities, difficulties, and needs. This is not a stage of self-advocacy, but rather prerequisites that require individuals with learning disabilities to become familiar with themselves and their characteristics. Children with learning abilities develop self-awareness partly intuitively and partly because of natural dialogue with their social environments. Self-awareness is not a unitary phenomenon. Individuals can be aware of different aspects of themselves at any given point in time, and deficits in self-awareness can be differently manifested at different times.

People with ASD are characterized by impaired self-awareness of their psychological self (also known as the theory of self or theory of mind). In contrast, awareness of the physical self is less impaired among people on the spectrum (Williams, 2010).

Thus, a fundamental contradiction becomes apparent: the prerequisites for effective self-advocacy are based on familiarity with oneself and one's characteristics, while the core difficulty of people with ASD pertains to self-awareness and theory of mind. This contradiction raises two questions:

- Can people with emotional and cognitive difficulties regarding self-awareness and self-definition advocate for themselves?
- Can people who have difficulties with language and communication skills advocate for themselves?

Since these difficulties are at the core of ASD, before self-advocacy is possible, another primary concept must be considered: self-disclosure.

Self-Disclosure

Effective self-advocacy requires a great deal of self-awareness, so the advocacy process must be preceded by a process of self-disclosure and learning to recognize the full range of one's own characteristics. Ideally, the self-advocacy process begins by establishing in early childhood the self-awareness and familiarity with oneself that are essential prerequisites for a successful self-advocacy process (Shore, 2006).

Because people with ASD have distinctive difficulties in self-awareness, self-definition, and communication skills, additional special components are required in imparting the dialogue skills needed in the self-advocacy process (Field & Hoffman, 1999). Skills needed for self-disclosure, which involve theory of mind and communication abilities, do not develop normatively in children with ASD; some researchers describe this as the essence of the disability (Baron-Cohen, 1995).

A comprehensive process of self-disclosure is preferably carried out in all five areas of development: language, communication, cognition, sensorimotor, and emotional.

The process of self-disclosure takes place with therapists, educational teams and parents and includes an unpacking of the child's[1] unique and full range of abilities, difficulties, and characteristics. In the process of self-disclosure, it is important to ensure that children do not describe themselves using negative terms, such as stupid, lazy, or a troublemaker. Instead, they should define their difficulties in various areas of development and functioning, such as sensory regulation, taking initiative, organization, thinking, need for consistency, learning, language, auditory processing, communication, and/or socialization. All of this should be discussed honestly and respectfully, without bias or value judgments.

It is important that the process of self-disclosure begins as early as possible (in preschool, kindergarten, or elementary school). The earlier this process begins, the more effectively the child and parents can internalize and integrate into their daily lives and discourse the terms and concepts that give concrete meaning to the complex

[1] Although the term "child" is used, this process applies to people of all ages with ASD.

whole of the child's abilities and challenges (Shore, 2006). Furthermore, the earlier that children receive explanations, as part of a process of self-disclosure, regarding their traits and how these differ from the norm, the more effectively and consistently they will be able to self-advocate in the future. The process of self-disclosure must be free of value judgments, while not whitewashing the reality. It is important to use language that the child understands; when possible, it is beneficial to use visual aids and concrete examples.

When parents take part in the therapeutic dialogue with their child, they can consistently and spontaneously apply and integrate the contents of the self-disclosure and the terms used to describe their child into their daily discourse, as incidents arise in real life (Field & Hoffman, 1999). When parents find ways to describe their child, using examples from daily life, and do so consistently throughout the treatment period, it will become easier for the child to internalize difficulties and generalize them into a coherent sense of "self."

In advanced stages of the self-disclosure process (as described below in the section on the ten stages of self-disclosure), children should be encouraged to apply a term or name to their diagnosis. It is highly recommended that this name be used initially by the parents in a conversation with their child.

Disclosure of Diagnosis of ASD

Recent studies have examined the effects of diagnosis disclosure on peer engagement and interactions for people with ASD. For example, there has been research on the effects of disclosure of a diagnosis of ASD in university settings, especially its relevance to the effects on college students' scholastic standing, academic achievements, and social abilities (Thompson-Hodgetts et al., 2020). The present chapter focuses on younger children, primarily in elementary school through high school. One question addressed pertains to whether disclosing an ASD disorder in school reduces peers' stigmatizing attitudes toward a classmate with ASD or if disclosure negatively affects the perception of the student.

White et al. (2020) studied the stigmatization of adolescents (ages 11–16) in the UK. The authors tested the effect of disclosure on the social and emotional distance pupils wanted to maintain from a fictional classmate and found that disclosure of the autism diagnosis did not affect social or emotional distance. Newheiser and Barreto (2014) found that disclosing a stigmatized identity frees the person from the pressure of secrecy and improves the person's feeling of authenticity. Acceptance of a diagnostic label of autism legitimizes the person's differences, provides a positive sense of self, and gives a sense of common identity with other people with ASD (Mogenson & Mason, 2015). It has been suggested that more knowledge about autism leads to a more positive feeling toward the person diagnosed with ASD (Sasson & Morrison, 2019).

In addition to studies about the effects of self-advocacy on school-aged children, on their classmates, and their self-perception, new tools have been developed to help adolescents with ASD develop a sense of self. One of these is the Transition Tool Kit offered by Autism Speaks, which aims to help people with ASD self-advocate, speak up for themselves, negotiate and ask for what they need, know their rights and responsibilities, and use the available resources.

A related issue is the question of how students with ASD make sense of themselves in the school setting. Williams et al. (2019) identified three aspects of experience that contribute to how students with ASD see themselves as different than their peers: difficulties linked to ASD, interpersonal relationships, and the accessibility of the school environment.

A case study examined the disclosure of ASD diagnosis on peer interactions of a child with ASD in a summer camp (Fan et al., 2022) and found that peer engagement and reciprocal interactions improved following the diagnosis disclosure. The author suggested a protocol for rehabilitation via a disclosure protocol accompanied by an explanation of autistic behaviors. However, the author noted that the intervention had not been evaluated in other contexts.

Family Decision: What Diagnosis to Give Their Child

Many parents do not want to "label" their child. They assume that people should accept other individuals' differences. In an ideal world, this may be true, but giving a label or diagnosis is sometimes the only way to receive essential services for the child (Freedman, 2010).

Recently, around the world, various terms have been used to describe this disorder. In addition to the definition of autism spectrum disorder in the DSM-5 (American Psychiatric Association, 2013), other terms are commonly used, such as social communication disorder, communication disorder, social disorder, autistic disorder, child with autism, and pervasive developmental disorder (PDD). Parents may spend weeks, months, and even years debating which term they feel comfortable with. This stage is not easy for parents who are required, sometimes for the first time, to admit that their child is on the autism spectrum. Disclosing the disability and giving it a name presents parents with dilemmas regarding whether they should tell their child and the other family members, including siblings, who may have heard the word "autistic" used as a derogatory term by their peers (Campbell, 2006).

Freedman (2010) gave several reasons why it is important to tell children that they are on the autism spectrum and to give their disability a name. First, knowledge helps children understand and accept themselves and avoid feeling that they are "not normal." Second, knowledge makes children feel that they are part of a population of people who are similar to them. Third, knowledge encourages children to advocate for themselves and explain to others their unique abilities and difficulties, which enables others to understand and accept them.

The often lengthy process of choosing a term that suits the parents' position may take place within an instructional dialogue between the parents and the primary therapist. Parallel to this is a dialogue with the child that takes place both in the therapeutic framework and with the family, during which they discuss the various definitions and conceptualizations of the child's full range of abilities and difficulties.

The Importance of Dialogue in Self-Advocacy Processes

Given that self-advocacy has been defined as speaking for oneself and representing one's interests, people must be in an evolving dialogue with themselves and their social environment in order to self-advocate effectively. They must develop skills and insights that enable them to explain their difficulties and needs to other people and to deal with the attitudes of those around them (Kozminsky, 2005). Self-advocacy requires direct, daily, reality-based, and structured dialogue for children to develop the skills necessary for understanding themselves. Children with ASD must be taught these social skills and how to interpret nonverbal communication in a structured, cognitive, and experiential way.

The emotional, linguistic, communicative, and cognitive infrastructure for self-advocacy is acquired through dialogue between the child and parents, caregivers, and teachers in family, therapeutic, and educational. This should integrate people who relate to the child in all the various life realms:

- Nuclear family: both of the child's parents and any siblings, each according to their age and developmental level;
- Extended family: grandparents, aunts, uncles, and cousins;
- Therapeutic/educational team: director/principal, teachers, psychologist, school counselor.

The development of this infrastructure enables children to implement the process on two main communicative levels:

1. Knowing *what* to say in self-advocacy: the relevant content and appropriate language;
2. Knowing *when* and *how* to self-advocate: understanding the best time, method, and pragmatic context for communicating one's needs or explaining the motivations for one's behavior.

This dialogue creates mutually considerate, understanding, and trusting relations between the person being integrated into the community and the receiving community or individuals within it (Shore, 2006). The long-term processes of self-disclosure and self-advocacy take place along four axes of dialogue, sometimes occurring consecutively and sometimes overlapping.

1. Therapeutic dialogue with the child: Clinical dialogue between the child and primary therapist, in the treatment room, may take place with an individual child, pairs of children, or in a group. In this way, children become aware of their full range of unique cognitive, sensory, social, and verbal-communicative characteristics and establish theory of mind self-awareness, including personal preferences, tendencies, ways of coping, and conduct in daily life.

2. Guidance dialogue with the family: This work takes place with and within the nuclear family. Dialogue between parents and their child uncovers the child's full range of distinctive characteristics and conceptualization of the child's disability. The family must decide on a term describing their child's disability that they find acceptable (communication disorder, social communication disorder, autism, etc.). Later in the process, the dialogue may be expanded to incorporate other household members and the extended family, each according to age and ability.
3. Integrative dialogue with relevant professionals: This includes all relevant educational, therapeutic, paramedical, and medical staff members.
4. Advocacy dialogue with the community: This dialogue takes place with communities that have been identified as significant in the person's life at the current stage, including the extended family, classroom, social group, workplace, and social relationships. Educational directors, teachers, and the advisory/therapeutic team (psychologists and counselors), and employers (for adults) should be involved in this dialogue.

Given that people with ASD generally have difficulty initiating social interactions, a variety of interventions have recently been developed that encourage them to take initiative (Grosberg & Charlop, 2014; Koegel et al., 2012, 2014). Advocacy is particularly difficult for them since it requires initiating interactions in which they must explain their difficulties and the adaptations to the social environment they need for their needs to be met. Despite these significant difficulties, the dialogue component of advocacy is essential.

Children on the spectrum often engage in maladaptive and sometimes manipulative behaviors, such as crying, yelling, throwing objects, or disruptions that are intended to stop or change environmental situations that they perceive as unfavorable (Gustafsson & Paplinski, 2004). Some of these behaviors are defined as "conduct disorders" or "self-stimulatory behaviors," but, in fact, they are mechanisms for self-organization emerging from the child's partial awareness of the disturbing stimulus (for example, noise in the environment) and the behaviors are responses to the disturbance (for example, covering their ears or growling). Clinical experience shows that repeatedly mirroring back to children with ASD the behaviors they engage in to regulate environmental disturbances (such as auditory sensitivities) enables them to formulate dialogic texts to make the environmental stimuli appropriate for their sensory systems.

Collaboration and Partnership in Processes of Self-Disclosure and Advocacy

As mentioned, the process, as presented so far, takes place on four axes. A condition for the success of the process is the participation of all the parties involved in the process (parents, therapists, educators, and counselors). In this way, all parties share a common interest. Each influences and is influenced by the matrix of interrelationships. They must work together and in agreement regarding the importance of the process and their willingness to carry it out (Schoeters et al., 2005). Such partnerships include the following aspects:

1. A shared schedule.
2. A common language and shared use of relevant content and terminology. For example, if a child's parents prefer the term "communication disorder" over the term "autism," all partners in the process should use the preferred terminology with sensitivity and take care not to deviate from it.
3. A shared platform for all partners to inform the others about where they are in the steps of the process, and to consult one another on questions and dilemmas that arise in the process. Such platforms include email groups and/or regular meetings throughout the process.
4. Agreement regarding who will coordinate the process (case manager).

Self-Disclosure and Self-Advocacy: An Applied Program

This section presents an implementation plan with steps for self-disclosure and self-advocacy. The plan is divided into two stages: (a) a ten-step protocol for self-disclosure, (b) a five-step protocol for self-advocacy. The structure of the program allows all partners in this complex process to speak a common language, for example, "We are currently at step nine, and have not yet talked with the child about his unique areas of knowledge. This means that we skipped step four. We need to go back and address the stage we skipped."

The Protocol of Ten Steps of Self-Disclosure for Children with ASD

Reflecting on the self-disclosure process is suitable for children at all levels of functioning. This depends, of course, on their current linguistic and cognitive level and emotional capacity. The contents of self-disclosure can be conceptualized through spoken words, writing, symbols, or images, and may be short or complex. The modes of conceptualization can be modified and adapted to changes in the child's development and abilities in all developmental areas and at any given time.

The long-term process of self-disclosure can be structured into ten steps, some of which overlap and some of which occur in sequence.

1. Definition and conceptualization of abilities and difficulties based on events in the treatment environment.
2. Definition and conceptualization of abilities and difficulties based on events in the home environment.

3. Definition and conceptualization of abilities and difficulties based on events in the educational environment.
4. Emphasis on distinctive areas of interest, competence, and expertise.
5. Integration of all the child's identified abilities and difficulties (verbal/visual).
6. Parents' conceptualization of the child's set of abilities and difficulties under a diagnostic term.
7. Primary therapist's conceptualization of the child's set of abilities and difficulties under a diagnostic term.
8. Comparison with other children with ASD (peers in the social environment or as seen in videos, films, and television programs).
9. Providing the child with opportunities for emotional–cognitive processing (denial, anger, sadness, raising questions).
10. Conceptualization of the set of abilities and difficulties under a diagnostic term according to the primary educational figure, for use exclusively in the educational framework.

Once children have been told that their particular set of abilities and difficulties has a diagnostic name according to their parents (step six) and primary therapist (step seven), it is important to consistently use this diagnostic name in situations that arise naturally at home and in the therapeutic space. That is, the disability and its relevant term should not be presented to the child in a one-time event or a private secret not to be discussed further.

The earlier that parents and caregivers describe to children their distinctive characteristics, needs, strengths, and difficulties, the better they will be able to carry out a self-advocacy process. Likewise, the more clearly and distinctly children are told that their difficulties do not stem from "stupidity" or "laziness," but rather that they represent a recognized diagnosis with a name and that others also suffer from it, the better they will be able to carry out the self-advocacy processes throughout their development and into adult life (Shore, 2006).

The Protocol of Five Steps of Self-Advocacy for Children with ASD

For self-advocacy actions undertaken by children with ASD to be as successful as possible, two parameters must be considered: environmental readiness and child readiness. According to the socio-ecological model (Wehmeyer et al., 2010), these two parameters should be the focus. Children must be encouraged to reach their full potential, and the environment must also be adapted to allow for the most successful intervention.

Environmental Readiness

It is of utmost importance to prepare the environment for the advocacy activities of children and adolescents with ASD. The social environment includes everyone who encounters the child. At school, this includes children in the same classroom and other classrooms; the teachers and other educational staff members, such as the principal, counselors, and psychologists; and even people working in the local education system. This preparation requires considerable thought and organization and may take a significant length of time, even years. It is not possible to promote children's self-advocacy without undertaking serious work to build an infrastructure in the systems surrounding the child and the family (Field & Hoffman, 2002).

In many cases, children and their parents are justifiably afraid to announce the diagnosis to the community, whether the term used is autism, autism spectrum, communication disorder, PDD, or others. It is necessary to instill in the community the emotional, cognitive, and perceptual tools to listen to the child with openness and understanding.

Brown and Zefadia (2010) proposed a preparatory program for a public elementary school in Efrat, Israel. The program, spanning 2–3 years, was intended to help children with ASD successfully integrate into the school. The program included self-awareness activities for children on the autism spectrum and other children in the group into which they were being integrated. All the children were given an opportunity to reflect on the difficulties they faced and their special skills. As a result of this process, the children understood that everyone has unique characteristics—those with an ASD diagnosis as well as those without. Brown and Zefadia noted several factors that contributed to the success of the integration program, which, notably, also contributed to the success of the advocacy activities.

- The regular education staff and special education staff must take shared responsibility for children with ASD.
- It is necessary to provide information to teachers and therapists about the characteristics of children with ASD, as they do not always have adequate experience and training to support these children. Educational and therapeutic staff members need explanations of the abilities, difficulties, and special needs of children with ASD.
- A positive and accepting climate must be created in the school. Support and encouragement from the principal, school staff, and students greatly influence the success of self-advocacy activities.

Wolfberg et al. (2012) developed intervention models, based on current theories and research, to support children with ASD as they play and form friendships with neurotypical children in integrated school, home, and community settings. A "demystification" intervention called "friend to friend" assists children with ASD in making friends by developing their peers' awareness, understanding, acceptance, and empathy by clarifying the characteristics of children on the autism spectrum (Wolfberg et al., 2012). These researchers described the social void that can exist between children with ASD and other children in their classrooms. This may happen because neurotypical children lack understanding of and appreciation for the special ways in which children with ASD communicate, connect, think, and play. Therefore, it is essential to support the educational system with the intention of helping all children gain an understanding of autism.

To emphasize the importance of preparing the environment for advocacy, Wolfberg et al. (2008) related an incident in which a university invited a 27-year-old man with ASD to give a lecture to a class of students majoring in special education. At the end of his talk, one student said she had a child with ASD in her class and asked how she could help this child do better in school. The man replied that she could help the child understand autism, but, equally importantly, help the other children in the class understand autism.

Child Readiness

Therapeutic dialogue with children that focuses on self-disclosure, together with dialogue with the parents to offer them guidance, and dialogue between the parents and their child, provides the foundation for children's ability to self-advocate and ask that the social and physical environment be adapted to their needs. In the past, due to the various difficulties experienced by the child, advocacy was carried out by other people, such as teachers, parents, or occasionally a close friend, ostensibly on behalf of the child (Abernathy & Taylor, 2009). It is essential that any self-advocacy be conducted in the presence of the child, with the participation of the child, and, as much as possible, by the child.

The inverse of this statement is equally significant: self-advocacy cannot be conducted in the child's absence. Any formal conversation concerning a child with ASD (such as teachers or counselors talking with students, or a parent talking with other children) that takes place without the presence and participation of the child in question may not be considered an act of self-advocacy. Such conversations may be categorized under other concepts, such as protecting, reporting, or updating. These activities (and others) are certainly relevant, but they are not self-advocacy. In this context, it is useful to recall the motto on the Autistic Self-Advocacy Network's website: "Nothing About Us Without Us" (ASAN, n.d.).

Once a child has a developmental infrastructure and has carried out processes of self-disclosure, and after an infrastructure has been established in the community to promote acceptance of the child, the child can initiate and maintain a dialogue with the community and self-advocate for his or her needs to be met. This is age-dependent and develops over time.

Barnard-Brak and Fearon (2012) examined the variables that most strongly influence the participation of students with ASD in their individualized education programs (IEPs). The researchers found that students who participated in self-advocacy processes showed higher engagement and participation in their IEPs, indicating the importance of developing self-advocacy skills for adolescents with ASD.

The First Advocacy Conversation

Introducing oneself and one's disability for the first time to a class of neurotypical peers is an important step toward the child's successful integration (Campbell, 2006). As will be described below, this first advocacy conversation will take place after a lengthy process of preparing all partners—the community, including the authority in the community, the family, and the child.

The initial advocacy conversation may be initiated by the child, the child's parents, the primary caregiver leading the process, or the authority figure of the educational framework. In any case, the conversation must be coordinated with all the involved parties who are in contact with the child. All self-advocacy conversations, and certainly the first one, can be highly complex due to the involvement of multiple people, each with different needs, including:

- The community members; they may respond in various ways, such as with questions, comments, personal sharing, mockery, or expressions of embarrassment.
- The community authority figure responsible for ensuring and protecting the needs of the child with ASD, as well as the needs of the community at large, in terms of the resources of time and the inclusion and attention of the community members.
- The child with special needs.

In addition, the child's family members involved in the process, especially the parents, often relate to the child's self-disclosure with excitement and concern about what may happen. Even if the child's parents are not present at the first advocacy conversation, they are highly significant partners, and their perspectives and needs must be considered. If the child has siblings who can be an appropriate audience for the child's self-advocacy process, it is recommended that the child conduct the first speaking exercise at home with siblings and/or extended family members. In this way, when children first explain their diagnosis, unique characteristics, and needs from the physical and social environment in a protected, sympathetic, and well-adapted environment, they can practice the words of advocacy, including unexpected situations, such as questions or comments from the recipients. The first advocacy conversation requires preparation for the child, the community (who constitute the audience for the advocacy content), and the primary community authority figures (teachers, youth group or activity counselors, etc.).

Preparing the Community

This involves general preliminary discussions held in the primary community of affiliation (classroom, club, etc.) about special needs and differences among the children in the class, such as glasses, hearing aids, or crutches. They should also discuss tolerance in accepting differences. Preparing the community for an advocacy conversation increases the willingness of others in the group to share their own difficulties. It inspires tolerance and acceptance of differences and unique behaviors in general and toward the child in question. Further, it encourages the community to take responsibility for proposing solutions and reasonable adjustments.

The educational staff must be prepared for the holding of the advocacy encounter. First, there should be coordination between the educational staff and the child in terms of the time and space resources available for the process. Second, the expectations of the child, the child's parents, and the educational staff should be aligned. Third, the authority figures should know and accept the child's preferred personal terminology.

Preparing the Child

The primary caregiver, in collaboration with the parents and the authority figure (teacher, counselor, etc.), is responsible for preparing the child for the conversation with the community. The preparation involves several areas.

(a) **Language preparation.** This includes the content the child wants to introduce; the set of characteristics, challenges, and needs the child wants to describe; and the texts and formulations that can be used to introduce the content. The guiding principle is to explain autism in simple and neutral terms that are not value-based or judgmental.
(b) **Cognitive preparation.** This involves how the child wants to organize the material; expectations regarding the event and the reactions of the audience; and the degree of flexibility required for various situations during the discussion. This preparation focuses on planning, flexibility, adaptation, and creativity based on what is happening.
(c) **Communicative preparation.** This pertains to pragmatic adaptation to the recipient audience in terms of the length and complexity of the presentation, the appropriateness of the degree of exposure, the child's manner of standing before the class, and the voice volume when speaking to a classroom audience, among other issues.
(d) **Preparing visual/audio aids.** The resources that the child will use should be available as needed, including pages with personal information and information about the audience, and video/audio presentations with the necessary devices (i.e., tablet, communication board).

(e) **Preparing the physical resources**. This includes all resources that will be available to the child, especially time (when and for how long), and location (where the conversation will take place).

Preparing children for their first self-advocacy conversation helps them plan and carry it out step by step, observe difficulties from the perspectives of community members, and deal with personal difficulties in various ways. The more familiar a child is with the resources needed for self-advocacy, the greater the chances that the child will also self-advocate in other contexts: in other classrooms, with other teachers, and with friends and family members in other social contexts.

The conversation and its content gain validity when conducted in the presence of the relevant authority figure. In the home, the authority figures are the parents, and self-advocacy at home should not take place with other authority figures present. In the classroom, the authority figures are the teacher and/or school counselor, and the parents should not be present for this conversation (Campbell, 2006).

Advocacy seems to proceed in spiral movement, characterized by actions repeated at different times, in different areas of life, and, as the person matures, in different periods of the life cycle (Kleinert et al., 2010). Below are the five stages of self-advocacy in children.

1. Involve the child and family members in the diagnosis and in identifying the full range of the child's characteristics.
2. Prepare the educational team for the self-advocacy encounter.
3. Hold general and ongoing conversations in the classroom about the special needs and exceptions of the students in the classroom (glasses, hearing aids, crutches, etc.).
4. Acquire the necessary visual/audio aids for the advocacy process (i.e., augmentative and alternative communication [AAC] tablet, laptop, or other devices).
5. Enable the child to hold an advocacy meeting/event.

Examples of texts from the first self-advocacy talks.

Shahar, Grade 4: "I want to tell you about myself today. As you have seen, I have some different behaviors, and I want to tell you why. My skin is very sensitive. I know that children don't mean to bother me, but when they touch me, I feel uncomfortable, so I have to sit at the table by myself. It is also very difficult for me to hear when people talk to me quickly, or when there's noise, even a little noise, in the classroom. It is hardest for me to hear if people talk to me from behind. That's why sometimes I cover my ears or make noises. The noises I make are only me making noise for myself, they aren't noises for you. So please don't think I'm weird when I make noises. It's just because I have a hard time hearing."

Eitan, grade 6: "Sometimes I need time alone. Anat, my teacher, calls it 'timeout'. I need to be quiet and alone during this time. Sometimes during this time, I jump, or make noises, or wave my arms. Please don't laugh at me. It helps my body relax so I can go back to class and study with you."

Amit, grade 6: (Amit types on a screen, and the text is read by his classmates).

"I understand things I read and hear, even if I hardly speak. It's very difficult for me to speak. That's why I type on the computer. Don't think I'm stupid because I don't speak. I know the entire solar system by heart, all the planets and their moons, their order in the solar system, and their sizes. Sigal, the communication clinician, says I have high intelligence even if I don't speak much."

The best ways to make self-advocacy successful need additional research. As Campbell (2006) noted in his article on the process of changing children's perceptions of autism, little is known about the effects of who says what, how, and to whom (the target audience).

Distinctiveness of the Process in Different Cultures

It must be remembered that self-disclosure and the willingness to define and verbally conceptualize one's abilities, and particularly one's difficulties, are interrelated with the values of the culture to which the family belongs. In the United States, for example, there is a high level of willingness to do so, and significant attention is given to this issue in the literature and in community systems (Zager et al., 2012). There are many intervention methods, and a wide variety of teaching materials designed for educators to use in helping children and adolescents with ASD and encouraging them to self-advocate (Wehmeyer & Schalock, 2001). However, in some cultures, it is common to talk about disabilities and difficulties in a condescending manner or to completely avoid any discussion or mention of disabilities (Zhang et al., 2010).

This is not a judgmental stance toward one cultural preference or another. Rather, it is noted here to emphasize and increase the sensitivity required in the process of disclosure and advocacy in general and in various specific cultures. It should be remembered that in different cultures, the stages for self-disclosure and self-advocacy will be different; some will be longer, some will not occur at all. However, this is a synergistic process in which the whole is greater than the sum of its parts.

The Autistic Self-Advocacy Network (ASAN) offers inclusive advocacy processes to provide support and services to individuals with autism, and simultaneously to educate communities with the goals of improving public perception of the disability, influencing public policy, increasing community engagement, and encouraging inclusion and respect for the neurological diversity that is characteristic of this disability (ASAN, n.d.).

Conclusion

This chapter presented the processes of self-disclosure and self-advocacy of children with autism in dialogue with themselves and their communities. Self-advocacy is preceded by a long process of self-disclosure that lasts months or even years. Self-disclosure forms the foundation and is accompanied by tools for the advocacy dialogue and the ability to advocate for one's needs in front of the community to which one belongs.

Self-awareness is not a unitary phenomenon. It is possible to be aware of different aspects of oneself at different times. Therefore, there is a need to routinely practice self-advocacy, which proceeds in a spiral throughout one's life. With the transition to adulthood and being in public places where greater adaptation and independence are required, such as academic institutions, workplaces, and public service institutions, it is important that people with ASD know how to advocate for the full range of rights to which they are legally entitled.

At the same time, more thought should be given to advocacy processes within nuclear families, extended families, and the community. Consideration should be given to the factors that hinder and promote parents' self-advocacy and their special needs as parents (and family members) of a child with ASD, and the implications of these processes for the family's ability to cope.

It is important that both processes, self-disclosure and self-advocacy, take place as part of a comprehensive system (therapeutic, family, and educational) that supports children as they learn about themselves and talk about themselves to their family, classmates, community, and world at large. This should be done in collaboration and partnership with all the relevant entities in the community in which the process takes place. The discussion above clarifies that involving the family in the process is a necessary, integral aspect that impacts the process and the child's progressive ability to express messages for self-advocacy in relevant contexts.

Self-advocacy can be viewed as a process undertaken by an individual vis à vis a group, which influences, nourishes, and benefits the individual. However, this observation is incomplete. The process may be hindered if it does not consider the benefit to the community. It is more accurate and valuable to view the self-advocacy process as a dialogue between an individual with ASD and the community to which the person belongs, and also as a dialogue between one community and the larger society in which it exists. The self-advocacy processes of people with ASD affect not only each individual's development, but the entire community: family, school, and even the society and country in which they live.

References

Abernathy, T. V., & Taylor, S. (2009). Teacher perceptions of students' understanding of their own disability. *Teacher Education and Special Education, 32*(2), 121–136. https://doi.org/10.1177/0888406409334084

American Psychiatric Association. (2013). *Diagnostic and statistical manual of mental disorders* (5th ed.). American Psychiatric Publishing.

Autism Self-Advocacy Network [ASAN]. (n.d.). *What we believe: Our motto: What is "Nothing about us without us"?* ASAN. https://autisticadvocacy.org/about-asan/what-we-believe/

Barnard-Brak, L., & Fearon, D. D. (2012). Self-advocacy skills as a predictor of student IEP participation among adolescents with autism. *Education and Training in Autism and Developmental Disabilities, 47*(1), 39–47. https://www.jstor.org/stable/23880560

Brown, R., & Zefadia, M. (2010). Model leshilluv yeladim im ASD betifqud gavoah bekhittah regilah: Bet hassefer Asah Khayyal, Efrat [A model for integrating children with high-functioning ASD into a regular classroom: The Asa Khayyal school in Efrat]. In S. Lowinger (Ed.), *Tiqshoret: Tippul biyiladim im beayot tiqshoret begilae bet hassefer hayyesodi [Communication: Treating children with communication problems at the elementary school age]* (pp. 211–234). Ach Publishing.
Baron-Cohen, S. (1995). *Mindblindness: An essay on autism and theory of mind.* MIT Press.
Campbell, J. (2006). Changing children's attitudes toward autism: A process of persuasive communication. *Journal of Developmental and Physical Disabilities, 18*(3), 251–272. https://doi.org/10.1007/s10882-006-9015-7
Fan, L., Shire, S., Couture, M., Zwaigenbaum, L., & Thompson-Hodgetts, S. (2022). *The influence of disclosure on peer engagement and interactions for a child with autism in summer camps: A within-case mixed methods study* [Master's thesis]. University of Alberta. https://doi.org/10.7939/r3-bk9g-1h91
Field, S., & Hoffman, A. (1999). The importance of family involvement for promoting self-determination in adolescents with autism and other developmental disabilities. *Focus on Autism and Other Developmental Disabilities, 14*(1), 36–41. https://doi.org/10.1177/108835769901400105
Field, S., & Hoffman, A. (2002). Preparing youth to exercise self-determination: Quality indicators of school environments that promote the acquisition of knowledge, skills, and beliefs related to self-determination. *Journal of Disability Policy Studies, 13*(2), 113–118. https://doi.org/10.1177/10442073020130020701
Freedman, S. (2010). Self-awareness skill sets. In S. Freedman (Ed.), *Developing college skills in students with autism and Asperger's Syndrome* (pp. 47–65). Jessica Kingsley Publishers.
Grosberg, D., & Charlop, M. (2014). Teaching persistence in social initiation bids to children with autism through a portable video modeling intervention (PVMI). *Journal of Developmental and Physical Disabilities, 26*(5), 527–541. https://doi.org/10.1007/s10882-013-9362-0
Gustafsson, L., & Papliński, A. (2004). Self-organization of an artificial neural network subjected to attention shift impairments and familiarity preference: Characteristics studied in autism. *Journal of Autism and Developmental Disorders, 34*, 189–198. https://doi.org/10.1023/B:JADD.0000022609.31371.4d
Kleinert, J. O., Harrison, E. M., Fisher, T. L., & Kleinert, H. L. (2010). "I can" and "I did"—Self advocacy for young students with developmental disabilities. *Teaching Exceptional Children, 43*(2), 16–26. https://doi.org/10.1177/004005991004300202
Koegel, R. L., Bradshaw, J. L., Ashbaugh, K., & Koegel, L. K. (2014). Improving question-asking initiations in young children with autism using pivotal response treatment. *Journal of Autism and Developmental Disorders, 44*(4), 816–827. https://doi.org/10.1007/s10803-013-1932-6
Koegel, L. K., Vernon, T. W., Koegel, R. L., Koegel, B. L., & Paullin, A. W. (2012). Improving social engagement and initiations between children with autism spectrum disorder and their peers in inclusive settings. *Journal of Positive Behavior Interventions, 14*(4), 220–227. https://doi.org/10.1177/1098300712437042
Kozminsky, L. (2005). *Speaking for themselves, self-advocacy of learners with learning disabilities.* Yesod Publisher.
Mogensen, L., & Mason, J. (2015). The meaning of a label for teenagers negotiating identity: Experiences with autism spectrum disorder. *Children, Health and Well-Being: Policy Debates and Lived Experience, 37*, 83–97. https://doi.org/10.1002/9781119069522.ch7
Newheiser, A. K., & Barreto, M. (2014). Hidden costs of hiding stigma: Ironic interpersonal consequences of concealing a stigmatized identity in social interactions. *Journal of Experimental Social Psychology, 52*, 58–70. https://doi.org/10.1016/j.jesp.2014.01.002
Pocock, A., Lambros, S., Karvonen, M., Test, D. W., Algozzine, B., Wood, W., & Martin, J. (2002). Successful strategies for promoting self-advocacy among students with LD: The LEAD group. *Intervention in School and Clinic, 37*(4), 209–216. https://doi.org/10.1177/105345120203700403

Sasson, N. J., & Morrison, K. E. (2019). First impressions of adults with autism improve with diagnostic disclosure and increased autism knowledge of peers. *Autism, 23*(1), 50–59. https://doi.org/10.1177/1362361317729526

Schoeters, L., Schelfhout, P., Roets, G., Van Hove, G., Townson, L., Chapman, R., & Buchanan, I. (2005). Partnership working between university researchers and self-advocacy organizations: A way forward for inclusion? in England and 'Fine feathers make a fine bird' in Flanders. *Journal of Intellectual Disabilities, 9*(4), 345–357. https://doi.org/10.1177/1744629505059178

Shore, S. (2006). The secrets of self-advocacy: How to make sure you take care of you. *Autism Advocate, 44*, 4. https://phxautism.org/wp-content/uploads/secrets-of-self-advocacy.pdf

Thompson-Hodgetts, S., Labonte, C., Mazumder, R., & Phelan, S. (2020). Helpful or harmful? A scoping review of perceptions and outcomes of autism diagnostic disclosure to others. *Research in Autism Spectrum Disorders, 77*, Article 101598. https://doi.org/10.1016/j.rasd.2020.101598

Townson, L., Macauley, S., Harkness, E., Docherty, A., Dias, J., Eardley, M., & Chapman, R. (2007). Research project on advocacy and autism. *Disability and Society, 22*(5), 523–536. https://doi.org/10.1080/09687590701427669

Wehmeyer, M. L., Shogren, K. A., Smith, T., Zager, D., & Simpson, R. (2010). Research-based principles and practices for educating students with autism: Self-determination and social interactions. *Education and Training in Autism and Developmental Disabilities, 45*(4), 475–486. https://www.jstor.org/stable/23879754

Wehmeyer, M. L., & Schalock, R. L. (2001). Self-determination and quality of life: Implications for special education services and supports. *Focus on Exceptional Children, 33*(8), 1–16.

Wehmeyer, M., & Smith, T. E. C. (2012). Promoting self-determination and social inclusion: A review of research-based practices. In D. Zager, M. Wehmeyer, & R. Simpson (Eds.), *Educating students with autism spectrum disorders: Research-based principles and practices* (pp. 227–246). Routledge.

White, R., Barreto, M., Harrington, J., Kapp, S. K., Hayes, J., & Russell, G. (2020). Is disclosing an autism spectrum disorder in school associated with reduced stigmatization? *Autism, 24*(3), 744–754. https://doi.org/10.1177/1362361319887625

Williams, D. (2010). Theory of own mind in autism: Evidence of a specific deficit in self-awareness? *Autism, 14*(5), 474–494. https://doi.org/10.1177/1362361310366314

Williams, E. I., Gleeson, K., & Jones, B. E. (2019). How pupils on the autism spectrum make sense of themselves in the context of their experiences in a mainstream school setting: A qualitative metasynthesis. *Autism, 23*(1), 8–28. https://doi.org/10.1177/1362361317723836

Wolfberg, P., Bottema-Beutel, K., & DeWitt, M. (2012). Including children with autism in social and imaginary play with typical peers. *American Journal of Play, 5*(1), 55–80.

Wolfberg, P., McCracken, H., & Tuchel, T. (2008). Fostering peer play and friendships: Creating a culture of inclusion. In K. D. Buron & P. Wolfberg (Eds.), *Learners on the autism spectrum* (pp. 182–207). Autism Asperger Publishing.

Zager, D., Wehmeyer, M., & Simpson, R. (Eds.) (2012). *Educating students with Autism Spectrum Disorders: Research-based principles and practices*. Routledge.

Zhang, D., Landmark, L., Grenwelge, C., & Montoya, L. (2010). Culturally diverse parents' perspectives on self-determination. *Education and Training in Autism and Developmental Disabilities, 45*(2), 175–186. https://www.jstor.org/stable/23879805

Chapter 9
Identity Development in Autism: A Collaborative Journey

Noorit Felsenthal-Berger

Abstract This chapter presents a decade-long case study of dyadic therapeutic intervention with Ori, a young boy diagnosed with high-functioning autism spectrum disorder (ASD), and his parents. Drawing on Greenspan and Wieder's developmental individual-difference relationship-based (DIR) model, the therapy aimed to decipher Ori's emotional world, enhance parent–child communication, establish secure attachment, and expand his self-reflection. While initially focusing on the parent–child dyad, the treatment flexibly shifted to primarily individual therapy for Ori in later years, always maintaining parent involvement and ongoing connection with educational settings. Key therapeutic themes included coping with anxieties and fears, navigating identity between belonging and loneliness, and the significant role of an imaginary character, Hannah Zelda/Sheindel. Hannah Zelda served as a unique therapeutic partner, enabling Ori to express challenging emotions and gain a different perspective. This integrative, long-term intervention highlights the profound developmental capabilities of children with ASD through collaborative work, fostering Ori's growth into a sensitive, functional young adult who actively finds his place and continually discovers new abilities. The case underscores the success achievable through cooperative, flexible therapeutic partnerships.

Keywords Dyadic therapy · Parent–child relationship · Emotional development · Social integration · Imaginary character · Anxiety coping · Identity formation

Introduction

This chapter describes a case study of a decade-long dyadic therapeutic process between a treating psychologist (me), a young boy (Ori) diagnosed with high-functioning autism spectrum disorder (ASD), and his parents. Such dyadic interventions usually begin in early childhood, often when the child is in elementary

---

N. Felsenthal-Berger (✉)
Educational Psychology Service, Municipality of Jerusalem, Jerusalem, Israel
e-mail: norfelb@gmail.com

S. Lowinger and S. Pearlman-Avnion (eds.), *Collaborative Care and Partnerships in Autism Diagnosis and Treatment*, Autism and Child Psychopathology Series,
https://doi.org/10.1007/978-3-032-07009-8_9

school. Various forms of dyadic therapy have been designed to help parents understand their child, form connections, establish secure attachment, expand mentalization, and improve parent–child communication in situations involving stress, trauma, vulnerability, and developmental challenges (Allen & Fonagy, 2006; Lieberman & Van Horn, 2008; Stern, 1995).

In the current case, which continued through Ori's childhood and early adolescence, the therapeutic goals included developing mutual family discourse, assisting the parents in deciphering Ori's emotional world, and expanding his ability to engage in self-reflection as he matured. Professional discretion in such interventions is based on awareness of the difficulties that children and youth with ASD have in understanding and sharing their emotional world and their tendency to mindblindness (Baron-Cohen, 1995). The mutual integrative dialogue between the child and parents in this dyadic therapy enabled them to decipher his inner emotional world, improve and expand communication, and establish secure attachment.

The theoretical basis for the treatment drew on Greenspan and Wieder's (2006) developmental individual-difference relationship-based (DIR) model for therapy with children with ASD and their parents. The model broadens what is considered normative in the developmental stages. The therapy takes place within the parent–child relationship, by relating to the child's world and experiences and translating them into a coherent self-narrative. The DIR model interweaves the child's unique profile and current developmental stage with the significant relationships in the child's life. The treatment discussed in this chapter addressed the three advanced stages of Greenspan's developmental scale (stages 7, 8, and 9), which deal with connecting ideas to feelings, expanding the capacity for reflection, and understanding oneself and others.

There is some similarity between the DIR model and models of family therapy for adolescents dealing with depression that strive to develop parent–child attachment and work collaboratively with the adolescents and their parents (Diamond, 2005). As a child matures, the need for separation and independence increases, and the dyadic model must be reassessed to enable flexibility between joint family meetings and individual meetings with the adolescent or young adult.

An additional aspect of the treatment described in this chapter was an ongoing connection between the therapeutic partners and the educational settings in which the child studied. As the therapy provided a safe space for expressing and understanding emotional experiences, there was a need to connect those experiences to the expanding environment in which the child was learning and developing. Throughout the treatment, connections were maintained with the various social circles and systems in which Ori and his parents were involved. This integrative dialogue gave rise to mutually influencing partnerships that assisted his growth and development.

Yet another central long-term partner in the treatment was an imaginary character created by Ori (Fein, 2015). During some therapy sessions, the boy dressed as an ultra-Orthodox Jewish woman, whom he named Hannah Zelda (later also called Hannah Sheindel), who took the role of a counsellor. Stepping into her shoes enabled Ori to engage in insightful discourse about various challenges and daily dilemmas. This character existed between worlds and thus helped him regulate, gain strength, and reflect. It became apparent that immersion in this character served as a bridge between his inner and outer realities. This was a significant tool for Ori to express himself and allowed the therapeutic partners to understand and enter his world. The character is part of a Chanuka children's song; she is a religious character although Ori is from a secular background and in her way she bridged the gap between different worlds.

Case Study

I have been engaged in a weekly dyadic therapeutic intervention with Ori and his parents for ten years. When we first met, he was in third grade. Today, he is successfully doing national service at the National Library in Jerusalem.

While in kindergarten, Ori was diagnosed as being on the high-functioning end of the autism spectrum. He received therapeutic support based on the DIR method while in kindergarten and early elementary school. At first, the therapy sessions I conducted with Ori involved the parent–child dyad, but in recent years it has shifted to primarily individual therapy with Ori, with meetings including the parents as needed. Throughout his schooling, Ori has been integrated into regular educational settings in the public school system in Jerusalem, Israel. There has been ongoing contact between his parents, me, and the educational staff.

In the early years of therapy, the emphasis was on expanding play routines and using play to address everyday situations. Over time, the therapy integrated discourse to help Ori develop narratives about himself. This process showed the progress and development that a child with high-functioning ASD can achieve through collaborative work that involves the child and all the important others in his life. It is a hopeful story of development achieved through continuous work using multiple integrated therapeutic tools. The main message is that there is no limit to what becomes possible when therapeutic work is undertaken in an appropriately cooperative manner.

In this chapter, first, I present the therapeutic journey we undertook together in chronological order. Subsequently, I analyze five central themes that emerged from the therapeutic process: (1) the meaning of long-term dyadic therapy, (2) the connection between the therapeutic setting and the external reality, (3) coping with anxieties and fears, (4) an identity that lies between belonging and loneliness, and (5) the unique character of Hannah Zelda as a partner in the therapy. The analysis is supported by direct quotes from conversations with Ori and his parents.

Beginning of the Treatment: Contact and Expanding Play

When we met, Ori was a cute, smart, and talkative boy. He had social difficulties at school, especially with reciprocity during play and conversation. He dealt with anxieties about various issues. When Ori was in third and fourth grade, we gradually expanded his imaginary play into full scripts that included reciprocity and stories as part of the game. The treatment goals were to help Ori find his place, socially, and cope with his anxieties. One of his anxieties was the annual class trip. Together, we discussed what he thought were the most positive and negative scenarios possible for the trip. We imagined disasters along with positive fantasies.

We brought in the concept of "Riddikulus" from the Harry Potter books, which were favorites of his, so their language was familiar and connected to his life. In the Harry Potter books, Harry and his classmates at the wizarding school use the "Riddikulus" magic charm to deal with fear by making it ridiculous, invoking humor, and sharing their fear with other people to get help. For years, this term helped Ori face his challenges by looking at his fears with shared humor, flexible thinking, and creativity that broke down stereotypes and roadblocks. This helped him go on the class trip and have a positive experience.

During the therapy sessions toward the end of fourth grade, Ori created and dressed up as the character of an ultra-Orthodox Jewish woman he called Hannah Zelda. The name was taken from a Hanukkah song with lyrics mentioning "Hannah Zelda, my beloved wife" as well as from two compassionate and caring educational figures at Ori's school, his teacher and assistant, who were both named Hannah. The real-life assistant Hannah, an elderly Orthodox Jewish woman, was an important attachment figure for Ori, a kind of benevolent grandmother figure who supported him and believed in his abilities. The imaginary Hannah Zelda appeared in our therapy sessions for many years, taking on different forms and roles as she developed.

The Move: Coping with a New Home and Community

When Ori was entering fifth grade, his family moved from Jerusalem to a small suburban community outside the city. The move involved adjusting to a new home and a new school. At the end of fourth grade, we began to prepare for the planned move with Ori during therapy, alongside the family's preparations for the move. The local school in which he was to be enrolled claimed that the issue of integration was part of its mission and there were even signs hung in the entrance of the school building with motivational statements about integration. It was decided that our therapy would continue, although it involved travel, in order not to create too many changes at once.

The transition year was complicated for Ori and his family on a personal level. From the beginning, the family encountered rejection from the local community. At the class picnic, the other parents distanced themselves from the "strangers," and Ori and his family felt isolated at the event. Their feeling of alienation was perpetuated when Ori's parents were not allowed to contact the teaching assistant or speak at a parents' meeting about Ori's integration. His new homeroom teacher did not know how to help him integrate or what to expect. She did not understand his abilities and made belittling statements. For example, when Ori called himself a "human GPS," she perceived this as arrogance and said he was "getting above himself." She did not understand his sensory sensitivity either, which was sometimes expressed in outbursts in response to noise in the classroom or rambunctious games during breaks. The children in the class mocked Ori, and the school staff lacked concern and sympathy.

During this time, the character of Hannah Zelda developed in the therapy. Ori dressed up in a dress and a wig in the treatment room. At first, his parents reacted with discomfort, but I realized that this character had a role to play and a narrative that was important for us to hear. This was Ori's way of explaining his experiences during the therapy that he was unable to communicate directly. Ori needed a way to bridge his experience of alienation and isolation and to seek understanding. During this playacting in the therapy room, Hannah Zelda emerged as a victimized character, a new immigrant from Canada who had not succeeded in integrating into Israeli society and who was bullied by her peers. Clearly, through Hannah Zelda, Ori was telling us about his emotional experiences in school.

Around this time, other characters developed in the therapy. One was a snail who wrote the *Berlitz* Hebrew–English dictionary that helped Hannah Zelda learn Hebrew and helped others understand what she said. Another character, named Danny Rodney, was a tyrannical dictator who imposed his will without negotiation or explanation and whose solution to differences is to eliminate them. As Ori's isolation at school increased, Danny Rodney's influence during the therapy increased. At one point, Ori acted as the Danny Rodney character outside the therapy room, during a drama class at school. The teachers were horrified by this fictional character. They called a meeting to discuss Ori's condition, at which the possibility of psychotic behavior was raised. The staff members were unable to see this as a distress response and request for help by a boy who felt misunderstood.

After numerous unsuccessful attempts to work with the school, Ori's parents decided to move the family back to Jerusalem at the end of the school year. In the last few months of that school year, Hannah Zelda returned to therapy as a more complex character who was not simply a victim but discussed options, choices, and emotions as well as her ability to have an influence over them. In addition to the tool of the "Riddikulus" magic, Ori dealt with his school experiences and the teachers' mockery by putting on trial fictional characters who represented people at school. In an imaginary court, Ori could express the difficulties he underwent, validate his sense of insulation, laugh at the term "inappropriate" that they used against him, and reclaim his feelings and experiences. At the end of that year, Ori was accepted to the Jerusalem Experimental School for sixth grade. There, he was able to begin a process of rehabilitation and finding his place.

Rehabilitation and Growth at a School that Exhibited Flexibility

This section describes Ori's experience at the Jerusalem Experimental School and the processes that took place within the educational system and during the therapy.

From this, it is possible to observe and learn what behaviors help students with ASD integrate into the classroom and community.

Before the beginning of the school year, preliminary conversations were held between his parents and the school staff. Ori's new homeroom teacher visited the family at home, which Ori felt established a connection; as he said, "My teacher met my cat, too." This facilitated his process of entering and integrating into the classroom. A joint WhatsApp group was created through which Ori's parents, the school staff, and I could communicate and share our thoughts as necessary regarding our joint work with him.

The school's position was flexible, and they did not ignore Ori's challenges. By creating personal connections, they gradually helped him find ways to address his difficulties in sports and math classes. The school principal acknowledged Ori's special abilities as a "human GPS" and appointed him to a committee that planned the arrival of the school buses and shuttles. It became clear that Ori belonged to this school and was not there only for a trial period. When Ori went on the annual class trip, which lasted several days and nights, he was provided with food adapted to his special sensitivities, and an assistant accompanied him. Ori became secure enough to talk about himself and decided to tell the class about his social difficulties and communication disability. The decision emerged from a joint process in therapy and with the school staff. Ori decided when and what he wanted to share.

During this time, in the therapy room, Ori built a "Flexible School" structure that could stand on different sides and change shape. Hannah Zelda became a teacher at the Flexible School and continued to appear in the therapy sessions, now pushing a baby in a stroller. Hannah Zelda faced challenges as an Orthodox teacher at the Flexible School, but she became an integration teacher, and rather than being a victim, she helped her students by drawing on her own experience.

Danny Rodney became an "enlightened ruler" then, over time, disappeared from the therapy sessions. The issue of Ori's autistic identity as part of his general identity was explicitly addressed in treatment, and Ori came to terms with his unique characteristics, strengths, and difficulties. He recognized what helps him and what things he could influence. At school, he found his place, socially, in a directed filmmaking group that highlighted his areas of interest and abilities.

Onset of Puberty

Ori entered seventh grade in the Experimental School's new middle school and continued in this framework throughout high school. As he transitioned from elementary to middle school, there were changes in class composition, and Ori had to readjust to new students and teachers.

The shared WhatsApp group between me, his parents, and the staff continued to function, and at this age, Ori joined the group so he could be a partner in this process, and we could communicate directly with him. Ori continued to deal with fears and anxieties, such as learning English, and even a fear of chickens. We manage to overcome these fears by acknowledging them, building a shared plan of gradual exposure with a supportive adult, and using shared laughter and humor, inspired by the "Riddikulus" charm from Harry Potter.

The therapeutic relationship became a mutual dialogue. Ori was preoccupied with questions of identity and finding a social place, academics, and family issues. His ability to reflect developed significantly. He continued to dress up as Hannah Zelda in some therapy sessions, the costume and role play allowing for another perspective. Hannah Zelda became a well-rounded character with a family and children. She advised Ori on various issues, for example his crippling difficulty with learning English. The character would arrive, as for a consultation, and tell him, "You're not stupid, you're smart, but you don't always know it." Ori wrestled with questions about what he was good at, what he needed help with, how to overcome challenges, and how to find his social place. He developed a close friendship with a classmate. Ori processed and discussed these issues during the therapy.

When the COVID-19 pandemic broke out and schools moved to remote learning, we discussed the advantages and disadvantages of social distancing, namely, loneliness versus protection from disease. During the pandemic, Ori wrote a book about the character of Hannah Zelda, her family, and her life history. He interviewed me and his parents and asked us to reflect on the character of Hannah Zelda and he wrote about what this character meant to him. He titled the book *Mary Poppins in a Headscarf*, expressing the support that the character of Hannah Zelda provided for him. He printed several copies and gave them to close friends. At one point, he decided to change her name to Hannah Sheindel; *sheindel* is a Yiddish word meaning "beautiful."

Toward the end of high school, Ori wanted to expand his social circles, so he joined the local branch of a communist youth movement. He made significant social connections and successfully participated in movement activities. That same year, Ori developed and experimented with romantic relationships, which we also discussed in therapy. In his final year of high school, we discussed questions about his future, such as whether to do army service or national service, and what would be most appropriate for him. Questions of identity and belonging in the context of ASD arose (Bagatelle, 2007; Belek, 2018).

Young Adulthood

At the end of 12th grade, after successfully passing his final exams, Ori began a year of national service at the National Library of Israel, located in Jerusalem. The decision to do national service was not easy, but eventually Ori began working in the scanning department at the National Library as part of a program called Otzma, whose goal is to assist people with ASD while doing national service. The position at the National Library suited Ori very well. He found working at the library fulfilling, created a meaningful connection with his supervisor, displayed great responsibility, and formed connections with other library employees. Ori felt that he had found a rewarding place in his world.

Nevertheless, difficulties arose in the context of identity and group affiliation. Ori did not feel a sense of belonging with the Otzma program support group or with those in the program who had studied in special education settings. At the same time, he did not fit in with the regular national service group. Ori defined himself as "falling between the chairs" and not belonging to either group. His ongoing difficulty in finding his place repeatedly emerged in the therapy.

Ori began learning to drive. As with many new experiences over the years, this decision aroused anxiety and ambivalence. Initially, Ori wanted to avoid the challenge because anxiety gave rise to a feeling of paralysis. He underwent a process of overcoming the anxiety, using approaches like those we had used from the early stages of his therapy. Ori's ability to communicate, explain himself, and reflect on the things that help him has expanded significantly over the years. Passing the driving test was challenging, especially after a failure that renewed his struggle with anxiety. Ori got his driver's license and gained experience driving outside the city, including a drive of several hours to the Sea of Galilee to meet his best friend from school and spend time with the members of his friend's youth group.

Ori explored options for the upcoming year, including academic studies and additional places to do national service. Eventually, he decided to do a second year of national service at the National Library. The library staff highly valued him and wanted him to stay so they offered him opportunities for advancement and development. He described the library as a positive place that is a microcosm of the surrounding reality. He established personal contacts with the library staff and even with readers and researchers who came there.

Currently, Ori is thinking about his future. He wants to continue his education and move out of his parents' home. He is seeking information and visiting different campuses. He is interested in various fields, including history, geography, the Middle East, and urban planning. His social challenges still exist, and we are working to help him find a sense of belonging among a group of peers.

Central Themes in Therapy

Five themes emerged as the building blocks of the therapy over time, which will be discussed in this section: (1) long-term dyadic therapy, (2) ongoing connection between the inner and external reality, (3) coping with anxieties and fears, (4) identity between belonging and loneliness, and (5) the character of Hannah Zelda as a partner in the therapy.

Dyadic Therapy

Dyadic parent–child therapy was the long-term therapeutic approach. In the past several years, the focus shifted to individual therapy with Ori and parent–child dyadic sessions as needed. It is based on Greenspan and Wieder's (1998, 2006) DIR therapeutic approach to integrated parent–child therapy for dealing with communication disabilities, in which the parents are active partners who can integrate the child's daily experiences outside the therapy room. The emphasis is to draw on the child's experiences and expand the scope of dialogue to increase reciprocity and mutual understanding.

Stern (1995) and Lieberman and van Horn (2008) emphasized the ability of dyadic therapy to affect the parent–child bond in real time, enabling it to be expanded and fine-tuned, to deepen the sense of secure attachment. It provides an opportunity for the parents and child to work on mutual understanding and mentalization, and (as age appropriate) to help the child understand the perspectives of the parents and significant others in various situations.

Dyadic therapy was chosen due to its emphasis on strengthening the bond between Ori and his parents and to provide insights into his inner world and experiences. Children and adolescents with ASD often have trouble regulating their emotional responses and they are often misunderstood by others in their social environment. The treatment deciphered his emotions and connected them to the challenges of everyday life. This therapy deepened the mentalization of Ori and his parents, created secure attachment, expanded Ori's narrative about himself, and improved his ability to have an impact and self-agency over his story, in partnership with his parents.

Ori's parents attested that the dyadic therapy created partnership, commitment, and a family culture that could not have been created with any other therapeutic model. Other models may create parallel systems and a subsequent breakdown of power relations. The dyadic therapy created a protected space with rules in which the family could engage in joint problem-solving with the therapist, enabling thoughts and dialogue about courses of action.

The joint meetings created the possibility of deciphering the situation during crises, the origin of which was often difficult to understand. As Ori matured, he was given greater control over the situation and had greater self-agency in therapeutic space. At each stage, the dyadic fit was re-examined with flexibility regarding choices. Greenspan's principle to "follow the child's lead" was maintained throughout the treatment.

Ori's father noted that the dyadic therapy also influenced his professional development as a teacher and his relationships with his students and their parents. Ori said he appreciated the coordination and partnership in the dyadic therapy, which offered the possibility of an immediate response, without an intermediary. He said that he has matured with age, and the dyad has become more equal.

Ongoing Connection Between the Inner and Outer Reality

The therapy provided a space in which Ori's emotional experience could be understood, deciphered, and validated. There was a constant connection with the outer reality, mainly at Ori's school, an environment in which he had to learn to cope. Interconnected tools and a therapeutic partnership were therapeutic cornerstones that enabled Ori's progress and the success of the therapy. There was a two-way process of understanding his emotional experiences and connecting them to the school, while simultaneously understanding what was happening at school and connecting those events to his emotions. The therapy could be likened to an accordion that contracts and expands.

Throughout the treatment, Ori was integrated into a regular classroom setting (not special education). The treatment addressed the challenges of integration and included ongoing contact with the educational staff who supported Ori at school. The treatment included tools that linked his inner world and the external reality, with Ori's parents, and between the family system and the educational system. I believe that the success of the treatment was due to the joint use of tools that enabled the integration of all of Ori's worlds and their mutual influences.

When a therapeutic partnership functioned, with shared thinking and problem-solving, including communication with his parents and the educational team (for example, through the WhatsApp group), things went well. When the partnership was disrupted, there was a general deterioration in Ori's emotional and social state.

Ori's parents said that they decided to integrate him into regular education starting from kindergarten out of a desire to help him function in normal society. I asked what had been helpful in the integration process, and they noted systems in which people were ready to learn and relate to his abilities, interests, and strengths, and did not give up on helping him overcome his difficulties. They emphasized that educational systems in which integration was successful were those that had a personal approach and customized support system that created connections, such as through home visits. The staff at such schools took responsibility and listened to the students' parents so they could overcome obstacles together.

An example of the differing approaches to integration in the two educational systems Ori encountered pertained to his extraordinary navigational ability. In one school, he was told he was "getting above himself," while in the second, he was included in a committee for planning a transportation system. This shows the difference between fear and minimizing his abilities versus giving him the space and leverage to find meaning in the school environment. Another example was seen in the communication styles of the various parties. One system prohibited daily contact with the aide, holding meetings only when a crisis erupted. The second system held regular meetings and communicated through a WhatsApp group between all the involved parties, including the student himself.

In my interview with Ori, he said that throughout his schooling, he took it for granted that he would be integrated into regular educational settings. He saw himself as part of the school culture. He felt seen by the staff and knew he always had someone to turn to. He had contact with children who were not "mainstream." He said that the school's flexibility helped him.

As a psychologist, I saw the connection with the educational system as an integral part of the treatment. This included discussions about his school experiences during the sessions and ongoing contact with the educational team, based on becoming acquainted with each other and thinking together. The therapeutic setting is also important to improve understanding and deepening of the child's inner world and relationships. At the same time, the connection with the system is essential for progress.

Coping with Anxieties and Fears

One of the challenges of the treatment was dealing with Ori's persistent anxieties and fears. Over time, our therapeutic approach was clarified and could be discussed directly with Ori as he matured. Children and youth with ASD often deal with anxieties and fears as they attempt to cope with and decipher a world that is not completely understandable to them and with people who often misunderstand them. Many children and youth with ASD also have sensitivity to noise or other sensory stimuli. Being overwhelmed by anxiety can lead to paralysis and avoidance of triggering stimuli.

Throughout the years of therapy, Ori dealt with various anxieties such as going on the annual field trip every year, academic subjects he had difficulty with, noise during recess, sports lessons, a fear of animals (chickens and dogs), and more recently, driving lessons and passing the driving test. My pet Labrador retrievers gave us opportunities to work directly with Ori to overcome his fear of dogs. We progressed from careful exposure outside to approaching the animal to a wonderful friendship with dogs, each of which has its own character. Ori was helped by the "Riddikulus" charm, the ability to mock and laugh at fear, while approaching and controlling it by taking small steps with the support of a trusted adult. In this way, Ori was able to cope with most of his challenges while gaining a sense of control over the situation.

Identity Between Loneliness and Belonging: Falling Between the Chairs

One of the themes that emerged in the therapy and occupied Ori over the years was the feelings of loneliness versus belonging. These issues arose from the beginning of the therapy when he was in the third grade and intensified significantly when he moved outside of Jerusalem. We continued to deal with it throughout his adolescence and young adulthood. One of the primary challenges for children and adolescents with ASD is finding a social group where they truly feel they belong. The difficulty intensifies with the complexity of social coping during adolescence.

In his teenage years, Ori found a social group in the communist youth movement. When he began his national service at the National Library, he was part of the Otzma group for special education students. He wanted to find a place and a sense of belonging, but felt that he fell between the "regular" group and the special education group. He did create a meaningful and positive sense of belonging with library staff members and several of his peers. Ori processed his feelings of difference and belonging through the character of Hannah Zelda, and this helped him find solutions.

Ori learned about ASD and considered autism to be part of his identity, but not as defining his entire identity. Other people could better understand his abilities and difficulties in the context of his diagnosis; at the same time, it was important for Ori to maintain control over when and with whom he shared the diagnosis. The most significant messages of the treatment were that he could have self-agency, explain himself, make choices, and generally create the narrative of his life.

The Character of Hannah Zelda/Sheindel

Ori created an imaginary character, an ultra-Orthodox woman named Hannah Zelda, later renamed Hannah Sheindel. He would dress up in a wig and clothes kept at the clinic for that purpose, and at one point, she arrived with a stroller and a doll. In this section, I analyze her development and what she represented in the eyes of Ori and his parents. On a theoretical level, it is difficult to categorize Hannah Zelda as an alter ego or imaginary friend, and she has characteristics of both. At first, his parents were unsettled by her appearance. She seemed bizarre to them. However, I felt we should listen to what Ori said through her voice, as she became a significant channel for him.

Initially, she was a humorous character named for a woman in a song and for his teacher and assistant, both named Hannah. Hannah Zelda spoke about her experiences as a new immigrant who was bullied. This enabled Ori to indirectly share feelings that he could not express directly. After the family moved back to Jerusalem, Hannah Zelda transformed from a victim figure to a teacher and change agent at the "Flexible School." She became a knowledgeable and supportive figure. In his teens, Ori wrote a biography about her titled *Mary Poppins in the Headscarf*, indicating her role as a companion and enabler. Ori would occasionally "invite" Hannah Zelda for consultations on issues he was struggling with. Then Ori would disguise himself as Hannah Zelda and have her converse with his parents and therapist. She became a moderating and supportive advisory figure in the therapy, enabling Ori to mentalize his struggles. Stepping into her shoes gave Ori a different perspective on issues that were troubling him.

Prior to writing this article, I "interviewed" Hannah Zelda. Through her, Ori said she was a vehicle for him to express things he didn't want to say or didn't know how to express. She said things that he would have had difficulty saying directly to his parents, or that he would have trouble explaining. As Hannah Zelda, he would refer to Ori in the third person, which allowed him to calmly observe himself from the outside, even in stressful situations. Speaking in Hannah's voice, he said that at first, Ori's parents treated Hannah as strange, but over time, they learned to accept her and understand that she helped Ori: "We understood together that I was a tool for expressing painful things."

Hannah Zelda, a figure enabling reflection and mentalization, believes in Ori's abilities. She views autism as a different way of experiencing the world, not a disability. She does not see autism as rooted in limitations and does not think that Ori's autism limits him. Rather, she says, adjustments and attention may be needed to help him. She said she hoped that eventually Ori would find a place that suits him at the library or at a university, that he would have friends, a romantic partner, and a job.

Conclusion

These wishes expressed hopeful attitudes as the therapy drew to a close. Over the course of ten years, I worked with Ori and his parents in a partnership in which everyone contributed and simultaneously influenced and was influenced by each other. The connections made in this therapeutic partnership helped Ori to develop into a sensitive, curious, and responsible young adult who learns and functions in the community, is valued, continually discovers new abilities, and thinks about his future.

This case study documents how children with ASD can progress through treatment that helps them understand their inner world and cope with the constant challenges of their daily reality. The description of this decade-long therapeutic case illustrates the developmental abilities of children with ASD and the possibility of influencing their development through a meaningful, integrative intervention. Inspiring growth and development occurred as a result of the long-term parent–child dyadic therapy, coupled with ongoing contact with the educational system, enabled connection with the child's complex and interesting emotional world, which included an imaginary character who played a significant role in it.

This perspective can be applied in a broad context. The meaningful journey and connections allowed a child with ASD to navigate finding his place in the world while dealing with his challenges and communication difficulties. I thank Ori, his parents, and Hannah Zelda/Sheindel for the opportunity to accompany them on this inspiring journey.

References

Allen, J. A., & Fonagy, P. (2006). *Handbook of mentalization-based treatment*. John Wiley.
Bagatelle, N. (2007). Orchestrating voices: Autism, identity and the power of discourse. *Disability and Society, 22*(4), 413–426. https://doi.org/10.1080/09687590701337967
Baron-Cohen, S. (1995). *Mindblindness: An essay on autism and theory of mind*. MIT Press.
Belek, B. (2018). Autism and the proficiency of social ineptitude: Probing the rules of "appropriate" behavior. *Ethos, 46*(2), 161–179. https://doi.org/10.1111/etho.12202
Diamond, G. S. (2005). Attachment-based family therapy for depressed and suicidal adolescents. In J. Lebow (Ed.), *Handbook of clinical family therapy* (pp. 17–41). Wiley & Sons.
Fein, E. (2015). Making meaningful worlds: Role-playing subcultures and the autism spectrum. *Culture, Medicine, and Psychiatry, 39*(2), 299–321. https://doi.org/10.1007/s11013-015-9443-x
Greenspan, S. I., & Wieder, S. (1998). *The child with special needs: Encouraging intellectual and emotional growth*. Perseus Books.
Greenspan, S. I., & Wieder, S. (2006). *Engaging autism: Helping children relate, communicate and think with the DIR floortime approach*. Da Capo Lifelong Books.
Lieberman, A. F., & Van Horn, P. (2008). Psychotherapy with *infants and young children: Repairing the effects of stress and trauma on early attachment*. Guilford.
Stern, D. N. (1995). *The motherhood constellation: A unified view of parent-infant psychotherapy*. Routledge.

Chapter 10
Shared Experiences Across Time: Effects on Growth and Development

Arava Mizrahi-Zinman

Abstract This chapter explores the crucial role of meaningful shared experiences in the development of autistic children, emphasizing their unique ways of organizing the world that can lead to challenges in interpersonal interactions. It proposes a cognitive framework for therapeutic interventions by examining how autistic children develop these experiences across three temporal spaces: the shared future (goals, intentions), the shared present (engaging in activities), and the shared past (autobiographical memories). The chapter stresses that while consistent experiences and emotional dialogue are vital for all children, autistic children often face difficulties in areas such as aligning intentions with others, coordinating actions in real-time, and forming coherent autobiographical memories. Drawing on concepts like event representation (scenarios) and joint intentionality, the chapter illustrates these challenges and the therapeutic approach through the case study of Roi. Strategies employed include utilizing familiar routines, sensorimotor engagement, verbal conceptualization, and tangible documentation (e.g., memory boxes/memoirs) to foster connection, predictability, and the development of a continuous sense of self. This approach aims to bridge gaps in shared meaning and support social development by weaving together experiences across time.

Keywords Shared experiences · Temporal spaces · Autobiographical memory · Joint intentionality · Social development

A. Mizrahi-Zinman (✉)
Department of Communication Sciences and Disorders, Ono Academic College, Kiryat Ono, Israel
e-mail: arava@nux.ai

Kesher Project, Ministry of Education, Jerusalem, Israel

S. Lowinger and S. Pearlman-Avnion (eds.), *Collaborative Care and Partnerships in Autism Diagnosis and Treatment*, Autism and Child Psychopathology Series,
https://doi.org/10.1007/978-3-032-07009-8_10

Introduction

Every child's development is influenced by consistent and meaningful experiences and emotional dialogue with significant others in their lives. While the development of autistic children, like that of their neurotypical peers, is shaped by cumulative significant relationships, they often experience and organize their world in distinctive ways, offering perspectives that differ from neurotypical norms. These differences can result in challenges when navigating interpersonal interactions, as their experiences can feel fragmented or lack coherent connections.

Shared moments of connection with autistic children can be precious, elusive, and therefore highly sought-after. Individuals working closely with autistic children recognize the profound impact these moments can have. These shared experiences are pivotal because most early learning occurs through human interaction during the first years of life, a period when foundational cognitive and social skills are formed. Therefore, establishing such experiences is a central and essential goal in the treatment of autistic children, as it creates opportunities for authentic connection and mutual understanding while respecting each child's individuality (Greenspan & Wieder, 2006; Steinman & Dromi, 2007).

Meaningful shared experiences are not confined to the present; they also exist in the past and future. This chapter explores how autistic children develop meaningful shared experiences across these three temporal spaces: past, present, and future.

1. **Shared Future**: The ability to share goals, intentions, and action plans, fostering a meaningful shared future (Sebanz et al., 2006; Tomasello et al., 2005; Warneken et al., 2012).
2. **Shared Present**: The ability to engage in shared activities, creating a meaningful present (Adamson & Bakeman, 2006; Stern, 2002; Trevarthen, 2008).
3. **Shared Past**: The ability to form autobiographical memories, enabling shared meaning of the past (Fivush, 2011; Williams & Conway, 2009).

These temporal spaces are crucial for social development. They help children connect meaningful events with actions, sensations, thoughts, and feelings, of their own and others. By participating in such experiences, children gradually build an understanding of themselves, of others, of relationships, and of how to navigate the world around them.

While the existing literature has examined each of these temporal spaces individually, this chapter brings them together as a unified clinical framework, highlighting their interdependence in shaping shared meaning for autistic children. By exploring how these dimensions interact in everyday experiences, the chapter offers a perspective that may support both theoretical understanding and practical reflection. In doing so, it lays the groundwork for clinical application—offering guiding principles for how therapy sessions can be structured to help autistic children move meaningfully between past, present, and future experiences.

The chapter first presents a theoretical basis for children's ability to represent events. Next, I will discuss how the three temporal spaces exist within the experiences and events in which children take part. These spaces will be illustrated through a clementine-picking event that took place during the care of Roi, a five-year-old child with high-functioning autism. At the end of the theoretical section, Roi's case is presented to demonstrate how these three spaces were expressed in different ways over the years during which he was treated.

Children's Ability to Represent Events

Humans have the unique ability to represent events in their memory (Schank & Abelson, 1977/2013, 1995/2014). Over time, they develop knowledge about those events and build a representation of them, which serves as a script or general scenario. The ability to represent knowledge through scenarios makes cognitive processes more efficient and economical. People organize their knowledge and memory about the world as a sequence of events and stories and use them to interpret and understand their experiences. For example, if someone is asked which kitchen items are needed to make orange juice, most would not recall a structured list, such as are given in recipe books. Instead, details are deduced from remembered scenarios and representations of making orange juice: first, the orange must be cut, so a knife and a cutting board are needed; then the fruit must be squeezed using a juicer; finally, the juice must be poured into a glass to drink. The equipment needed emerges, not from categorical sorting, but within the framework of a meaningful script that follows a sequence of interconnected actions. Further, people do not make orange juice the same way every time; it can be done with an electric juicer, a manual juicer, or squeezed by hand, but people have a general and flexible representation of the event, and some steps or variables may be left blank. Representations of events help people understand what is happening around them. They enable people to operate in a familiar environment and anticipate what will happen in what order, the purpose of the event, who will play which roles, what objects will be used, cause-and-effect, and what social relationships will be involved.

Representations help people understand and interpret events they have not yet experienced. For example, the first time someone makes lemonade, they can draw on the knowledge gained from making orange juice. The first time someone attends a picnic, they draw on the knowledge acquired from the dinner scenario and arrive with a set of expectations, some of which will be fulfilled and some of which will not be fulfilled. Operating within a familiar representation allows more cognitive resources to be directed toward learning.

Nelson (1986, 1989) incorporated Shank and Abelson's conclusions into her research on child cognition. Nelson argued that the field, at her time, focused on what children do not know and are unable to do. Nelson thought that research on child cognition should focus on what children do understand about what is happening around them. Nelson studied how children represent familiar events and content and how their knowledge changes as they gain new experiences. She found that children, as early as in their first year of life, construct mental representations of a particular scenario based on repeated experiences and events in their daily lives. These mental representations facilitate learning, as repeated experiences allow children to build on previous knowledge and allocate resources to learning new things.

The first comprehensive program to use cognitive event scripts from daily routines as a framework for therapeutic intervention with children was developed as part of the Kesher Project in Israel (Dromi, 2018; Dromi & Ringwald-Frimerman, 1996; Dromi et al., 2003, 2009). The idea that experiences should be embedded within a clear framework of structured events is gradually gaining traction, both in general education and more specifically in therapeutic work with children on the autism spectrum.

When implementing this framework in interventions with autistic children, it must be remembered that many of them are not able to organize every experience into a stable set of meanings and succeed in coordinating their bodies and minds during joint activity (Sebanz & Knoblich, 2021; Sebanz et al., 2006).

Often, during professional visits to kindergartens for autistic children, I observe activities initiated by educational therapists in which events are used to create meaningful shared experiences. For example, I observed a group activity that revolved around making potato pancakes. This activity was an event scenario as defined by Schank and Abelson (1977/2013) and later by Nelson (1986): a sequence of events in time and space that lead toward a goal. The children carried out the kindergarten teacher's instructions with the mediation of accompanying educational therapists. They watched the teacher's demonstrations and performed a relatively complex series of actions: peeling and grating potatoes, then mixing and seasoning them. They participated in a joint event and carried out a sequence of actions toward a specific, shared goal. Nevertheless, one could sense that something fundamental was missing, creating an impression of a widening gap between what the educational therapists and the kindergarten teacher were trying to achieve and what happened. Understanding and knowledge are embedded through a shared experience, not by achieving results. Although the children successfully made potato pancakes, the real goal of the activity—creating a meaningful learning experience with others—may have been missed. To better understand these missed opportunities for shared meaning-making, we can examine the challenges the children may have faced through the lens of the three temporal dimensions of experience: future, present, and past.

Future: Were the children making potato pancakes together able to represent and predict the sequence of actions to be realized and the goal to which these actions would lead? Were they able to form mental representations of collaborative actions and of intentions and goals shared with others?

Present: To what extent were the children able to coordinate their actions with those of other children? Could they coordinate their thoughts and physical behavior? Could they share affective and cognitive meanings? Could they share their feelings and emotions with each other?

Past: What did the children remember about what happened? Did they only remember sensorimotor sensations and facts (such as the order of actions to accomplish the goal)? Could they include autobiographical memories of their own experiences and those they shared with others? Were their memories embedded in accompanying emotions and thoughts? Were they able to talk about and process their memories? If so, how?

Shared Future: The Ability to Share Goals, Intentions, and Action Plans

The activity in the kindergarten provided clear goals: making and eating potato pancakes. The children had to understand the purpose and intention of their actions as individuals and as part of a group. This can be challenging for autistic children who may find it difficult to understand and be attentive to others' intentions. The children were engaged in a well-defined sequence of actions, including peeling, grating, mixing, and seasoning, to achieve their shared objective. This collaborative effort necessitated working with others, emphasizing the importance of teamwork and coordination. It raised important questions. Was the goal evident to the children? Did they fully grasp how their individual and collective actions contributed to achieving the shared objective? Understanding the purpose of their actions and the overarching plan was crucial, as it aided in predicting future steps.

Participating in joint activities with shared goals and plans requires children to have the ability to predict future events for themselves and others, interactions between them, and the overall outcomes of their coordinated efforts. If given a structured social framework that provides meaningful context and careful scaffolding, children can communicate and share goals and plans, practice collaboration, and develop more accurate and adaptable predictive abilities in complex social situations.

Tomasello's pioneering work focused on the origins of social thinking, language, and cooperation, and provides an important foundation. According to the evolutionary account proposed by Tomasello (2005, 2009, 2014), humans have motivations and cognitive abilities to collaborate and achieve collective objectives, a unique feature that distinguishes them from other primates.

Tomasello introduced the concept of *joint intentionality*, which I refer to in this chapter as *shared action plans*. This refers to the ability to share intentions and coordinate actions with others to achieve a common goal. This capacity, which begins developing in early childhood, involves coordinating attention with other people to share goals, intentions, and psychological states, ultimately fostering cooperative actions (Brownell et al., 2006; Cerullo et al., 2021; Gilbert, 2009). This capacity is underpinned by three key abilities that emerge during these formative years (Pacherie, 2011; Sebanz & Knoblich, 2021; Sebanz et al., 2006; Warneken et al., 2012). The first is the ability to see themselves as agents with a purpose. The second is the ability to see other people as separate agents with their own goals, intentions, and action plans. The third is the ability to work collaboratively on shared goals, intentions, and action plans.

Tomasello (2005) defined four stages of a goal-oriented activity:

1. Goal: Formulating a mental representation of a change in the environment (e.g., opening a closed box).
2. Intention: Choosing a plan of action to achieve the goal and selecting an approach (e.g., using a key to open the box or breaking it).
3. Realization: Implementing the plan of action to achieve the goal (e.g., realizing the purpose by using the key).
4. Control: Perceiving the environment after the plan's implementation and assessing whether the goal was achieved or if another plan is needed (e.g., if the key doesn't fit or it is not possible to break the box).

Each participant's goal and action plan must be related to the other participants' purposes and action plans. Participants must respond to each other, share ideas about achieving the goal together, and can coordinate intentions in a mutually clear way.

Autistic Children's Ability to Participate in Joint Actions with Shared Goals

The topic of joint action with shared goals among people with autism has not been well explored. Only a handful of studies have addressed it (Cerullo et al., 2021). These studies indicate that the capacity of autistic children to participate in joint actions and coordinate efforts with others to achieve shared goals can be challenging. While these studies found that autistic children were able to recognize themselves and others as independent agents with distinct intentions and plans, their intentions did not always align with those of others (Fulceri et al., 2018; Liebal et al., 2008). Even when they were attentive toward others' intentions and shared goals, the studies found they had difficulty bridging this with coordination and attunement during collaborative efforts in real-time (Colombi et al., 2009; Fitzpatrick et al., 2013).

Boria et al. (2009) found that while autistic children can recognize the immediate goals of others' actions, such as grasping an object, they often struggle to infer the broader intentions or reasons behind the action. Such findings reveal challenges in grasping the "why" behind observed actions. In peer-to-peer contexts, autistic children performed better in tasks with nonsocial partners, such as computer-based systems, than during interactions with peers (Bar Yehuda & Bauminger-Zviely, 2024). This underscores how the added social demands of peer collaboration amplify coordination challenges. Trevisan et al. (2021) examined joint action and found that under child–child conditions, autistic children showed poorer action coordination and less synchronous movement, but their performance improved markedly in child–adult interactions, underscoring the importance of scaffolding and support from adults who provide clear instructions, step-by-step guidance, and structured environments that reduce ambiguity and foster alignment of actions.

Another body of research that can shed light on the challenges faced by autistic children in representing and sharing joint actions with others is predictive coding theory (see NeuroLaunch, 2024). According to the theory of predictive coding (also called predictive processing), the human brain constantly generates predictions based on sensory information and updates these predictions based on new experiences. It generates and updates models to anticipate sensory inputs, comparing these predictions with actual experiences to minimize discrepancies. This mechanism allows for efficient perception, learning, and interaction with the environment.

In autistic children, predictive coding processes may function differently. Research indicates that individuals with autism may assign atypical precision to sensory inputs and prediction errors, leading to challenges in forming accurate predictions about the world. This can result in difficulties in adapting to new situations and complex social and sensory situations. Social interactions, which require rapid predictions and understanding of others' intentions and behaviors, can be particularly affected by these differences (Ganglmayer et al., 2019). This underscores the importance of tailored interventions to address predictive challenges.

Roi was my patient for five years. His case is described in detail later in the chapter. This section describes a clementine-picking scenario that served as a framework for a meaningful shared experience between him, his mother, and me. Roi would come to treatments with one of his parents. Near the clinic there was a clementine tree and his father would pick himself a clementine to eat while waiting for the session to start. On one visit, Roi came with his mother. I suggested we go outside and pick a clementine to take to his father. This goal seemed meaningful to Roi, and he excitedly broke into a run across the yard. Although he had not previously picked clementines by himself, this activity was not new to him. Roi understood and could predict what would happen based on previous experiences in which he had reached objects in high places (experiences that he enjoyed, like hanging up a hammock or catching helium balloons) and watching his father picking clementines. Roi had a general representation of the event from which he could build a set of expectations and interpret the actions of the other participants.

This point is significant when thinking about treatments for autistic children who tend to avoid changes and new situations that cause them anxiety and tend to act in repetitive and limited ways. New activities that are embedded in their daily routines and are based on familiar previous events can help them feel a sense of security and stability. Roi was able to undertake actions that were familiar to him, and he agreed with my suggestion that we should pick the clementine together. This defined a shared goal for Roi, his mother, and me.

First, we all looked at the tree, searching for the lowest clementine that would be easy to reach. Roi's mother found one on a low branch and pointed to it to get our attention. Roi followed her finger point and intention. He then began to jump in an attempt to reach it. I watched his action and started jumping too and reaching my hands toward the clementine. He watched me and continued to jump energetically, stretching his arm. In this way, we communicated our common goal. We tried to understand each other's plan of action and shared intentions.

Shared Present: The Ability to Engage in Shared Activities to Create a Meaningful Present

The question of how people share meanings, ultimately shaping the distinctive world we inhabit, has fascinated philosophers, theorists, and researchers for centuries and remains a topic of exploration and debate. Humans have the remarkable ability to share and preserve the essence of experiences, actions, events, and ideas, forming the foundation of our personal and collective memories. These shared meanings are embedded in language, culture, and social norms, all of which have evolved over time.

When does this capacity to share experiences begin? Some researchers suggest that this ability is present from birth. Even in the first weeks and months of life, infants engage in dyadic patterns, participating in shared content and meaning with their parents. They alternate making sounds, smiles, looks, and movements, building a dynamic and emotionally rich dialogue characterized by predictable patterns. This mutual regulation of interactions fosters bonding, emotional connection, and the development of increasingly complex communication. The early ability, nurtured within the intimate parent–child relationship, forms the bedrock for more complex forms of shared understanding as the child develops (Beebe et al., 2000; Shai & Fonagy, 2013; Stern, 1985, 2002, 2010; Tomasello & Carpenter, 2007).

Trevarthen's research (2008) offered a profound understanding of how shared meaning begins to emerge in infancy. He illuminated how infants and parents co-create actions within a shared interactive space, continuously adjusting to one another. Turn-taking, he showed, is not merely about alternating sounds or movements with similar timing, rhythm, emotional tone, and similar levels of arousal. Turn-taking is not only about acting in turns—it's about listening to each other and being open to influence. Turn-taking is about truly observing and embracing the other's actions, allowing themselves to be shaped by the partner's actions, and responding with variations that reflect and build upon what the other has expressed. Without this kind of mutual listening, Trevarthen might have observed only monotonic exchanges—not a living symphony of interaction. These evolving, responsive exchanges form a dynamic and adaptive process that gives rise to shared creations of coherent narratives with a beginning, middle, and end.

Mutual creations persist throughout childhood, evolving as children develop communicative skills and begin to sustain episodes of triadic interactions during which they share objects and events with a social partner (Bakeman & Adamson, 1984). As children progress in mastering language, they increasingly infuse symbols into episodes of joint engagement (Adamson et al., 2004), broadening their focus to encompass words and references to events that extend beyond the immediate context (Adamson & Bakeman, 2006). This progression is crucial for developing joint intentions, as children start to understand and participate in shared goals and collaborative activities.

Children constantly face the challenge of sustaining mutual interactions that involve taking turns, co-creating experiences, maintaining attentiveness, and responding to one another, not only through their emotions and sensorimotor actions, but also through their desires, intentions, thoughts, and beliefs. These elements are expressed both verbally and non-verbally, creating a kind of musical symphony that is also a mental one. A symphony that enables the exchange of complex ideas and the building of shared meanings, underpinning the fluidity and connection of joint activities.

The Ability to Engage in Shared Activities with Shared Meanings in Autistic Children

Among autistic children, processes of early interaction and shared meaning formation may diverge significantly from those observed in children with typical development. Young children exhibiting signs of autism spectrum disorder demonstrate delays or disruptions in joint attention and coordinated engagement. Autistic children often have less accurate and less frequent alignment of their motor and dialogue behaviors with interaction partners (McNaughton & Redcay, 2020). This is compounded by atypical processing in sensorimotor systems and a decreased tendency to adapt to others' actions, leading to disrupted rhythm, intensity, and timing during exchanges (Cerullo et al., 2021). Adults' scaffolding efforts may not consistently elicit reciprocal responses, resulting in fragmented interactions rather than the dynamic flow typical of mutual regulation (Bottema-Beutel et al., 2014).

Autistic children often spend less time in coordinated joint engagement that involves actively integrating attention between a partner, objects, and events, as compared to their typically developing peers. They often spend more time in object-focused engagement with limited interaction with partners (Adamson et al., 2009). Language-infused joint engagement, crucial for expanding communication scope, is notably less frequent in autistic children, mainly due to difficulties in integrating symbols and shared references into their interactions (Bottema-Beutel et al., 2014).

Additionally, deficits in social orienting, such as reduced attention to facial expressions and gestures, hinder the ability to engage in meaningful synchrony with others. Autistic children often exhibit atypical temporal coordination during joint actions, further impeding the attunement of shared emotions and complex communication (Bowsher-Murray et al., 2022). These patterns suggest a fundamental difficulty in achieving the integrated interplay required for joint action and co-created meaning.

Despite these challenges, targeted interventions have demonstrated promise in supporting these developmental domains. Approaches focusing on emphasizing interpersonal synchrony and enhancing joint attention through supported engagement have been shown to improve social communication outcomes (Greenspan & Wieder, 2006; Kasari et al., 2010).

After Roi, his mother, and I defined a shared goal together, Roi came up with something: an idea for how to achieve it. His plan of action was to jump. I stood beside him and was attentive to his idea, as expressed through his actions. I jumped alongside him and raised my hands. This was my way of showing Roi that I was listening to him and being influenced by his actions.

Roi noticed what I was doing and how it corresponded with his own movements. He jumped again with even more energy, stretching his arms as far as he could, adjusting his activity to coordinate with mine. Still, this didn't help us reach our goal. I tried to climb the tree but slipped. Roi, influenced by my idea and behavior, watched me closely and then tried to climb as well—but he also slipped.

Then Roi had a new idea. He asked me to pick him up. I listened to him but explained that I wasn't willing to do that because my back hurt. Instead, I suggested that he pick me up. It was my way of responding to his idea with a playful variation. He agreed and tried to lift me but couldn't. His mother joined him, and together we fell to the ground and got a little dirty. We were laughing yet also felt helpless in the face of the stubborn clementine.

While lying on the ground, I pointed out a small branch nearby. We tried to knock down the clementine with it but didn't succeed. Roi's mother followed my idea and behavior. She found a longer branch. She proposed a new plan that included all of us. She asked Roi and me to help her lift the branch. We held it together, and as a team, managed to knock the clementine to the ground.

The three of us were happy and proud—we had achieved our goal. We had succeeded not only in coordinating our physical actions and sensorimotor movements, but also in attuning to each other's ideas, thoughts, intentions, desires, and emotions. We shared meaning through this process—meaning that formed a coherent narrative with a beginning, a middle, and an end.

For autistic children the ability to share common meanings is complex (Slade, 2009). Often, the connection is lost or severed, and something that had been meaningful becomes meaningless within seconds. The ability to maintain shared meaning requires awareness of the various threads that connect the participants and sustain joint activity. In this scenario, our shared goal was undoubtedly such a thread. The shared goal of picking the clementine was meaningful to Roi and served as a thread that maintained the connection between Roi, his mother, and me.

The clear and concrete goal helped Roi organize his mental representation of what was happening. Once there was a clear shared goal, Roi was able to hold onto the idea that we were doing something together. Understanding what was happening and having some control over it enabled him to direct his resources toward the ongoing joint activity and to learn during it.

The goal was not the only thread that connected the three of us. There was also an established emotional relationship between us. Further, his mother and I understood what interests Roi, what excites him, and what is meaningful to him. As his partners in the interaction, we were able to adjust our actions to match his level of affect, excitement, and stimulation.

Other threads that connected us were the sensorimotor experiences of jumping, climbing, trying to lift me, and swinging the long, heavy stick. These enabled Roi to experience movements and sensations, also for his vestibular system, which were tailored to his sensorimotor needs. It would have been extremely difficult for Roi to stay focused during an activity undertaken in a room or at a table, without the satisfaction provided by these sensorimotor experiences. The multi-sensory activity enabled him to move, touch, smell, see, hear, and finally even taste the clementine; that was the first time he had ever eaten a citrus fruit. This supported his ability to process, understand, and represent what was happening around him. The sensorimotor interaction supported and deepened the mental interaction between us, which made the shared experience richer and more meaningful.

In addition to the shared purpose, emotional connection, and sensorimotor experience, there were verbal threads that maintained a meaningful connection. The dialogue between Roi, his mother, and myself helped us represent the shared meaning of the experience and our opinions and feelings, which preserved our common goal. These were also cognitive threads that tied Roi to us: the challenge, curiosity, and anticipation.

Shared Past: The Ability to Form and Share Autobiographical Memories

The poet Avot Yeshurun said: "A person walks on his memories; they are his shoes." Memories are a central component of our sense of identity. We carry them everywhere, and in many ways, they also carry us. Memories provide stability and security as we navigate the world. Studies emphasize that memory and sense of self are mutually nourishing and reinforce each other through ongoing interactions. In this way, they are of crucial importance for the way we communicate and conduct ourselves in the world (Fivush, 2011, 2019; Lind, 2010; Ross et al., 2020).

Autobiographical Memory

Tulving (1983) identified three types of memory, corresponding to distinct types of consciousness: procedural, semantic, and episodic. Procedural memory governs motor skills. This type of memory operates automatically and remains latent, as individuals typically do not consciously think about the specific components of the action (e.g., which muscles are engaged while cycling). Semantic memory consists of general knowledge independent of personal experience or context, such as mathematical formulas, historical dates, or the names of world capitals. The third type, episodic memory, is mostly autobiographical. This is the only type of memory directly connected to an individual's past. It involves explicit recollections of an event that occurred at a specific time and place for a particular individual. Episodic memory can include non-autobiographical elements (such as a sequence of actions), but its deeply personal contextual nature allows for the creation of rich and emotionally significant memories about the self (Pasupathi & Wainryb, 2010; Williams & Conway, 2009). This type of memory is anchored in various contexts, such as the person's sensations and thoughts during an event, and personal significance derived from emotions, motivations, and goals shaped through interactions with others. Unlike the first two types of memory, episodic memory is explicit, enabling a continuous sense of self over time: "I was there" and "I did that." Autobiographical memory links past events into a cohesive life story, connecting the past, present, and future. Such memories are essential for self-definition and emotional regulation, contributing to identity formation and maintaining continuity over time (Fivush, 2011; Holland & Kensinger, 2010; Ross et al., 2020; Williams & Conway, 2009).

Autobiographical memory develops during early childhood, often from the second year of life, through social interactions and cognitive advancements including the maturation of basic memory systems, an understanding of temporal sequences, language acquisition, the ability to create and comprehend narratives, and the emergence of a separate sense of self (Hoerl & McCormack, 2005; Howe et al., 2003; Newcombe et al., 2007; Simcock & Hayne, 2002). This is marked by the emergence of the *cognitive self*, which is a sense of oneself as a distinct individual capable of anchoring events to personal identity. Around this time, children achieve developmental milestones such as mirror self-recognition and the understanding of self-referential pronouns (e.g., me, mine), which establish the foundation for encoding experiences as "my" memories (Howe et al., 2003). Around age four, a significant cognitive shift occurs as children transition from merely "knowing" an event happened to consciously "remembering" it (Nelson, 1992). This development, termed *autonoetic awareness*, enables richer and more structured autobiographical recollection enhancing the child's capacity for autobiographical consciousness.

While the initial onset of these memories is rooted in individual cognitive advances, language acquisition, and social interactions, particularly with caregivers, play a pivotal role in elaborating and preserving these memories. Language is not merely a way to express autobiographical memory. It is fundamental in providing the structure and organization characteristic of autobiographical memory (Nelson & Fivush, 2004). The development of language skills allows children to engage in dialogue with others about their past experiences. They become more skilled at creating organized representations of past events, allowing memories to become communicable and meaningful. Research on childhood memories indicates that parents more frequently talk with their children about the past and future from the third year of life. Both the quantity and the type of conversations about shared events have been found to contribute to the further development of children's memories. A significant contribution to the creation of lasting memories has been linked to how parents encourage their children to develop narratives and process their experiences into stories (Fivush, 2011).

Dialogue about autobiographical memories invites the use of language to describe mental states: emotions (e.g., "Dad was happy"), motives and goals (e.g., "I wanted to pick the clementine for Dad"), and thoughts (e.g., "I thought I could lift it"). Each participant in the dialogue can describe the event from their perspective. In this way, conversations about memories help children evaluate different viewpoints and integrate their personal meaning with a complex understanding of others' motives and mental states. Language enables children to articulate and share their memories, fostering a deeper understanding of both their own experiences and the perspectives of others (Fivush, 2019).

Autobiographical memory is closely intertwined with sensorimotor experiences and sensory inputs, which serve as elements for memory encoding and retrieval. Sensory inputs create vivid memory traces, especially in the context of early, repeated, and emotionally salient events (Ianì, 2019). Sensorimotor experiences contribute to a multi-modal memory network, integrating physical sensations with cognitive processing and feelings to create rich and accessible memories (Dijkstra & Post, 2015; Willander et al., 2015). The co-activation of sensory and emotional systems makes memories tied to sensory experiences more likely to be retained. These connections highlight the importance of sensory and motor engagement in supporting the development of a robust autobiographical memory system during early childhood (Bauer, 2007).

Autobiographical Memory Abilities in Autistic Children

Studies on memory in individuals with autism show that, while their semantic memory often functions well, their episodic autobiographical memory tends to be weaker than in neurotypical individuals (Goddard et al., 2007, 2014). Clinical reports indicate that many autistic individuals struggle to reflect on their inner world (McDonnell et al., 2017). Although some may have an exceptional ability to recall every detail of a past event, they may lack a connection to the self that experienced the event. They often produce fewer memories of specific, contextually rich experiences (Rhode, 2012). These difficulties have significant implications, as the inability to organize past experiences in memory in relation to the self makes it challenging for individuals with autism to update, consolidate, and refine their personal identity.

This difficulty in creating autobiographical memory and forming a cohesive present identity makes it difficult to imagine oneself in future hypothetical scenarios (Brown et al., 2012; Crane & Goddard, 2008; Lind & Bowler, 2009; Tanweer et al., 2010). Lack of social memory exacerbates these difficulties. While individuals with autism may excel in non-social memory tasks, their ability to encode, retain, and retrieve memories embedded in social contexts is often diminished (Brezis et al., 2014).

Challenges in autobiographical memory among autistic individuals are closely tied to difficulties in self-referential processing, executive functioning, and the ability to construct a coherent narrative. McDonnell et al. (2017) noted that many autistic children exhibit difficulty in processing and integrating relational information and this results in fragmented memory retrieval and an emphasis on isolated details rather than the broad context of an event. Zamoscik et al. (2016) found that autistic individuals are more likely to recall early childhood memories that are characterized by a strong sensory focus, as compared to neurotypical individuals. These memories are rich in visual, tactile, and auditory details, reflecting a sensory-based memory processing mechanism. While their heightened sensitivity to sensory input can lead to vivid recall of specific elements, it can also make it harder to filter relevant information, complicating the integration of sensory memories into coherent autobiographical narratives.

These findings suggest a vicious cycle: a weaker sense of self leads to difficulties in organizing and retrieving autobiographical memories, which, in turn, hinder the development of a coherent sense of self, further reinforcing the challenge of organizing and recalling memories. This circular difficulty colors the way autistic children experience the world and attribute meaning to events. Dialogues about past experiences are crucial for the development of autobiographical memory. Therefore, recalling shared experiences and engaging in dialogue about these memories with the child is a vital aspect of therapeutic work (Fivush, 2011; Larkina & Bauer, 2012).

When referring to past events, autistic children tend to refer to primarily semantic aspects: who was there, when it happened, what they did, where they were, what happened before, and what happened afterward. A challenge in therapeutic practice is maintaining the therapist–child connection as vital, meaningful, and mutual, not only during current interactions but also in memories of the past. Therapists must revive and cultivate memories based on semantic facts, so they become personal, specific memories of a meaningful shared experience between the child and another person. In this way, we may be able to help the child build a sense of continuity internally and within the relationship.

Our role is to illuminate for the child not only the details of the event, but primarily the components of the personal experience: each participant's feelings, desires, intentions, thoughts, and authentic personal experiences during the event in the past and in the present, as it is being discussed.

My belief is that recalling shared experiences should be an integral part of the child's therapeutic routine. We should link a specific shared experience in the present to events in the recent or distant past and future events yet to occur. This includes events that the therapist and child each experienced separately as well as events they shared.

With many of the children I treat, we create a "memory box" or diary in which we put mementos from our shared experiences, such as writings, pictures, drawings, and photographs. We include objects that have significant value and represent experiences we have had together: the carton from the milk we fed to cats, the peel from an orange we ate, a small bottle with residue from the soap we used to wash a doll. Tangible documentation of events is of great importance in treating autistic children. Images, films, or objects are not as ephemeral as words or movements. In a sense, these means of documentation freeze a past event and allow us to observe the objects and thus revisit and discuss the past event in the future.

The choice of medium for documentation should be meaningful from the child's perspective. The goal is to evoke not only the memory of the event but primarily elements of the personal experience that the event created. For some children, pictures are meaningful, and for others, objects are more significant. Some children can make a drawing of an event, and this will be meaningful documentation for them. For others, smelling, tasting, or touching something will remind them of the experience. We need to find a place for all of these in the therapeutic space, reflecting each child's personal experience.

For Roi, visual and verbal channels significantly helped him process past experiences, so Roi, his parents, and I made a shared memoir. We drew pictures of shared experiences, pasted photos in, and added text to tell our stories. This was not a ritual or regular activity; sometimes Roi was interested in the memoir book and sometimes less so. He kept the notebook at home and would bring it to every session. Sometimes there were entire sessions when he wanted only to leaf through the pages, to find the picture of the cat we fed, the photo of the toy car that broke while we were playing with it, the tape we used to fix a torn page of the book. Sometimes we added documentation of new experiences, either soon after the event or later, for a longer period.

A few days after the session when we picked clementines together, Roi's mother called me in a panic. The clementine we picked for his father had been left in the bag where the diary was kept. The fruit rotted and caused extensive damage to the notebook. At first, I was overcome with disappointment, but I quickly realized that this unplanned event could constitute a significant shared space for our developing relationship. I told her not to do anything, to leave everything as it was, and to put the diary in the bag to the next session as if nothing had happened. Roi arrived at our next meeting full of enthusiasm. His mother had printed out photographs she had taken of us picking the clementines, and he wanted to paste them into our journal. When we took the notebook out of the bag, the three of us discovered the extent of the damage the clementine had caused.

This incident in the treatment room of finding the damaged notebook gave us a different and unexpected shared experience of disappointment and sorrow that something significant to the three of us had been destroyed. We set out on a new shared event with a shared goal—rescue the diary. We tore out each page, cleaned them, stretched a rope, and hung them to dry. We decided to make a new diary, this time in a binder with each page inside a plastic sleeve so that "never, never, never, will anything like this ever happen to our diary again." There is no doubt that this was a significant shared experience for Roi, no less than picking the clementines had been.

Roi: Case Study

This chapter presents the theoretical basis for three temporal spaces in shared events, representing the future, present, and past through intentions, experiences, and memories. These were illustrated by describing a scenario of picking clementines during Roi's treatment. In describing his case, I show how these spaces were expressed and developed over the years of his treatment.

Roi's parents sought treatment from me when he was three years old due to communication difficulties. They said that when he was about one year old, they became concerned that he was not developing properly. They felt that he did not understand what was said to him, and he did not respond to his name. He was interested in and played mainly with objects but showed little interest in interactions with people around him. They described Roi as a toddler who protested by crying, enjoyed cuddling with his parents, and found comfort in their arms when he was distressed, especially when they rocked him. They said that he would spin hoops and balls repeatedly. He was especially fond of wind chimes and would play with them for a long time: moving them, listening to the sounds they made, and shaking the strings on which the bells were tied.

At the age of one and a half years old, Roi was integrated into a therapeutic rehabilitative educational setting. At the age of two, after being diagnosed with autism spectrum disorder, he began attending a communication kindergarten. When he was four years old, he began studying in a regular educational setting with the guidance of an integrative teacher.

I treated Roi when he was between the ages of three to eight. At the beginning of the therapeutic intervention, he spoke in simple sentences and could use distinct language to express basic desires and personal needs. He also used repetitive and stereotypical language. He demonstrated a certain degree of ability to pay attention to and express interest in another person regarding specific objects, especially books. He enjoyed listening to an adult read to him and would recite the text along with the reader. He liked playing ball with others.

In terms of intentionality, when Roi came to therapy, he saw himself as an agent with goals and intentions in the world. He knew how to act purposefully toward people and used verbal communicative intentions including protesting, requesting an object, action, or continued activity. He acted deliberately toward objects, giving the impression that he could hold in mind a plan of action (which Tomasello called intentionality), for example, climbing on a chair to get a toy on a high shelf. Roi understood, at least to some extent, that the people around him were separate from him, and might have their own goals.

However, it was evident that Roi had difficulty taking part in mutual and joint activities such as playing together. Roi could use intentional communication to request a game that interested him, but he had difficulty communicating his intentions to influence a relationship or joint activity or being influenced by another person's communicative intentions and attempts to influence the interaction.

The temporal space of the present occupied a particularly prominent place in the early stages of therapy. However, the future and the past were also evoked to some extent from the beginning of therapy. The present was the basis on which significant experiences were built, and later our shared intentions and memories grew from these, representing the future and past.

At the beginning of treatment, the present time was expressed by establishing initial circles of communication. In the first months of treatment, it was evident that it would be difficult to build a repertoire of socially and emotionally meaningful joint activities that would allow for interpersonal communication and not cause Roi to disengage. During treatment, Roi would often go in and out of the room. He would focus on the numbers on electronic devices and used toys in the room in a repetitive manner. My attempts to connect with Roi's experiences or his interest in objects and numbers were mostly unsuccessful, as were my attempts to establish dyadic interactions in the therapy room based on sensory experiences.

A breakthrough in treatment occurred when we changed the setting and held the sessions in a nearby playground. This enabled us to construct a repertoire of joint dyadic activities centered on sensorimotor interaction, which were more suitable for Roi than the activities that were possible in the room. Roi enjoyed running around the playground with me or one of his parents chasing him. Gradually this evolved from simply running away to a game of tag. The pleasure of escaping turned into excitement about one of the adults catching him and lifting him up. It was apparent that these interactions between the participants were more effective, better adapted, and used more motor skills than those that could have been done inside. When Roi ran, his movements were full of joy and laughter. He would repeatedly check that the adult was following him. The excitement, and growing anticipation for the moment when the adult would catch him reflected Roi's intention for the encounter. It was clear that the activity had become familiar to him, and he was able to predict what was about to happen based on previous similar shared experiences. Gradually, we successfully developed variations of the activity. What began with the adults catching Roi and lifting him into the air evolved into rolling together on the grass, and eventually into a game where Roi rode the adult like a horse. Roi appeared to remember the sequence of these joint activities and began to anticipate them. He seemed to anticipate physical sensations, such as the moment his father would catch him or the feeling of being lifted into the air. He seemed to predict how strong the touch would be or how quickly they would move. Roi also appeared to predict the social and emotional responses the game might evoke—whether it would be fun for him, or how joyful and excited his father might be.

Over time, he became increasingly able to adapt to changes within the familiar activity and even began to initiate them by himself. This growing flexibility was also evident between sessions, as Roi began initiating joint games reminiscent of those played in the therapeutic space. These connections—within the activity itself and between treatment sessions—revealed the early emergence of Roi's awareness of the temporal spaces: past, present, and future. Slowly, meaningful experiences began to accumulate within familiar routines. The meaningful shared physical experiences we accumulated (in the present) formed the basis for Roi to use his memory abilities (of the past) to anticipate what was about to happen (in the future). Meaning, and especially shared meaning, served as an organizing principle for Roi. Predictive, repetitive routines with a clear sequence and purpose enabled him to anticipate the physical, cognitive, emotional, and social aspects of joint activity.

The multimodal sensorimotor inputs that Roi perceived during these experiences, including sights, sounds, smells, movements, touch, together with mental states like desires, intentions, emotions, and language used by him and others coalesced into a unified meaning. These activities were repeated every week, allowing Roi to remember them and represent them. Being able to successfully anticipate what was about to happen gave him a sense of control, security, and stability. He had partners who were significant to him and who shared his memories, reminded him of past events, and discussed how those events might affect the present. These experiences supported his communicative initiatives for joint interaction. Gradually, Roi was able to take part in activities that were similar but not entirely identical. Developing variations within familiar activities was a promising sign that Roi could retrieve memories of the past and use them flexibly in the present temporal space.

The joint activities in which Roi participated with the adult gradually developed from dyadic sensorimotor activities to triadic activities that included more complex game ideas related to objects (e.g., the hammock we hung together) and events (e.g., making pizza together). Language began to take a more prominent place in the interactions and became a means by which we were able to influence each other and share our thoughts, feelings, and desires. It also supported Roi's growing ability to plan and to remember, both key functions in shaping meaningful joint experiences.

In the following examples, I show how the activities in which Roi participated helped to establish the temporal space of the future in the therapy space. In this regard, the therapy focused on two objectives. The first objective was to arouse Roi's curiosity and attention to his interaction partner's goals and action plans. The second was to help Roi act in joint action plans and toward shared goals.

Several strategies were used to achieve the first objective of increasing his awareness of other people's goals and action plans. These strategies included expanding familiar routines, verbal conceptualizations, visual representations, varied action plans, and delaying the action.

First, I expanded upon the repetitive activities that were part of the treatment routine. For example, Roi liked to swing in a hammock at the beginning of each treatment and expected the hammock to be hanging in the room, ready for him. Then one session, I left the hammock lying on the floor. When Roi came in, he was surprised to see the change. He expected the hammock to be re-hung. This was an opportunity to draw his attention to my plan of action for hanging the hammock, such as bringing a ladder and climbing it. A photograph of the hanging hammock helped me show the purpose of my actions and supported our discussion. I succeeded in getting Roi's attention and made him curious about various possible action plans we could use to achieve our goals.

Another time, while playing with small toy cars that slide along a track, one car rolled into a narrow gap under the closet. Roi was frustrated and wanted the car back so he could continue playing. His mother and I tried different ways of getting the car out: with our hands, a pencil, and a ruler. None of these worked. Eventually, we got the car out with a broomstick. Each of these action plans was communicated to Roi verbally and through visual representations. For example, I made drawings to show Roi what was happening. In our discussions, we encouraged Roi to wonder about other people's actions, such as by asking, "Why do you think Mom brought the broom?" and suggest action plans by himself to achieve our goal.

Using the strategy of delaying the action also helped achieve the therapeutic objective. For example, once when Roi asked his mother for a drink of water, she didn't bring the bottle out immediately. She rummaged through her bag, looking for the bottle. This gave Roi an opportunity to observe his mother perform a deliberate action to achieve her goal. The pause in the action created a space that allowed Roi to wonder about the actions of people around him. The unfolding dialogue helped conceptualize thoughts about his mother's actions and the intentions behind them. We wondered together: Why haven't he gotten the bottle yet? Did Mom understand him? Is she looking for the bottle?

The second objective of the therapeutic intervention was to help Roi work with others on action plans toward shared goals. Several strategies were used to achieve this, including diverse action plans, drawing Roi's attention to the mutual work and coordination between participants switching roles. For example, we would hang the hammock from its high brackets in various ways, such as climbing a ladder, standing on a chair, or Roi's father lifting him onto his shoulders.

In another activity, we played with a helium balloon on a short string. We tried to reach the balloon in different ways, alone and together, using the shared knowledge we had gained from the experience of hanging the hammock. Roi's knowledge of experiences such as hanging the hammock (in the past) helped him anticipate people's actions in the new event of catching the balloon (in the future), to understand and grasp the common goal and realize it through mutual interaction (in the present).

In another game, his father would "fly" Roi on his feet like an airplane then drop to the floor, and Roi and I together would pull his father to his feet. Roi and I maintained a common goal and spontaneously developed various action plans during our interactions. We tried to lift his father by each of us holding one of his father's hands, or one of us pulling the father's hands and the other pushing against his back. Often it was more fun when we didn't succeed, and his father would pull Roi to him and hug and tickle him. Such joint activities required us to learn to match the intensity and rhythm of our movements to each other to successfully achieve our common goals.

Sometimes I would drop out of my expected role during an activity. For example, in one activity we carried a tub full of balls down a long hallway. I would sometimes let go of the tub and allow the balls to scatter around the room. In other cases, I intentionally acted out of sync when carrying out a joint action plan, such as lifting the tub so high that Roi could not comfortably hold it on his side or walking at a slower or faster pace than Roi's. This was another way to draw Roi's attention to my role in the event and our mutual coordination.

Switching roles was another helpful strategy. For example, we would build a tall tower together out of large, soft blocks, and then together we would knock them down and jump on them. We divided the roles among ourselves. One person placed the cubes on top of each other, and the other's role was to keep the tower from collapsing. We would switch roles so that each of us could experience the event from different perspectives. Switching roles helped Roi have a representation of his own actions and those of another person, and thus understand how, although each of us acts differently, we are all working to achieve the same goal.

The past temporal space developed alongside the spaces of the present and the future. Activities involving shared goals and joint action plans provided Roi with an organizing framework that supported his ability to encode and retain what had already occurred. Our dialogue was a central and fundamental factor in establishing memories of shared experiences. It allowed us to relate to past events and bring them up in shared discourse. The objective was to cultivate memories. These were based not only on semantic aspects of the experience (to make chocolate milk, we need milk, chocolate powder, a cup, and a spoon) but also on authentic, specific personal memories of the shared meaningful experience and the feelings and emotions we each had, individually and together.

When we celebrated the birthday of a doll, Roi wanted to set off fireworks because he enjoyed seeing the sparkling lights, but I said I didn't want to because I was afraid of fire. After debating this, we found a solution by lighting sparklers on the cake, but I stood far away at the other end of the room. We later recalled this, and thus embedded our memories with personal, autobiographical meanings that each of us attributed to them.

We addressed experiences from the recent past (e.g., the previous session) as well as events from the more distant past, months, and even years earlier. We connected past experiences to what was happening in the present time (in the therapy room) or what would happen in the future. For example, when we first made chocolate milk together, I told Roi that I once made chocolate milk for friends and accidentally used salt instead of sugar, which caused me great embarrassment. We used my autobiographical experience to relate to what was about to happen. We were careful not to get confused and made sure that we used sugar and not salt. The feelings, emotions, and autobiographical memories we shared deepened our connection. Using visual representations and mementos such as artifacts from the events helped us talk about it. Our diary of shared memories, in which we documented our experiences in writing, helped us to construct a narrative with a structure of a clear beginning, middle, and end.

Conclusion

Shared experiences shape and deepen our connections with others. The time Roi and I spent picking clementines together was meaningful, a meaning that lived not only in the present moment, but also in the future we imagined together and in the memories we shared of the past. The therapeutic setting was structured in a way that allowed Roi to make sense of the experience, infuse it with personal and interpersonal meaning, and shift fluidly between being present in the moment, reflecting on the past, and looking toward the future.

Roi's treatment ended after five years, when he was eight and a half years old. We dedicated our final session to a writing activity, which he loved. I brought an envelope and notes and suggested that we write on the notes things that we would miss from the therapy sessions. Roi was excited about this. He told me: "Arava, write that I will miss your pencil. Arava, write that I will miss your car. Arava, write that I will miss this eraser." I left the meeting confused and wondering how significant our shared experiences had been for him, and what meaning they held in his eyes.

A few weeks later, Roi sent me the following letter, offering his response to what had been left unspoken in our final session. I share this letter here with Roi's permission, as he kindly agreed to let it be read by you.

To Arava,

I have missed you ever since May. I really, really want to come back to you to do activities and write about a topic. Soon we'll come to visit you for a surprise. I think that… yes, I really, really love you. Do you love me too? Arava: I'm at the "Cherry on the Whipped Cream" summer camp. When you were a child, did you go to summer camp too? I think so. I hope our visit will be fun and exciting.

Arava, I loved the parting letters we wrote on April 28. I'll be back soon. I'm sure you are enjoying the lessons with the child who replaced me on Thursday at five o'clock. Come visit us too. I think that the email you write will be like parting letters. Do you think so too? I also think so.

Arava, say: Roi-lu-lu-lu-lu-lu-lu-lu-lu, I love you!

Ms. Mizrahi, I tell you that our lessons were nice!

I have to finish writing this email soon because I have a fever.

But I miss you so so so much!!!!!!!!!!!

Ms. Mizrachilulu, I'm crazy wazy about you!!!!!!!

I'll finish in four minutes

Listen to Mr. Excellent: I want to see many more new things that you will have in your room.

Arava, I really really wanna come back to you! I love you, I'm crazy wazy about you, I'm so excited — but my favorite thing is hugging you a ton!!!!!!!!

Listen, at the end, I have something important to say: I love you also in my heart.

Good luck

Kisses and hugs

Roi

I find this last letter that Roi wrote to me to be a fascinating testimony to his ability to succeed in integrating the three temporal dimensions: past, present, and future. In the letter, he takes pleasure in a playful sensorimotor game of sounds, inventing for the first time a creative and melodic nickname for me—one that echoes the way I used to call him during our sessions. He longs for meaningful, shared experiences from the past—such as our joint writing in the memory journal, which he enjoyed so much. He expresses curiosity about other children I might be treating in his place, shares his own experience of a summer camp visit, and wonders about my personal experience as a child. He refers to future events as well—like a letter he wishes I would write to him, or a possible reunion between us. He manages to hold all three temporal dimensions as meaningful and clearly experiences our connection as significant.

The Babylonian Talmud writes: "I have learned much from my teachers, more from my colleagues, and most of all from my students."

I thank Roi for all I have learned from him, and for the opportunity to share what I have learned with you.

References

Adamson, L. B., & Bakeman, R. (2006). Development of displaced speech in early mother–child conversations. *Child Development, 77*(1), 186–200. https://doi.org/10.1111/j.1467-8624.2006.00864.x

Adamson, L. B., Bakeman, R., & Deckner, D. F. (2004). The development of symbol-infused joint engagement. *Child Development, 75*(4), 1171–1187. https://doi.org/10.1111/j.1467-8624.2004.00732.x

Adamson, L. B., Bakeman, R., Deckner, D. F., & Romski, M. (2009). Joint engagement and the emergence of language in children with autism and Down syndrome. *Journal of Autism and Developmental Disorders, 39*(1), 84–96. https://doi.org/10.1007/s10803-008-0601-7

Bakeman, R., & Adamson, L. B. (1984). Coordinating attention to people and objects in mother–infant and peer–infant interaction. *Child Development, 55*(4), 1278–1289. https://doi.org/10.2307/1129997

Bauer, P. J. (2007). *Remembering the times of our lives: Memory in infancy and beyond.* Psychology Press.

Bar Yehuda, S., & Bauminger-Zviely, N. (2024). Social-motor coordination between peers: Joint action developmental trajectories in ASD and TD. *Journal of Autism and Developmental Disorders, 54*(3), 811–828. https://doi.org/10.1007/s10803-022-05851-1

Beebe, B., Jaffe, J., Lachmann, F., Feldstein, S., Crown, C., & Jasnow, M. (2000). Systems models in development and psychoanalysis: The case of vocal rhythm coordination and attachment. *Infant Mental Health Journal, 21*(1–2), 99–122.

Bowsher-Murray, C., Gerson, S., Von dem Hagen, E., & Jones, C. R. (2022). The components of interpersonal synchrony in the typical population and in autism: A conceptual analysis. *Frontiers in Psychology, 13*, 897015. https://doi.org/10.3389/fpsyg.2022.897015

Boria, S., Fabbri-Destro, M., Cattaneo, L., Sparaci, L., Sinigaglia, C., Santelli, E., Cossu, G. & Rizzolatti, G. (2009). Intention understanding in autism. *PloS One, 4*(5), e5596. https://doi.org/10.1371/journal.pone.0005596

Bottema-Beutel, K., Yoder, P. J., Hochman, J. M., & Watson, L. R. (2014). The role of supported joint engagement and parent utterances in language and social communication development in children with autism spectrum disorder. *Journal of Autism and Developmental Disorders, 44*(9), 2162–2174. https://doi.org/10.1007/s10803-014-2092-z

Brezis, R. S., Galili, T., Wong, T., & Piggot, J. I. (2014). Impaired social processing in autism and its reflections in memory: A deeper view of encoding and retrieval processes. *Journal of Autism and Developmental Disorders, 44*(5), 1183–1192. https://doi.org/10.1007/s10803-013-1980-y

Brown, B. T., Morris, G., Nida, R. E., & Baker-Ward, L. (2012). Brief report: Making experience personal: Internal states language in the memory narratives of children with and without Asperger's disorder. *Journal of Autism and Developmental Disorders, 42*(3), 441–446. https://doi.org/10.1007/s10803-011-1246-5

Brownell, C. A., Ramani, G. B., & Zerwas, S. (2006). Becoming a social partner with peers: Cooperation and social understanding in one- and two-year-olds. *Child Development, 77*(4), 803–821. https://doi.org/10.1111/j.1467-8624.2006.t01-1-.x-i1

Cerullo, S., Fulceri, F., Muratori, F., & Contaldo, A. (2021). Acting with shared intentions: A systematic review on joint action coordination in autism spectrum disorder. *Brain and Cognition, 149*, 105693. https://doi.org/10.1016/j.bandc.2021.105693

Colombi, C., Liebal, K., Tomasello, M., Young, G., Warneken, F., & Rogers, S. J. (2009). Examining correlates of cooperation in autism: Imitation, joint attention, and understanding intentions. *Autism, 13*(2), 143–163. https://doi.org/10.1177/1362361308098514

Crane, L., & Goddard, L. (2008). Episodic and semantic autobiographical memory in adults with autism spectrum disorders. *Journal of Autism and Developmental Disorders, 38*(3), 498–506. https://doi.org/10.1007/s10803-007-0420-2

Dijkstra, K., & Post, L. (2015). Mechanisms of embodiment. *Frontiers in Psychology, 6*, 1525. https://doi.org/10.3389/fpsyg.2015.01525

Dromi, E. (2018). Otisam: Massa lahavanat haretsef [*Autism: A journey toward understanding the spectrum]*. Niv Press.
Dromi, E., Eden, S., Zdunaysky-Erlich, S., Ringwald-Frimerman, D., & Levy-Eitan, H. (2009). Tiqshoret vesafah baggil harakh: Hitrakhesh kemodel lehitarevut khinnukhit [*Communication and language in early childhood: The scenario as a model for educational intervention*]. Maalot.
Dromi, E., Fox, A., Ringwald-Frimerman, D., & Tzohar, N. (2003). Yissum tokhnit "qesher" began hayyeladim [*Implementing the "Connections" program in kindergartens*]. Ma'alot.
Dromi, E., & Ringwald-Frimerman, D. (1996). Hitarevut tiqshoret vesafah liladim lequye shemiah. hashalav haqqedam mille [*Communication and language intervention for hearing-impaired children: The pre-verbal stage*]. Ramot Publishing.
Fitzpatrick, P., Diorio, R., Richardson, M. J., & Schmidt, R. C. (2013). Dynamical methods for evaluating the time-dependent unfolding of social coordination in children with autism. *Frontiers in Integrative Neuroscience, 7*, 21. https://doi.org/10.3389/fnint.2013.00021
Fivush, R. (2011). The development of autobiographical memory. *Annual Review of Psychology, 62*(1), 559–582. https://doi.org/10.1146/annurev.psych.121208.131702
Fivush, R. (2019). *Family narratives and the development of an autobiographical self: Social and cultural perspectives on autobiographical memory*. Routledge.
Fulceri, F., Tonacci, A., Lucaferro, A., Apicella, F., Narzisi, A., Vincenti, G., Muratori, F., & Contaldo, A. (2018). Interpersonal motor coordination during joint actions in children with and without autism spectrum disorder: The role of motor information. *Research in Developmental Disabilities, 80*, 13–23. https://doi.org/10.1016/j.ridd.2018.05.018
Ganglmayer, K., Schuwerk, T., Sodian, B., & Paulus, M. (2019). Do children and adults with autism spectrum condition anticipate others' actions as goal-directed? A predictive coding perspective. *Journal of Autism and Developmental Disorders, 50*(6), 2077–2089. https://doi.org/10.1007/s10803-019-03964-8
Greenspan, S. I., & Wieder, S. (2006). *Engaging autism: The floortime approach to helping children relate, communicate, and think*. Perseus Books.
Gilbert, M. (2009). Shared intention and personal intentions. *Philosophical Studies, 144*, 167–187. https://doi.org/10.1007/s11098-009-9372-z
Goddard, L., Howlin, P., Dritschel, B., & Pattel, T. (2007). Autobiographical memory and social problem-solving in Asperger Syndrome. *Journal of Autism and Developmental Disorders, 37*(2), 291–300. https://doi.org/10.1007/s10803-006-0168-0
Goddard, L., Dritschel, B., Robinson, S., & Howlin, P. (2014). Development of autobiographical memory in children with autism spectrum disorders: Deficits, gains, and predictors of performance. *Developmental Psychopathology, 26*(1), 215–228. https://doi.org/10.1017/S0954579413000904
Hoerl, C., & McCormack, T. (2005). Joint reminiscing as joint attention to the past. In N. Eilan, C. Hoerl, T. McCormack, & J. Roessler (Eds.), *Joint attention: Communication and other minds: Issues in philosophy and psychology* (pp. 260–286). Clarendon Press.
Holland, A. C., & Kensinger, E. A. (2010). Emotion and autobiographical memory. *Physics of Life Reviews, 7*(1), 88–131. https://doi.org/10.1016/j.plrev.2010.01.006
Howe, M. L., Courage, M. L., & Edison, S. C. (2003). When autobiographical memory begins. *Developmental Review, 23*(4), 471–494. https://doi.org/10.1016/j.dr.2003.09.001
Ianì, F. (2019). Embodied memories: Reviewing the role of the body in memory processes. *Psychonomic Bulletin & Review, 26*(6), 1747–1766. https://doi.org/10.3758/s13423-019-01674-x
Kasari, C., Gulsrud, A. C., Wong, C., Kwon, S., & Locke, J. (2010). Randomized controlled caregiver-mediated joint engagement intervention for toddlers with autism. *Journal of Autism and Developmental Disorders, 40*(9), 1045–1056. https://doi.org/10.1007/s10803-010-0955-5
Larkina, M., & Bauer, P. J. (2012). "Family stories" and their implications for preschoolers' memories of personal events. *Journal of Cognition and Development, 13*(4), 473–504. https://doi.org/10.1080/15248372.2011.591295

Liebal, K., Colombi, C., Rogers, S. J., Warneken, F., & Tomasello, M. (2008). Helping and cooperation in children with autism. *Journal of Autism and Developmental Disorders, 38*(2), 224–238. https://doi.org/10.1007/s10803-007-0381-5

Lind, S. (2010). Memory and the self in autism: A review and theoretical framework. *Autism, 14*(5), 430–456. https://doi.org/10.1177/1362361309358700

Lind, S., & Bowler, D. M. (2009). Recognition memory, self-other source memory, and theory-of-mind in children with autism spectrum disorder. *Journal of Autism and Developmental Disorders, 39*(9), 1231–1239. https://doi.org/10.1007/s10803-009-0735-2

McDonnell, C. G., Valentino, K., & Diehl, J. J. (2017). A developmental psychopathology perspective on autobiographical memory in autism spectrum disorder. *Developmental Review, 44*, 59–81. https://doi.org/10.1016/j.dr.2017.01.001

McNaughton, K. A., & Redcay, E. (2020). Interpersonal synchrony in autism. *Current Psychiatry Reports, 22*(3), 12. https://doi.org/10.1007/s11920-020-1135-8

Nelson, K. (1986). *Event knowledge: Structure and function in development*. Erlbaum.

Nelson, K. (Ed.). (1989). *Narratives from the crib.* Harvard University Press.

Nelson, K. (1992). Emergence of autobiographical memory at age 4. *Human Development, 35*(3), 172–177. https://doi.org/10.1159/000277149

Nelson, K., & Fivush, R. (2004). The emergence of autobiographical memory: A social cultural developmental theory. *Psychological Review, 111*(2), 486–511.

NeuroLaunch. (2024, August 11). *Autism and predictive brain function: Neural processing in neurodiversity.* NeuroLaunch. https://neurolaunch.com/autism-and-the-predictive-brain/

Newcombe, N. S., Lloyd, M. E., & Ratliff, K. R. (2007). Development of episodic and autobiographical memory: A cognitive neuroscience perspective. *Advances in Child Development and Behavior, 35*, 40–89.

Pacherie, E. (2011). Framing joint action. *Review of Philosophy and Psychology, 2*(2), 173–192. https://doi.org/10.1007/s13164-011-0052-5

Pasupathi, M., & Wainryb, C. (2010). On telling the whole story: Facts and interpretations in autobiographical memory narratives from childhood through midadolescence. *Developmental Psychology, 46*(3), 735–746.

Rhode, M. (2012). Whose memories are they and where do they go? Problems surrounding internalization in children on the autistic spectrum. *International Journal of Psychoanalysis, 93*(2), 355–376. https://doi.org/10.1111/j.1745-8315.2011.00507.x

Ross, J., Hutchison, J., & Cunningham, S. J. (2020). The me in memory: The role of the self in autobiographical memory development. *Child Development, 91*(2), e299–e314. https://doi.org/10.1111/cdev.13211

Schank, R. C., & Abelson, R. P. (2013). *Scripts, plans, goals, and understanding: An inquiry into human knowledge structures.* Psychology Press (Original work published in 1977). https://doi.org/10.4324/9780203781036

Schank, R. C., & Abelson, R. P. (2014). Knowledge and memory: The real story. In R. S. Wyer (Ed.), *Knowledge and memory: The real story: Advances in social cognition, Vol. VIII* (pp. 1–85). Psychology Press (Original work published in 1995). https://doi.org/10.4324/9781315806594

Sebanz, N., Bekkering, H., & Knoblich, G. (2006). Joint action: Bodies and minds moving together. *Trends in Cognitive Sciences, 10*(2), 70–76. https://doi.org/10.1016/j.tics.2005.12.009

Sebanz, N., & Knoblich, G. (2021). Progress in joint-action research. *Current Directions in Psychological Science, 30*(2), 138–143. https://doi.org/10.1177/096372142098442

Shai, D., & Fonagy, P. (2013). Beyond words: Parental embodied mentalizing and the parent–infant dance. In M. Mikulincer & P. R. Shaver (Eds.), *Mechanisms of social connections: From brain to group* (pp. 185–203). American Psychological Association. https://doi.org/10.1037/14250-011

Simcock, G., & Hayne, H. (2002). Age-related changes in verbal and nonverbal memory during early childhood. *Developmental Psychology, 39*(5), 805–814.

Slade, A. (2009). Mentalizing the unmentalizable: Parenting children on the spectrum. Journal of Infant, *Child and Adolescent Psychopathology, 8*(1), 7–21. https://doi.org/10.1080/15289160802683054

Steinman, M., & Dromi, E. (2007). Tiqshoret, safah vedibbur etsel yeladim tseirim im lequyot al haretsef haotiseti: Haarakhah al pi haggishah hahitpattekhutit-tivit veeqronot betikhnun hahitarevut [Communication, language, and speech in young children with disabilities on the autistic spectrum: Assessment according to the natural-developmental approach and principles in planning intervention]. In S. Lowinger (Ed.) *Tiqshoret: Tippul byiiladim im beayot tiqshoret begilae bet hassefer hayyesodi [Communication: Treating children with communication problems at the elementary school age*] (pp. 93–160). ACH Publishing House.

Stern, D. N. (1985). *The interpersonal world of the infant.* Karnac.

Stern, D. N. (2002). *The first relationship: Infant and mother.* Harvard University Press.

Stern, D. N. (2010). *Forms of vitality: Exploring dynamic experience in psychology, the arts, psychotherapy, and development*. Oxford University Press.

Tanweer, T., Rathbone, C. J., & Souchay, C. (2010). Autobiographical memory, autonoetic consciousness, and identity in Asperger Syndrome. *Neuropsychologia, 48*(4), 900–908. https://doi.org/10.1016/j.neuropsychologia.2009.11.007

Tomasello, M. (2005). Beyond formalities: The case of language acquisition. *The Linguistic Review, 22*(2–4), 183–197. https://doi.org/10.1515/tlir.2005.22.2-4.183

Tomasello, M. (2009). *Why we cooperate.* MIT Press.

Tomasello, M. (2014). *A natural history of human thinking*. Harvard University Press.

Tomasello, M., & Carpenter, M. (2007). Shared intentionality. *Developmental Science, 10*(1), 121–125. https://doi.org/10.1111/j.1467-7687.2007.00573.x

Tomasello, M., Carpenter, M., Call, J., Behne, T., & Moll, H. (2005). Understanding and sharing intentions: The origins of cultural cognition. *Behavioral and Brain Sciences, 28*, 675–735. https://doi.org/10.1017/S0140525X05000129

Trevarthen, C. (2008). The musical art of infant conversation: Narrating in the time of sympathetic experience, without rational interpretation, before words. *Musicae Scientiae, 12*(1), 15–46. https://doi.org/10.1177/1029864908012001021

Trevisan, D. A., Enns, J. T., Birmingham, E., & Iarocci, G. (2021). Action coordination during a real-world task: Evidence from children with and without autism spectrum disorder. *Development and Psychopathology, 33*(1), 65–75. https://doi.org/10.1017/S0954579419001561

Tulving, E. (1983). *Elements of episodic memory.* Clarendon Press.

Warneken, F., Gräfenhain, M., & Tomasello, M. (2012). Collaborative partner or social tool? New evidence for young children's understanding of joint intentions in collaborative activities. *Developmental Science, 15*(1), 54–61. https://doi.org/10.1111/j.1467-7687.2011.01107.x

Williams, H. L., & Conway, M. A. (2009). Networks of autobiographical memories. In P. Boyer & J. V. Wertsch (Eds.), *Memory in mind and culture* (pp. 33–61). Cambridge University Press.

Willander, J., Sikström, S., & Karlsson, K. (2015). Multimodal retrieval of autobiographical memories: Sensory information contributes differently to the recollection of events. *Frontiers in Psychology, 6*, 1681. https://doi.org/10.3389/fpsyg.2015.01681

Zamoscik, V., Mier, D., Schmidt, S. N., & Kirsch, P. (2016). Early memories of individuals on the autism spectrum assessed using online self-reports. *Frontiers in Psychiatry, 7*, 79. https://doi.org/10.3389/fpsyt.2016.00079

Effective Collaboration: Parents, Teachers, and Therapists

Chapter 11
Parental Involvement, Parent–Teacher Relationships, and Development of Children with Autism Spectrum Disorder

Hadas Mekayten and Shiri Pearlman-Avnion

Abstract This study examined how early parental involvement in interventions and the quality of the parent–teacher relationship are related to and predict the development of children with ASD, simultaneously assessing their joint contribution. The research involved 69 parents and 69 kindergarten teachers of children with ASD in Israel, utilizing questionnaires to measure parental involvement dimensions, parent–teacher trust and communication, and child development in areas such as language, sociability, sensory/cognitive awareness, and physical health/behavior. The findings revealed a complex picture. While general parental involvement did not directly predict overall child development, specific parental involvement subscales, such as interest/presence and communication patterns, showed significant positive correlations with certain developmental areas, like physical health/behavior and language. From the parents' perspective, the quality of their relationship with teachers positively correlated with and predicted their child's overall development, including language/communication, sociability, and physical health/behavior. Teachers' responses did not yield these significant correlations or predictive power. The study confirmed its main hypothesis: early parental involvement and the quality of the parent–teacher relationship, when considered together, significantly predict the development of children with ASD, accounting for approximately 9% of the variance. These results underscore the importance of a collaborative and coordinated approach between parents and educators to foster optimal development in children with ASD.

Keywords Autism spectrum disorder · Parental involvement · Early intervention · Parent–teacher relationship · child development

H. Mekayten
Psychological-Educational Services, Katzrin, Israel

S. Pearlman-Avnion (✉)
Tel-Hai College, Kiryat Shmona, Israel
e-mail: shiripearlmanavnion@yahoo.com

S. Lowinger and S. Pearlman-Avnion (eds.), *Collaborative Care and Partnerships in Autism Diagnosis and Treatment*, Autism and Child Psychopathology Series,
https://doi.org/10.1007/978-3-032-07009-8_11

Introduction

Autism spectrum disorder (ASD) is a neurodevelopmental disorder characterized by persistent and significant deficiencies and limitations in social interactions, activities and interests, communication, and exhibition of repetitive behaviors (American Psychiatric Association, 2013; Oono et al., 2013). Symptoms range from mild to significant disability, with or without developmental delay (Chao et al., 2018). Cognitive functioning ranges from giftedness and fluent speech to extreme limitations and inability to speak, and from independent performance to the need for constant individual attention (Coulter, 2009). Biological studies have confirmed the heterogeneity of this disorder and linked ASD to hundreds of genes (Johnson et al., 2013; Schaaf & Zoghbi, 2011) and myriad neurobiological mechanisms (Ebrahimi-Fakhari & Sahin, 2015). Therefore, treatment for ASD must address a wide range of developmental areas (Wallace & Rogers, 2010), and the therapeutic plan and goals must be individualized (Ginosar, 2019).

Diagnosis of ASD has been consistently rising around the world and currently stands at approximately 1 in 89 children in Europe (Troisi et al., 2020), 1 in 54 in the United States (Maenner et al., 2020), and recently 1:36 (Centers for Disease Control & Prevention, 2023). In Israel, diagnosis of ASD has also been increasing, and current estimates are like those in Europe (Segev et al., 2019).

Development of Children with ASD

Child development is a dynamic process in which children move from complete dependence on caregivers during their infancy to independence in various life areas by late childhood (Fernald et al., 2009). Children with mild, moderate, or severe developmental delays may not achieve expected milestones for their age (World Health Organization [WHO], 2007). Neuropsychological development is strongly affected, both positively and negatively, by environmental factors (Fernald et al., 2009; Koizumi, 2004).

Early Intervention

The average age of diagnosis of ASD in the United States is four years old (Christensen et al., 2019). Although the disorder can be detected as young as 14 months and diagnostic stability is high by 18 months (Landa, et al., 2013; Landa et al., 2018), children exhibiting signs of ASD are seldom diagnosed at this age (Ozonoff et al., 2015).

If the syndrome is diagnosed early, parents, educators, and therapists can promote the child's optimal development and functioning (WHO & UNICEF, 2012). The second year of life is developmentally critical because brain plasticity at this age enables the creation and organization of neural connections as children learn and respond to their experiences and environment (Courchesne et al., 2011; Dawson, 2008; Dawson et al., 2012; Kolb & Gibb, 2011; Lewis et al., 2014). While atypical connections may form at this stage, it is also an appropriate stage at which to impact the developmental trajectory in a positive direction (Dawson, 2008; Moulton et al., 2016). Early childhood is a time of rapid physical and cognitive changes, including the development of intelligence, personality traits, and social behavior (Fernald et al., 2009; Küçükturan & Akbaba Altun, 2017).

The variation in developmental outcomes among children with ASD puts pressure on parents to find effective intervention programs (Clark et al., 2017). Intensive and early interventions have been shown to bring about greater developmental gains in various adaptive domains (including IQ) and reduction of symptoms, even to the point that the child no longer shows evidence of the disorder, as compared to interventions initiated at later ages (Howard et al., 2005; Rogers et al., 2012; Sallows & Graupner, 2005; Smith et al., 2015). Young children exhibiting clear symptoms of ASD who received early treatment presented significantly fewer symptoms of ASD later as compared to children who showed fewer symptoms in their initial assessment and whose families postponed treatment (Orinstein et al., 2014).

Parental Involvement in Early Intervention

Every educational and therapeutic process requires cooperation with the parents to achieve maximum results (Badi'ah et al., 2020). In specific, the relationship between parents' involvement in early treatment and children's development has been established in previous studies (Badi'ah et al., 2020; Farrell, 2009; Koizumi, 2004; Siller & Sigman, 2008). Thus, parents of children with ASD should be treated as valued and respected partners as they navigate the services available to their children (Carbone et al., 2010; Russa et al., 2015). Placing the family at the center of interventions for children with special needs recognizes their primary role and responsibility in providing daily, long-term care (Ingber & Dromi, 2011).

Intervention is most effective when the family prioritizes it and integrates it into their daily routines, such as by creating common interests (objects and activities) with their children who are learning to imitate their environment (Farrell, 2009). In this way, children and parents can synchronize and focus their intentions, enabling the children to communicate and express themselves better (Siller & Sigman, 2008), given that atypical synchronization in social interactions is common among people with ASD (Fitzpatrick et al., 2018). When parents and children experience reciprocal communication, the children's verbal ability tends to improve, and the severity of their symptoms diminishes (Warren et al., 2010). Additionally, children with ASD who exhibit positive behaviors may encourage greater parental interaction and involvement (Benson et al., 2008).

Parental involvement in the therapeutic program can improve their child's development (Forry et al., 2011). Properly structured interventions facilitate beneficial interaction between parents and children (Dawson, 2008; Dawson et al., 2012; Osborne et al., 2008). When parents mediate the therapeutic intervention, the severity of their children's symptoms can be reduced, and their cognition and sociability improved (Nevill et al., 2018).

Parental involvement includes communicating with the therapeutic team, updating them about the child's functioning, and expressing interest in the process. Involved parents visit the treatment center, participate in sessions, request training from the therapeutic team, implement their instructions, and offer ideas to improve the treatment and services provided. They seek the team's advice when making decisions about diagnostic and evaluation processes (Ingber, 2004; Sharabi & Marom-Golan, 2018).

However, parents of children with ASD often experience high levels of stress, which may limit their ability to be actively involved in their children's treatment (Wang et al., 2020). Support from significant others, such as extended family members and close friends, can moderate this stress and, therefore, is positively related to parental involvement in the treatment program (Yan et al., 2022).

Parent–Teacher Relationships in ASD Interventions

The relationship between the parents and teachers of children with ASD is a new research field. To promote the children's progress, achievement, and well-being (Ritvo et al., 2018), parents and teachers should cooperate in defining therapeutic goals, selecting an intervention plan, and implementing it (Ginosar, 2019). Kindergarten teachers care for children in various realms: emotional, cognitive, social, and physical (Sevimli-Celik et al., 2011). They face the challenge of organizing a flexible and adaptable environment, especially when attempting to help children with ASD interact with their peer group (Boavida et al., 2018). Early interventions in which teachers, parents, and a professional multidisciplinary team collaborate can promote the development of children with ASD and reduce gaps between them and their peers (Caeiro & Franco, 2021; Guralnick, 2005, 2017; Küçükturan & Altun, 2017; Stoner et al., 2005). Involved parents can translate the skills taught at school into the home and help their children learn behaviors appropriate for their home and community (Chandran et al., 2019).

The quality of parents' relationship with teachers and therapists affects their satisfaction with the services provided. A healthy relationship and shared commitment to the child's development benefits not only the children but the parents and family as well (Sucuoğlu & Bakkaloğlu, 2018). Trust and communication are core factors affecting the quality of this relationship (Petrogiannis & Penderi, 2014). Parents and teachers with a strong relationship based on trust and communication can provide each other with important information that helps in defining diagnostic, educational, and treatment goals (Campbell & Kozloff, 2007).

Parents who are involved in their children's education tend to communicate more effectively with their children and have a feeling of competence and agency (Elicker et al., 2013; Serpell & Mashburn, 2011). Similarly, the teachers gain insights into the children's special needs and the challenges they face in their home life (Pirchio et al., 2013). The parent–teacher relationship is correlated with indicators of social skills, achievement, solving cognitive problems, and addressing the child's behavioral issues (El Nokali et al., 2010).

However, undefined boundaries regarding responsibility and authority may lead to challenges and dilemmas. Parents may not agree with the professional model that defines their relationship with the kindergarten teacher. Parents tend to focus on their own child's needs and behaviors in the peer group and the kindergarten teacher's attitude toward their child. The teacher must consider the needs of all the children in the class, mediate conflicts during lessons, and address inappropriate behavior in the classroom (Greenbaum & Fried, 2011; Rekalidou & Penderi, 2010). While this can lead to conflict, a trust-based relationship encourages constructive dialogue despite complex situations, tensions, and disagreements (Greenbaum & Fried, 2011). Further, children may consciously or unconsciously reflect their parents' views of their teachers, whether positive or negative. Teachers who see parents as passive observers endanger cooperation (Katzenelson, 2014).

The severity of symptoms among children with ASD may be affected by interactions with their kindergarten teachers (Dykstra et al., 2013). Children with limited cognitive and verbal skills communicate less with the kindergarten teacher, which, in turn, impacts the parent–teacher relationship (Swartz & Easterbrooks, 2014). When children exhibit lower social and academic skills and more severe behavioral problems, the parent–teacher relationship tends to suffer (Swartz & Easterbrooks, 2014). Positive parent–teacher relationships have been associated with more sensitive and supportive interactions between the child and the teacher (Serpell & Mashburn, 2011). High-quality therapeutic programs encourage communication between parents and teachers, enabling positive and effective relationships (Rentzou, 2011).

Educational Interventions for Children with ASD in Israel

Israel's Special Education Law, enacted in 1988, requires schools to offer educational and therapeutic responses to children with special needs, including ASD. Treatments include physiotherapy, communication clinics, occupational therapy, music therapy, preventive health care, and more. These services are provided by professionals who use recognized methods such as developmental-integrative therapy, cognitive-behavioral therapy (CBT), applied behavior analysis (ABA), and developmental individual-difference (DIR). The psychology branch of the Israel Ministry of Education and Culture is tasked with promoting the well-being and mental health of all students in the education system and provides educational psychology services for students, their parents, administrators, and the educational staff in schools and community organizations (Israel Ministry of Education & Culture, 2010).

Experimental Data, Aims, and Definitions

The purpose of the following study was to examine the extent to which parental involvement in early interventions and the quality of the relationship between parents and kindergarten teachers are related to and predict the development of children with ASD. Few previous studies have considered all three aspects simultaneously. The following definitions were used: *Early parental involvement* refers to parents' interest, presence, communication patterns, initiative, responsibility, active partnership, and social interaction in interventions for their young children with ASD (Ingber, 2004); *Communication pattern* refers to parents' relationship with the therapeutic team in terms of exchanging information, listening and talking to each other, and the guidance that the team gives the parents (Ingber, 2004); *Parent–teacher relationship* refers to trust and communication between the parent of a child with ASD and that child's preschool/ kindergarten teacher; and *Development of children* with ASD refers to the children's progress in the areas of speech/language/communication skills, sociability, sensory/cognitive awareness, and physical health/behavior. The *language and communication* subscale refers to the number of words the child can say, the ability to speak meaningfully, have a conversation, and more. The *physical health/behavior* subscale refers to incontinence, eating issues, sensitivity to noise, insisting on a rigid routine, and more.

This study hypothesized the following: 1. Early parental involvement will be positively and significantly related to the development of their children with ASD; 2. The quality of the parent–teacher relationship (trust, communication) will be positively and significantly correlated with the development of children with ASD; 3. Early parental involvement will predict the development of children with ASD; 4. The quality of the parent–teacher relationship will predict the development of children with ASD; 5. Early parental involvement and the quality of the parent–teacher relationship will predict the development of children with ASD.

The study participants included 69 parents of children diagnosed with ASD and 69 preschool/kindergarten teachers of those children. All the teachers in the sample were women. All the parents and teachers were of Israeli-Jewish nationality. The children studied in kindergartens across Israel. Since the kindergarten location was not found to be significant, it was not included in subsequent analyses.

Research tools included demographic questionnaires. Parents and teachers completed separate questionnaires on background demographic traits. The Family Involvement in Early Intervention Questionnaire, a 23-item family involvement questionnaire (Ingber, 2004; Ingber et al., 2010), was developed to examine the level and style of parental involvement in a family-centered program for young children with special needs. This tool was originally written in Hebrew. The parents ranked their responses on a 5-point Likert scale from 1 (not at all) to 5 (always), such that a higher score reflected a higher level of parental involvement. The questionnaire has five main factors: interest and presence (with an internal consistency of $\alpha = 0.55$), communication patterns (0.71), initiative and responsibility (0.76), active partnership (0.78), and social involvement (0.77). Internal consistency for the general index was 0.87. In the original study, the internal consistency measures of the factors were: interest and presence (0.71), communication pattern (0.69), initiative and responsibility (0.63), active partnership (0.62), and social involvement (0.53). The internal consistency of the general index was $\alpha = 0.82$. To evaluate the parent–teacher relationship, the Quality of Parent–Teacher Relationship Scale in Kindergarten (QPTRS-K) (Petrogiannis & Penderi, 2014) was used. In addition, the researchers selected 20 items from other recognized tools, such as a scale for evaluating the parent–child relationship (Elicker et al., 1997) and a scale for assessing the parent–teacher relationship (Vickers & Minke, 1995). The questionnaire items were back-translated to Hebrew by two translators. Parents and teachers ranked their answers on a Likert scale from 1 (do not agree at all) to 5 (strongly agree), such that a higher score reflected a more positive parent–teacher relationship. The questionnaire consists of two factors: trust/acceptance (internal consistency of $\alpha = 0.94$ according to both the parents' and the teachers' responses) and communication/responsiveness (internal consistency of 0.91 for the parents' responses and 0.92 for the teachers' responses). The internal consistency of the overall index was $\alpha = 0.90$ for both the parents and the teachers.

Finally, the Autism Treatment Evaluation Checklist, based on the Autism Treatment Evaluation Checklist (ATEC) (Rimland & Edelson, 1999), was developed to help researchers, parents, and professionals evaluate the long-term effectiveness of treatments for children and adults with ASD. The 77 items of the checklist are divided into four categories: speech/communication/language, sociability, sensory/ cognitive awareness, and physical health/behavior. For this study, the questionnaire was back-translated into Hebrew by two translators. Parents ranked the developmental change that occurred in their children due to the intervention program on a Likert scale from 1 (no improvement at all) to 5 (significant improvement), with the option to indicate 6 (not relevant). Internal consistencies were 0.97 for speech/ language/communication, 0.97 for sociability, 0.97 for sensory/cognitive awareness, and 0.94 for physical health/behavior. The internal consistency of the general index was $\alpha = 0.98$. In the original study, the Autism Research Institute presented the following unstandardized r-indices: $\alpha = 0.92$ for speech/language/communication, 0.84 for sociability, 0.87 for sensory/cognitive awareness, and 0.81 for physical health/ behavior. The internal consistency of the general index was 0.942.

Data collection started by sending a request to the Israel chief scientist and the college ethics committee, explaining the research questions and ensuring that all ethical issues would be observed, such as maintaining anonymity and using research tools appropriate for the study sample. After receiving approval from these two parties, a liaison put us in contact with teachers at special education kindergartens that specialize in assisting children with ASD, called "communication kindergartens". These schools were in the northern region of Israel, where the survey began.

We explained to the teachers the rationale of the research and what was requested of them. Those who agreed to participate were asked to explain the research to their students' parents and ask if they would be willing to participate. Teachers and parents made informed decisions regarding their participation. Parents and teachers who agreed to answer the questionnaires received a link through Qualtrics software, where they signed an informed consent form and completed the questionnaires during their free time and voluntarily. Participants were asked to respond to all questionnaire items. Questionnaire respondents were asked to recommend other potential participants. We sent explanatory letters to eligible participants (teachers and parents of children with ASD in special education kindergartens), thus building the sample using the snowball method.

Data Processing and Results

Descriptive statistics analysis and Cronbach's alpha reliability tests were performed for the measurement tools for the three central variables (parental involvement, parent–teacher relationship, and development of children with ASD) and their subscales. Pearson correlation analyses were performed to test the first two hypotheses. Multiple linear regression analyses were performed to test the third, fourth, and fifth hypotheses. To test intervening variables, Spearman and Pearson correlation analyses) were performed. All analyses were performed using IBM SPSS Statistics 25. The independent (predictor) variables were parental involvement in early interventions and the quality of the parent–teacher relationship. The dependent variable was the development of children with ASD.

Early Parental Involvement

The early parental involvement variable had a relatively high mean score and low standard deviation. The communication pattern subscale had the highest mean with the lowest standard deviation. The social involvement subscale had a significantly lower mean than the other parental involvement subscales and a relatively high standard deviation.

Parents' Perspectives on the Parent–Teacher Relationship

From the parents' responses to the questionnaires, the overall scale on the quality of the parent–teacher relationship had a high mean score. The mean for the subscale of trust in the teacher was slightly higher than the subscale for communication with the teacher.

Teachers' Perspectives on the Parent–Teacher Relationship

From the teachers' questionnaires, the quality of the parent–teacher relationship and its subscales had slightly lower means than the corresponding variables from parents' questionnaires. The mean for the subscale of trust in the parent was higher than the subscale for communication with the parent.

Development of Children with ASD

For the variable of the development of children with ASD, the mean score was relatively high. Among its four subscales, sociability had the highest mean and the lowest standard deviation. The language/communication subscale had the second-highest mean and the highest standard deviation, followed by sensory/cognitive awareness. The subscale physical health/behavior had the lowest mean score.

Family Demographics

A significant negative correlation was found between the parents' age and the subscale of parental interest and presence, such that the older the parent, the lower their level of interest and presence in the intervention for their child with ASD, and vice versa.

A significant negative correlation was found between the number of children in the family and the language and communication development of the child with ASD, such that the higher the number of children in the family, the lower the degree of improvement in the language and communication skills of the child with ASD, and vice versa.

Age of Diagnosis

The age at which the child was diagnosed with ASD had a significant negative correlation with the parental involvement subscale of initiative and responsibility, such that the younger the child's age at diagnosis, the higher the parents' initiative and responsibility in the intervention, and vice versa. The age of the child's diagnosis had positive and significant correlations both with the general scale of development and with the subscale of development of sensory/cognitive awareness, such that the earlier the child was diagnosed, the lower the level of development in general and sensory/cognitive development in specific, and vice versa.

Duration of Intervention

The duration of the therapeutic intervention had a significant negative correlation with the parental involvement subscale of active participation, such that the longer the therapeutic program lasted, the less the parents were actively involved, and vice versa. The duration of the therapeutic program had a significant positive correlation with the quality of the parent–teacher relationship according to the parents' responses and with its two subscales, trust in the teacher and the quality of communication with the teacher. The longer the therapeutic program continued, the better the parents' perception of the quality of the relationship with the teacher, including the degree of trust and the quality of communication, and vice versa. Program duration had a significant positive correlation with the subscale of physical health/behavior, such that the longer the treatment program, the greater the improvement in this index, and vice versa.

Correlations Among the Research Variables After Controlling for Demographic Traits Previously Found to Be Correlated in the Research

Hypothesis 1: Parental Involvement and the Development of Children with ASD

The first hypothesis predicted a positive relationship between parental involvement in early interventions and the development of children with ASD. A significant positive correlation between parental interest/presence and the child's development in terms of physical health/behavior. The variable of communication patterns has a significant positive correlation with language and communication development.

No significant relationship was found between the general variable of parental involvement in early intervention and the general variable of the development of children with ASD or with the four subscales for development: language and communication, sociability, sensory/cognitive awareness, and physical health/behavior. Thus, the first research hypothesis cannot be fully confirmed.

Hypothesis 2: Parent–Teacher Relationship and the Development of Children with ASD

The second hypothesis predicted a positive relationship between the quality of the parent–teacher relationship and the development of children with ASD. A significant positive correlation was found between the general variable of the quality of the parent–teacher relationship and the general variable of the development of children with ASD, as well as correlations with three of the four development subscales: language and communication, socialization, and physical health/behavior.

Parents' Perspectives

The subscale of parental trust in the teacher has a significant positive correlation with the general variable of development of children with ASD and with three of the development subscales: language and communication, socialization, and physical health/behavior. The subscale of parental communication with the teacher has significant positive correlations with the general variable of development of children with ASD and with three development subscales: language and communication, sociability, and physical health/behavior. Development of sensory/cognitive awareness was not significantly correlated with the quality of the parent–teacher relationship or either of its subscales: trust in and communication with the teacher.

Teachers' Perspectives

Analysis of the data from the kindergarten teachers' questionnaires found no significant correlations between the general variable of the quality of their relationship with the parents or with either of its two subscales: trust in and communication with the parents. No correlation was found with the general variable of development of children with ASD or any of its four subscales. Therefore, the second hypothesis was only partially confirmed. The parents' responses largely confirm it, with some qualification regarding the impact of the parent–teacher relationship on the children's sensory/cognitive development, but the teachers' responses did not uphold this hypothesis.

Hypothesis 3: Parental Involvement in Early Intervention Will Predict the Development of Children with ASD

According to our third hypothesis, early parental involvement will predict the development of children with ASD. A multiple linear regression analysis was conducted. The regression model for predicting the development of children with ASD by dimensions of parental involvement in early intervention was significant. The predictor variables explained approximately 24% of the variance of the dependent variable.

The variable of parental interest and presence had the most significant positive contribution in predicting the development of children with ASD. The next most significant variable was parents' initiative and responsibility, which had a negative correlation such that a higher level of parental initiative and responsibility predicted lower development of children with ASD. The other dimensions of parental involvement did not show any significant new and unique contribution in predicting the development of children with ASD beyond the impact of the two mentioned above. Thus, the third research hypothesis was confirmed.

Hypothesis 4: The Quality of the Parent–Teacher Relationship Will Predict the Development of Children with ASD

According to the fourth hypothesis, the quality of the parent–teacher relationship will predict the development of children with ASD. The regression model based on the data from the parents' questionnaires showed that the parent–teacher relationship significantly predicted the development of children with ASD. The two predictor variables explained about 9% of the difference in the dependent variable. However, neither predictor variable showed any significant and unique contribution to predicting child development, when each was controlled for.

The regression model based on data from the kindergarten teachers' questionnaires showed that the dimensions of the parent–teacher relationship did not significantly predict the development of children with ASD. Neither predictor variable made any significant new or unique contribution in predicting the development of children with ASD. Therefore, the fourth research hypothesis was partially confirmed.

Hypothesis 5: Parental Involvement in Early Interventions and the Quality of the Parent–Teacher Relationship Together Will Predict the Development of Children with ASD

According to the fifth hypothesis, early parental involvement and the quality of the parent–teacher relationship together will predict the development of children with ASD. The regression model for predicting the development of children with ASD was significant. Again, the predictor variables explained approximately 9% of the variance in the variable of the level of development of children with ASD. The predictor variable of the quality of the parent–teacher relationship showed a significant contribution after removing the parental involvement variable. The parental involvement variable alone did not show any additional significant contribution in predicting the dependent variable after removing the parent–teacher relationship variable. Despite the non-significant unique contribution of parental involvement, the two independent variables together predicted the development of children with ASD, confirming the fifth research hypothesis.

Discussion of the Results and Further Implications for Parental Involvement, Parent–Teacher Relationships, and Development of Children with Autism Spectrum Disorder

The study we presented examined how various dimensions of parental involvement in early interventions for their children with ASD and the quality of the relationship between the parents and the kindergarten teacher were correlated with and predicted various aspects of the development of their children with ASD. Unlike previous research in this field, the current study considered both independent variables simultaneously, presenting their joint contribution in affecting and predicting the development of these children.

Parental Involvement and Development of Children with ASD

The findings of this study highlight the complexity of this issue. Two of the five subscales in the early parental involvement variable were significantly and positively related to two of the subscales of the child development variable: parental interest/presence with the children's physical health/behavior development and parents' communication patterns with the children's language development.

According to the parents' reports, the quality of their relationship with their children's teachers is positively related to and predicts their children's development. However, analyses of the teachers' responses showed no significant correlation between their relationship with the parents and the children's development and did not predict it. Thus, early parental involvement is correlated with the development of children with ASD, but this variable alone is not significant in predicting the children's development; only in conjunction with the quality of the parent–teacher relationship (according to the parents' report). Therefore, it is the joint contribution of these two variables that significantly predicts the development of children with ASD.

The findings of this study support, to some extent, a complex picture of parental involvement in therapeutic interventions for their children with special needs, as presented by Ingber (2004). The factors of interest and presence and communication patterns were found to best represent parents' involvement in their children's education and therapeutic programs. The other three factors, active partnership, initiative and responsibility, and social involvement, explained some of the variation but were not as central as the first two.

Ingber and Dromi (2011) concluded that parental involvement ranges along a spectrum from passive to active and autonomous. Furthermore, while many parents agree that cooperating with the professional care team is important, they may have differing expectations of the intervention plan and ways of responding to it, and varying capacities for being involved in it. Some parents expect to be full partners in choosing the methods used in the intervention and express an explicit desire to take responsibility for their children's education, while other parents support the decisions of the therapeutic team and do not feel the need to be full partners in the process. Further, the researchers questioned whether parental involvement has a direct and measurable effect on children's development (Ingber & Dromi, 2011).

Impact of Demographic and Background Traits

The current study found that the parents' age was negatively related to their interest and presence in the intervention of their children. Also, the age at which the child was diagnosed is negatively related to the parents' initiative and responsibility. The duration of the therapeutic program provided to children in kindergarten is negatively related to parents' active partnership. Therefore, it is necessary to refer to the background traits of the parents and children and other factors that may affect the degree of parental involvement or the ability to measure it directly. For example, Yan et al. (2022) found a significant and positive relationship between parents of children with ASD receiving social support from friends and family and their involvement in interventions for their children. Similarly, Wang et al. (2020) found that the stress experienced by parents of children with ASD was negatively related to their involvement in the treatment program. The findings of the current study in the context of previous research show that the relationship between parents' involvement in the treatment program and children's development is not simple and requires complex analyses.

Parent–Teacher Relationship and the Development of Children with ASD

Analyses investigating our second hypothesis showed that according to the parents' responses, the quality of their relationship with the teacher had a significant and positive correlation with the development of their children with ASD overall and particularly with three of the four subscales: language and communication, sociability, and physical health/behavior. However, the teachers' responses showed no significant relationship between their relationship with the parents and the development of their students with ASD.

Although there has been little empirical research on interactions between parents and kindergarten teachers (Pirchio et al., 2013), the parent–teacher relationship is a cornerstone in the children's development, functioning, achievements, and mental health (Katzenelson, 2014). The family and educational system both wish to promote the child's welfare, and each recognizes the distinctive influence of the other, but efforts to cooperate do not always lead to agreement (Ritvo et al., 2018). Interactions between parents of children with special needs and the education staff are complex and emotionally intense, encompassing multiple concerns, feelings of guilt, frustration, blurring of boundaries and responsibilities, and more (Israel Ministry of Education and Culture, n.d.). The quality of the parent–teacher relationship depends on how each party perceives the essence, nature, and importance of their interactions; parents and educators may see themselves as partners and allies, or, in less favorable situations, the parents see teachers as service providers, and the teachers expect parents to remain passive observers (Katzenelson, 2014).

In most cases, parents want to communicate with kindergarten teachers about their child's behavior and the school's hygiene and safety rules, while kindergarten teachers contact parents to give them information about classroom programs and activities, to request help and support, or to inquire about the child's development (Papandreou et al., 2009). Parents tend to have a more optimistic and positive perception of their relationship with their children's kindergarten teacher, as compared to the teacher's perception (Petrogiannis & Penderi, 2014; Rentzou, 2011). Similarly, the present study found that the parents perceived the quality of their relationship with the teacher as promoting their child's development, whereas the teachers did not make this connection. This reflects parents' and teachers' different perceptions and expectations regarding their relationship, as noted in the previously mentioned studies. Parents who experience difficulties with their children may rely on the kindergarten teachers as professionals, whereas the teachers do not have this perception of the parents.

Other factors may be involved. For example, the current study found that the teacher's experience was significantly related to the quality of the parent–teacher relationship, according to both the parents and teachers. Therefore, the expectation that both the parents and teachers will see each other as partners in promoting children's development is complex. The findings of this study do not necessarily contradict this, even though the relationship was not found to be significant by the kindergarten teachers. Teachers and parents want to promote children's development, especially children in special education, so their recognition that the parent–teacher relationship is critical to the child's development should be mutual. Nevertheless, the perception of the relationship and its content may be defined differently by each party.

Early Parental Involvement Will Predict the Development of Children with ASD

This study found that early parental involvement predicts the development of children with ASD. This confirms previous findings that parental involvement in treatments for children with ASD is crucial at every stage of development and treatment (Azeem et al., 2016), especially in early childhood, (Mareoiu et al., 2015). More specifically this study found that parental interest and presence is the predicting variable that makes the most significant positive contribution.

In comparison of parents of children with ASD by gender, the mothers reported themselves as being more involved and having higher levels of interest and presence in their child's treatment plan in general, while the fathers were more likely to be involved with support services and professional therapists in specific (Sharabi & Marom-Golan, 2018). The current study's findings may have been affected by the fact that most of the surveyed parents (over 78%) were female.

Surprisingly, high level of parental initiative and responsibility predicted low development of children with ASD. To encourage active parental involvement in their children's therapy, there is a need for ongoing communication regarding the family's expectations and needs for meeting the challenges of raising a child with special needs (Ingber & Dromi, 2011). This involves making joint decisions about how interventions will be planned and implemented, defining the roles, responsibilities, and level of control of each party, and determining how the results will be evaluated. Ingber and Dromi (2011) proposed a model of parents according to their level of responsibility and initiative, from those who maintain a partnership with the therapist to those who see the therapist as having sole responsibility. Therefore, one must consider the parents' level of initiative and responsibility for the treatment plan and the relationship between the parents and the professionals who take care of their children in the therapeutic/educational framework.

Quality of Parent–Teacher Relationship Predicts the Development of Children with ASD

According to the parents' responses, the quality of their relationship with the teacher predicted their children's development. However, according to the teachers' responses, their relationship with the parents did not predict their students' development. This partially verifies a previous study conducted in an inclusive kindergarten in Turkey, which found that the surveyed mothers of children with special needs perceived their relationship with the teachers as a positive and critical factor in their children's development.

Additionally, our findings agree, albeit partially, with those of Petrogiannis and Penderi (2014), who developed the QPTRS-K questionnaire used in the current study, and who found positive and strong correlations between the perceptions of both the teachers and parents regarding the contribution of their relationship to the children's development. That study found that parents of children with special needs have a high motivation to cooperate with the teacher based on a belief that good relationships will help improve the child's functioning and development. In their comparison of the total scores for the scales and subscales, they found both the parents and kindergarten teachers perceived the quality of their relationship as making a positive contribution to the children's development, but the parents perceived it as a more significant factor (Petrogiannis & Penderi, 2014).

Early Parental Involvement and the Parent–Teacher Relationship Will Together Predict the Development of Children with ASD

The main research hypothesis, that early parental involvement and the quality of the parent–teacher relationship, taken together, will predict the development of children with ASD, was fully confirmed. Although the early parental involvement variable alone was not a significant predictor, when the two variables were combined, the model was significant, explaining about 9% of the variance in the index of child development.

This presented study found a negative relationship between parental initiative and responsibility and the age at which the child was diagnosed with ASD; that is, the parents' sense of initiative and responsibility is more significant when the child is diagnosed at a younger age. The parents may understand that kindergarten is a critical period in their child's development and therefore may be motivated to be involved in the intervention at this stage.

Further, the longer the duration of the therapeutic program, the more positive the parents' perception of the quality of their relationship with the kindergarten teacher. Children who are diagnosed early can receive a longer treatment program. Therefore, these findings taken together may indicate that parents who are aware that this is a critical period in child development take a higher level of initiative and responsibility in the kindergarten treatment program, which, in turn, improves their relationship with the teacher as the therapeutic program continues.

The findings of Azeem et al. (2016) that parental involvement in interventions for their children with ASD is correlated with positive behaviors and personality traits and a positive relationship with the educational staff, contributing to the child's development and well-being are in line with the findings of the current study. This indicates the significance of both parental involvement and the quality of the relationship with the teacher for the development of children with ASD.

However, each of these variables is complex. Every parent defines their level of involvement and the kind of relationship they want to have with the kindergarten teacher. Furthermore, each kindergarten teacher's perspective on their relationship with students' parents is individual. Therefore, the findings should be further assessed with other advanced data analysis methods.

Strengths and Limitations of the Study

The study's primary strength and contribution involves the simultaneous examination of the relationship between all three research variables. While previous studies have assessed the relationship between two of the research variables, to the best of our knowledge, none have looked at all three together in educational settings in general or therapeutic kindergarten programs for children with ASD or other communication disorders in specific. Therefore, this research enriched our knowledge in little-studied research areas.

The study had several limitations. First, participants answered self-report questionnaires, and their answers may have been biased according to their subjective world. Second, the study sample recruited using the snowball method cannot be considered representative, making it difficult to apply the conclusions to the general population. Third, internal consistency of less than 0.55 was found for the social involvement subscale in the original study (Ingber, 2004; Ingber et al., 2010), and for the parental interest and presence subscale in the current study. Fourth, the analysis was based on correlations, so no conclusions about cause-and-effect relationships can be drawn. Fifth, data were collected at one point in time only.

Practical Implications

The study we chose to present makes a significant contribution by showing that parental involvement in early interventions for their children with ASD and the quality of their relationship with the teacher together promote and predict children's development. Children with ASD experience a wide range of complex challenges. Teachers and parents play dynamic, crucial, and complex roles in helping these children reach their potential. This can cause emotions such as frustration, fear for the future, and exhaustion. This study offers cautious optimism regarding the contribution that people in the child's immediate environment can make. Parental involvement ranges from passive to active, reflecting diverse factors such as socioeconomic status, education level, the child's level of functioning, parental stress, various educational/therapeutic teams, and more. Moreover, because parents and teachers may have differing perceptions of the nature of their relationship, there is a need to coordinate their expectations, so each understands how to help the children and promote their development.

Future research may examine the research questions at multiple points in time to document the developmental process more accurately. Additional questionnaires could be included to examine other factors that may affect the results. In-depth interviews with parents and teachers could assess differences in their perceptions about the nature of their relationship. Finally, given the complexity of these variables and the lack of prior research on the interaction between them, more complex analyses, such as a path model or examination of mediating factors, could shed additional light on how parental involvement and the quality of the parent–teacher relationship make a joint contribution to the development of children with ASD.

References

American Psychiatric Association. (2013). *Diagnostic and statistical manual of mental disorders (5th. Ed.)*. APA. https://doi.org/10.1176/appi.books.9780890425596

Azeem, M. W., Imran, N., & Khawaja, I. S. (2016). Autism spectrum disorder: An update. *Psychiatric Annals, 46*(1), 58–62. https://doi.org/10.3928/00485713-20151202-01

Badi'ah, A., Mendri, N. K., Nugroho, H. S. W., & Handayani, W. (2020). The effect of parenting on the language development of autistic children. In *Proceedings of the International Conference on Science and Engineering, 3*, 509–515. https://doi.org/10.14421/icse.v3.554

Benson, P., Karlof, K. L., & Siperstein, G. N. (2008). Maternal involvement in the education of young children with autism spectrum disorders. *Autism, 12*(1), 47–63. 10.1177%2F1362361307085269

Boavida, T., Aguiar, C., & McWilliam, R. A. (2018). Early intervention and early childhood contexts. In M. Fuertes, C. Nunes, D. Lino & T. Almeida (Eds.), *Theory, practices and research in early intervention* (pp. 7–23). CIED/ Lisbon Higher School of Education.

Caeiro, A. P., & Franco, V. (2021). Kindergarten teachers' perspective on early intervention in autism spectrum disorders. *Journal of Intellectual Disability-Diagnosis and Treatment, 9*(3), 311–320. https://doi.org/10.6000/2292-2598.2021.09.03.7

Campbell, M., & Kozloff, M. (2007). Comprehensive programs for families of children with autism. In M. B. James & E. S. Charles (Eds.), *Handbook of parent training: Helping parents prevent and solve problem behaviors* (pp. 67–106). John Wiley & Sons.

Carbone, P. S., Behl, D. D., Azor, V., & Murphy, N. A. (2010). The medical home for children with autism spectrum disorders: Parent and pediatrician perspectives. *Journal of Autism and Developmental Disorders, 40*(3), 317–324. https://doi.org/10.1007/s10803-009-0874-5

Centers for Disease Control and Prevention. (2023). CDC: Autism rate rises to 1 in 36 children.

Chandran, H., Jayanthi, K., Prabavathy, S., Renuka, K., & Bhargavan, R. (2019). Effectiveness of video assisted teaching on knowledge, attitude and practice among primary caregivers of children with autism spectrum disorder. *Advances in Autism, 5*(4), 231–242. https://doi.org/10.1108/AIA-10-2018-0039

Chao, K. Y., Chang, H. L., Chin, W. C., Li, H. M., & Chen, S. H. (2018). How Taiwanese parents of children with autism spectrum disorder experience the process of obtaining a diagnosis: A descriptive phenomenological analysis. *Autism, 22*(4), 388–400. 10.1177%2F1362361316680915

Christensen, D. L., Maenner, M. J., Bilder, D., Constantino, J. N., Daniels, J., Durkin, M. S., Fitzgerald, R. T., Kurzius-Spencer, M., Pettygrover, S. D., Robinson, C., Shenouda, J., White, T., & Zahorodny, W., Pazol, K., & Dietz, P. (2019). Prevalence and characteristics of autism spectrum disorder among children aged 4 years—early autism and developmental disabilities monitoring network, seven sites, United States, 2010, 2012, and 2014. *MMWR Surveillance Summaries, 68*(2), 1–19. https://doi.org/10.15585%2Fmmwr.ss6802a1

Clark, M. L., Barbaro, J., & Dissanayake, C. (2017). Continuity and change in cognition and autism severity from toddlerhood to school age. *Journal of Autism and Developmental Disorders, 47*, 328–339. https://doi.org/10.1007/s10803-016-2954-7

Coulter, R. A. (2009). Understanding the visual symptoms of individuals with autism spectrum disorder (ASD). *Optometry & Vision Development, 40*(3), 164–175.

Courchesne, E., Mouton, P. R., Calhoun, M. E., Semendeferi, K., Ahrens-Barbeau, C., Hallet, M. J., Barnes, C. C., & Pierce, K. (2011). Neuron number and size in prefrontal cortex of children with autism. *JAMA, 306*(18), 2001–2010. https://doi.org/10.1001/jama.2011.1638

Dawson, G. (2008). Early behavioral intervention, brain plasticity, and the prevention of autism spectrum disorder. *Development and Psychopathology, 20*(3), 775–803. https://doi.org/10.1017/s0954579408000370

Dawson, G., Jones, E. J., Merkle, K., Venema, K., Lowy, R., Faja, S., Kamara, D., Murias, M., Greenson, J., Winter, J., Smith, M., Rogers, S. J., & Webb, S. J. (2012). Early behavioral intervention is associated with normalized brain activity in young children with autism. *Journal of the American Academy of Child & Adolescent Psychiatry, 51*(11), 1150–1159. https://doi.org/10.1016/j.jaac.2012.08.018

Dykstra, J. R., Sabatos-DeVito, M. G., Irvin, D. W., Boyd, B. A., Hume, K. A., & Odom, S. L. (2013). Using the language environment analysis (LENA) system in preschool classrooms with children with autism spectrum disorders. *Autism, 17*(5), 582–594. https://doi.org/10.1177/1362361312446206

Ebrahimi-Fakhari, D., & Sahin, M. (2015). Autism and the synapse: Emerging mechanisms and mechanism-based therapies. *Current Opinion in Neurology, 28*(2), 91–102. https://doi.org/10.1097/wco.0000000000000186

Elicker, J., Noppe, I. C., Noppe, L. D., & Fortner-Wood, C. (1997). *Parent-caregiver relationship scale (PCRS)* [Database record]. *APA PsycTests*. https://doi.org/10.1037/t49053-000

Elicker, J., Wen, X., Kwon, K., & Sprague, J. B. (2013). Early head start relationships: Association with program outcomes. *Early Education and Development, 24*(4), 491–516. https://doi.org/10.1080/10409289.2012.695519

El Nokali, N. E., Bachman, H. J., & Votruba-Drzal, E. (2010). Parent involvement and children's academic and social development in elementary school. *Child Development, 81*(3), 988–1005. https://doi.org/10.1111/j.1467-8624.2010.01447.x

Farrell, A. F. (2009). Validating family-centeredness in early intervention evaluation reports. *Infants & Young Children, 22*(4), 238–252. https://doi.org/10.1097/IYC.0b013e3181b8b1db

Fernald, L. C., Kariger, P., Engle, P., & Raikes, A. (2009). *Examining early child development in low-income countries: A toolkit for the assessment of children in the first five years of life*. World Bank. https://openknowledge.worldbank.org/bitstream/handle/10986/28107/NonAsciiFileName0.pdf?sequence=1

Fitzpatrick, P., Frazier, J. A., Cochran, D., Mitchell, T., Coleman, C., & Schmidt, R. C. (2018). Relationship between theory of mind, emotion recognition, and social synchrony in adolescents with and without autism. *Frontiers in Psychology, 9*, 1337. https://doi.org/10.3389/fpsyg.2018.01337

Forry, N. D., Moodie, S., Simkin, S., & Rothenberg, L. (2011). *Family-provider relationships: A multidisciplinary review of high-quality practices and associations with family, child, and provider outcomes*. U.S. Department of Health and Human Services. https://www.acf.hhs.gov/sites/default/files/documents/opre/family_provider_multi.pdf

Ginosar, N. (2019, September 6). "Kemo luleyan al khut" – Tippul behorut liyiladim im otizm vehitmodedut im temot paradoqesaliyyot ["Like an acrobat on a highwire": Therapy for parents of children with autism and dealing with paradoxical themes]. *Hebrew Psychology*. https://www.hebpsy.net/articles.asp?id=3860

Greenbaum, C. W., & Fried, D. (Eds.) (2011). *Relations between the family and the early childhood education system (preschool to grade 3)*. Israel Academy of Sciences and Humanities. https://education.academy.ac.il/SystemFiles/23022.pdf

גרניבאום, ז.צ'. ופריד, ד. (עורכים). (2011). *קשרי משפחה-מסגרת חינוך בגיל הרך (גן-ג'): מטות-מצב והמלצות*. הוועדה לנושא קשרי משפחה-מסגרת חינוכית בגיל הרך (גן-ג') וזיקתם להתפתחות הילד ולהצלחתו במערכת החינוך. האקדמיה הלאומית הישראלית למדעים. ירושלים: תשע"א. נדלה מתוך: http://education.academy.ac.il/SystemFiles/23022.pdf

Guralnick, M. J. (2005). An overview of the developmental systems model for early intervention. In M. J. Guralnick (Ed.), *The developmental systems approach to early intervention* (pp. 3–28). Baltimore: Brookes.

Guralnick, M. J. (2017). Early intervention for children with intellectual disabilities: An update. *Journal of Applied Research in Intellectual Disabilities, 30*(2), 211–229. https://doi.org/10.1111/jar.12233

Howard, J. S., Sparkman, C. R., Cohen, H. G., Green, G., & Stanislaw, H. A. (2005). A comparison of intensive behavior analytic and eclectic treatments for young children with autism. *Research in Developmental Disabilities, 26*, 359–383. https://doi.org/10.1016/j.ridd.2004.09.005

Ingber, S. (2004). *Involvement of parents in education and rehabilitation programs for hearing-impaired children in Israel: Assessment of parents and professionals.* Dissertation towards a Doctor of Philosophy degree, Tel Aviv University.

Ingber, S., Al-Yagon, M., & Dromi, E. (2010). Mothers' involvement in early intervention for children with hearing loss: The role of maternal characteristics and context-based perceptions. *Journal of Early Intervention, 32*(5), 351–369.

Ingber, S., & Dromi, A. (2011). Parental involvement in family-centered intervention programs for children with special educational needs. In C. W. Greenbaum & D. Fried (Eds.), *Relations between the family and the early childhood education system (preschool to grade 3): Status report and recommendations of the committee for the study of the relations between the family and the early childhood education system (preschool to grade 3) and their association with the child's development and achievement in the education system.* Israel Academy of Sciences and Humanities.

Israel Ministry of Education and Culture. (2010). *Educational activities in kindergarten: Guidelines for the educational team.* Ministry of Education, Division for Pre-Primary Education. https://meyda.education.gov.il/files/PreSchool/KavimManhim.pdf

Israel Ministry of Education and Culture. (n.d.). *Partnership between parents and educational teams.* Israel Ministry of Education. https://parents.education.gov.il/prhnet/special-education/parental-partnership/parental-partnership

Katzenelson, E. (2014). The relationship between parents and their children's education system. *Psychoactualia.* https://katzr.net/23fce4

Koizumi, H. (2004). The concept of 'developing the brain': A new natural science for learning and education. *Brain and Development, 26*(7), 434–441. https://doi.org/10.1016/j.braindev.2003.09.011

Kolb, B., & Gibb, R. (2011). Brain plasticity and behavior in the developing brain. *Journal of the Canadian Academy of Child and Adolescent Psychiatry, 20*(4), 265–276. https://www.ncbi.nlm.nih.gov/pmc/articles/PMC3222570/

Küçükturan, A. G., & Akbaba Altun, S. (2017). Motivations and barriers in promoting preschool education. *Educational Sciences: Theory & Practice, 17*(4). 1433–1450. https://doi.org/10.12738/estp.2017.4.0368

Johnson, N. L., Giarelli, E., Lewis, C., & Rice, C. E. (2013). Genomics and autism spectrum disorder. *Journal of Nursing Scholarship, 45*(1), 69–78. https://doi.org/10.1111/j.1547-5069.2012.01483.x

Landa, R. J., Gross, A. L., Stuart, E. A., & Faherty, A. (2013). Developmental trajectories in children with and without autism spectrum disorders: The first 3 years. *Child Development, 84*(2), 429–442. https://doi.org/10.1111/j.1467-8624.2012.01870.x

Landa, R. J. (2018). Efficacy of early interventions for infants and young children with, and at risk for, autism spectrum disorders. *International Review of Psychiatry, 30*(1), 25–39. https://doi.org/10.1080%2F09540261.2018.1432574

Lewis, J. D., Evans, A. C., Pruett, J. R., Botteron, K., Zwaigenbaum, L., Estes, A., Gerig, G., Collins, L., Kostopoulos, P., McKinstry, R., Dager, S., Paterson, S., Schultz, R. T., Styner, M., Hazlett, H., & Piven, J. (2014). Network inefficiencies in autism spectrum disorder at 24 months. *Translational Psychiatry, 4*(5), e388. https://doi.org/10.1038%2Ftp.2014.24

Maenner, M. J., Shaw, K. A., & Baio, J. (2020). Prevalence of autism spectrum disorder among children aged 8 years—autism and developmental disabilities monitoring network, 11 sites, United States, 2016. *MMWR Surveillance Summaries, 69*(4), 1–12. 10.15585%2Fmmwr.ss6904a1

Mareoiu, M., Bland, C., Dobbins, N., & Niemeyer, J. A. (2015). Exploring perspectives on childcare with families of children with autism. *Early Childhood Research & Practice, 17*, 1–13. https://files.eric.ed.gov/fulltext/EJ1072386.pdf

Moulton, E., Barton, M., Robins, D.L., Abrams, D.N., & Fein, D. (2016). Early characteristics of children with ASD who demonstrate optimal progress between age two and four. *Journal of Autism and Developmental Disorders, 46*, 2160–2173. 10.1007%2Fs10803–016–2745–1

Nevill, R. E., Lecavalier, L., & Stratis, E. A. (2018). Meta-analysis of parent-mediated interventions for young children with autism spectrum disorder. *Autism, 22*(2), 84–98. https://doi.org/10.1177/1362361316677838

Oono, I. P., Honey, E. J., & McConachie, H. (2013). Parent-mediated early intervention for young children with autism spectrum disorders (ASD). *Evidence-Based Child Health: A Cochrane Review Journal, 8*(6), 2380–2479. https://doi.org/10.1002/14651858.cd009774.pub2

Orinstein, A. J., Helt, M., Troyb, E., Tyson, K. E., Barton, M. L., Eigsti, I. M., Naigles, L., & Fein, D. A. (2014). Intervention for optimal outcome in children and adolescents with a history of autism. *Journal of Developmental & Behavioral Pediatrics, 35*, 247–256. https://doi.org/10.1097/DBP.0000000000000037

Osborne, L. A., McHugh, L., Saunders, J., & Reed, P. (2008). Parenting stress reduces the effectiveness of early teaching interventions for autistic spectrum disorders. *Journal of Autism and Developmental Disorders, 38*(6), 1092–1103. https://doi.org/10.1007/s10803-007-0497-7

Ozonoff, S., Young, G. S., Landa, R. J., Brian, J., Bryson, S., Charman, T., Chawarska, K., Macari, S. L., Messinger, D., Stone, W. L., Zwaigenbaum, L., & Iosif, A. M. (2015). Diagnostic stability in young children at risk for autism spectrum disorder: a baby siblings research consortium study. *Journal of Child Psychology and Psychiatry, 56*(9), 988–998. https://doi.org/10.1111%2Fjcpp.12421

Papandreou, M., Birbili, M., & Martidou, R. (2009). Parents' perceptions of the role of kindergarten and their involvement in children's education. In *OMEP European Regional Meeting and Conference 2009 Conference Proceedings* (pp. 437–452). Syros: OMEP. https://doi.org/10.21890/ijres.369197

Petrogiannis, K., & Penderi, E. (2014). The quality of parent–teacher relationship in kindergarten: A Greek study. *International Research in Education, 2*(1). https://doi.org/10.5296/ire.v2i1.4343

Pirchio, S., Tritrini, C., Passiatore, Y., & Taeschner, T. (2013). The role of the relationship between parents and educators for child behavior and wellbeing. *International Journal about Parents in Education, 7*(2), 145–155. http://eslplus.eu/documents/The_role_of_the_Relationship_between_Parents_and_Educators_for_Child_Behaviour_and_Wellbeing.pdf

Rekalidou, G. & Penderi, E. (2010). A collaborative action research project in the kindergarten: Perspectives and challenges for teacher development through internal evaluation processes. *New Horizons in Education, 58*(2), 18–33. https://files.eric.ed.gov/fulltext/EJ966648.pdf

Rentzou, K. (2011). Parent–caregiver relationship dyad in Greek day care centres. *International Journal of Early Years Education, 19*(2), 163–177. https://doi.org/10.1080/09669760.2011.609045

Rimland, B., & Edelson, S. (1999). *Autism Treatment Evaluation Checklist (ATEC)*. San Diego: Autism Research Institute. https://psycnet.apa.org/doi/https://doi.org/10.1037/t03995-000

Ritvo, B., Luke, E., & Berg, A. (2018). *Relationships, connection and educational partnership between the education staff and the students' parents*. Israel Ministry of Education, Psychological-Advisory Service. https://meyda.education.gov.il/files/shefi/horim/Mismach_Mediniut_2019.pdf

Rogers, S. J., Estes, A., Lord, C., Vismara, L., Winter, J., Fitzpatrick, A., Guo, M. & Dawson, G. (2012). Effects of a brief Early Start Denver Model (ESDM)–based parent intervention on toddlers at risk for autism spectrum disorders: A randomized controlled trial. *Journal of the American Academy of Child & Adolescent Psychiatry, 51*(10), 1052–1065. https://doi.org/10.1016%2Fj.jaac.2012.08.003

Russa, M. B., Matthews, A. L., & Owen-DeSchryver, J. S. (2015). Expanding supports to improve the lives of families of children with autism spectrum disorder. *Journal of Positive Behavior Interventions, 17*(2), 95–104. 10.1177%2F1098300714532134

Sallows, G. O., & Graupner, T. D. (2005). Intensive behavioral treatment for children with autism: Four-year outcome and predictors. *American Journal of Mental Retardation, 110*, 417–438. https://doi.org/10.1352/0895-8017(2005)110[417:ibtfcw]2.0.co;2

Schaaf, C. P., & Zoghbi, H. Y. (2011). Solving the autism puzzle a few pieces at a time. *Neuron, 70*(5), 806–808. https://doi.org/10.1016/j.neuron.2011.05.025

Segev, A., Weisskopf, M. G., Levine, H., Pinto, O., & Raz, R. (2019). Incidence time trends and socioeconomic factors in the observed incidence of autism spectrum disorder in Israel: A nationwide nested case–control study. *Autism Research, 12*(12), 1870–1879. https://doi.org/10.1002/aur.2185

Serpell, Z., & Mashburn, A. J. (2011). Family-school connectedness and children's early social development. *Social Development, 21*(1), 21–46. https://doi.org/10.1111/j.1467-9507.2011.00623.x

Sevimli-Celik, S., Kirazci, S., & Ince, M. L. (2011). Preschool movement education in Turkey: Perceptions of preschool administrators and parents. *Early Childhood Education Journal, 39*(5), 323–333. https://doi.org/10.1007/s10643-011-0473-x

Sharabi, A., & Marom-Golan, D. (2018). Social support, education levels, and parents' involvement: A comparison between mothers and fathers of young children with autism spectrum disorder. *Topics in Early Childhood Special Education, 38*(1), 54–64. 10.1177%2F0271121418762511

Siller, M., & Sigman, M. (2008). Modeling longitudinal change in the language abilities of children with autism: Parent behaviors and child characteristics as predictors of change. *Developmental Psychology, 44*(6), 702–1691. https://psycnet.apa.org/doi/https://doi.org/10.1037/a0013771

Smith, T., Klorman, R., & Mruzek, D. W. (2015). Predicting the outcome of community-based early intensive behavioral intervention for children with autism. *Journal of Abnormal Child Psychology, 43*(7), 1271–1282. https://doi.org/10.1007/s10802-015-0002-2

Stoner, J. B., Bock, S. J., Thompson, J. R., Angell, M. E., Heyl, B. S., & Crowley, E. P. (2005). Welcome to our world: Parent perceptions of interactions between parents of young children with ASD and education professionals. *Focus on Autism and Other Developmental Disabilities, 20*(1), 39–51. https://psycnet.apa.org/doi/https://doi.org/10.1177/10883576050200010401

Sucuoğlu, N. B., & Bakkaloğlu, H. (2018). The quality of parent–teacher relationships in inclusive preschools. *Early Child Development and Care, 188*(8), 1190–1201. https://doi.org/10.1080/03004430.2016.1261124

Swartz, M. I., & Easterbrooks, M. A. (2014). The role of parent, provider, and child characteristics in parent–provider relationships in infant and toddler classrooms. *Early Education and Development, 25*(4), 573–598. https://psycnet.apa.org/doi/https://doi.org/10.1080/10409289.2013.822229

Troisi, J., Autio, R., Beopoulos, T., Bravaccio, C., Carraturo, F., Corrivetti, G., Cunningham, S., Devane, S., Fallin, D., Fetissov, S., & Gea (2020). Genome, Environment, Microbiome and Metabolome in Autism (GEMMA) study design: Biomarkers identification for precision treatment and primary prevention of autism spectrum disorders by an integrated multi-omics systems biology approach. *Brain Sciences, 10*(10), 743. https://doi.org/10.3390/brainsci10100743

Vickers, H. S., & Minke, K. M. (1995). Exploring parent-teacher relationships: Joining and communication to others. *School Psychology Quarterly, 10*(2), 133.

Wallace, K. S., & Rogers, S. J. (2010). Intervening in infancy: Implications for autism spectrum disorders. *Journal of Child Psychology and Psychiatry, 51*(12), 1300–1320. https://doi.org/10.1111/j.1469-7610.2010.02308.x

Wang, H., Hu, X., & Han, Z. R. (2020). Parental stress, involvement, and family quality of life in mothers and fathers of children with autism spectrum disorder in mainland China: A dyadic analysis. *Research in Developmental Disabilities, 107*, Article 103791. https://doi.org/10.1016/j.ridd.2020.103791

Warren, S. F., Gilkerson, J., Richards, J. A., Oller, D. K., Xu, D., Yapanel, U., & Gray, S. (2010). What automated vocal analysis reveals about the vocal production and language learning environment of young children with autism. *Journal of Autism and Developmental Disorders, 40*(5), 555–569. https://psycnet.apa.org/doi/https://doi.org/10.1007/s10803-009-0902-5

World Health Organization [WHO]. (2007). *International Classification of Functioning, Disability, and Health: Children & Youth Version: ICF-CY*. World Health Organization. https://apps.who.int/iris/bitstream/handle/10665/42407/9241545429_tha+eng.pdf?sequence=7

World Health Organization [WHO] & UNICEF. (2012). *Early childhood development and disability: A discussion paper.* World Health Organization. Malta. http://apps.who.int/iris/bitstream/10665/75355/1/9789241504065_eng.pdf.

Yan, T., Hou, Y., & Deng, M. (2022). Direct, indirect, and buffering effect of social support on parental involvement among Chinese parents of children with autism spectrum disorders. *Journal of Autism and Developmental Disorders, 52*(7), 2911–2923. https://doi.org/10.1007/s10803-021-05170-x

Chapter 12
Enhancing Parental Involvement in High-Functioning Autism Interventions

Sigal Moyal and Susan Lowinger

Abstract This article underscores the critical and unquestionable role of parents in the successful treatment of young children with autism spectrum disorder (ASD). The literature emphasizes that parents are the most significant figures in a child's life, profoundly influencing their development and capacity to acquire new skills. While collaboration between therapists and parents is paramount, the study described in this chapter found that parental characteristics, emotional states, and behavioral patterns can significantly impede a child's progress. Thus, this chapter advocates for essential interventions with parents to equip them with skills such as executive function, self-regulation, and emotional management, enabling them to serve as effective models for their children. It details how parent-mediated interventions lead to improved child outcomes, enhanced skill generalization, and sustained treatment gains. The chapter also explores factors that compromise treatment effectiveness, such as parental disengagement and a lack of treatment continuity at home. Parents may lack the skills that the child is trying to improve, and thus fail to be good models for their children. The Interactive Play Intervention (IPI) model introduced here offers a structured framework for therapists and parents to identify and work on shared therapeutic goals, fostering deeply internalized change for both child and parent. This resource is indispensable for professionals and families aiming to optimize ASD treatment outcomes through robust parent-therapist collaboration.

Keywords Parental involvement · Therapist–parent collaboration · Parent-mediated interventions · Executive functions · Behavioral patterns · IPI model · Skill acquisition · Treatment effectiveness

---

S. Moyal (✉)
Ben Gurion University/Tel Aviv University, Jerusalem, Israel
e-mail: e6255744@gmail.com

S. Lowinger
Developmental Psychology, Kishurim Clinic, Jerusalem, Israel

S. Lowinger and S. Pearlman-Avnion (eds.), *Collaborative Care and Partnerships in Autism Diagnosis and Treatment*, Autism and Child Psychopathology Series,
https://doi.org/10.1007/978-3-032-07009-8_12

Introduction

The need for parents of young children with autism spectrum disorder (ASD) to be involved in the treatment is unquestionable. Collaboration between therapists and parents is essential for the success of the treatment. Parents play a key role and have a crucial influence on the child's improvement and ability to generate new skills.

However, various family traits may affect parental involvement and interfere with the child's process and delay their improvement. By offering understanding, support, and guidance, therapists can help parents cope with the treatment and be part of the process.

There is a lack of research on the need for interventions to assist parents regarding the skills that the child is trying to improve. Parents may lack these skills themselves and need to practice them so they can be good models for their children. The focus can be changed to working with parents on their awareness and understanding, and to help them practice social, cognitive, emotional, and behavioral skills, and help their child acquire these skills.

Parent–child dynamics are more important than therapist–child relationships since the parents are the most significant people in the child's life. The child's development is related to both biological and environmental factors. Parents can lead their children by providing education and especially by setting a personal example. Along with the child's character, the dynamics in the home affect the child's social functioning. Children absorb their parents' behavior, imitate the patterns to which they are exposed, and build ways of responding that are reinforced by the social environment. The innate character traits of the child are inseparable from those of the parents. Parents must deal not only with the child's autism but also with the consequences of their own behavior patterns. Even if significant work is invested in the treatment of children with ASD, incorrect behavioral patterns on the part of the parents may prevent the child from reaching his or her true potential.

Therefore, interventions with the parents are essential so they can go through a joint process with their child on specific goals related to social interaction. Working with parents on acquiring skills such as executive function, self-regulation, mental rigidity, perfectionism, and dealing with difficulties, alongside the child's process of acquiring these skills, is highly significant for the child's success.

The Importance of Collaboration Between Therapists and Parents

Treatment for ASD typically involves interventions aimed at improving children's adaptive skills and reducing their symptoms. Parent-mediated interventions and parent training in these areas have been receiving increasing support (Diggle & McConachie, 2003; McConachie et al., 2005; Sofronoff et al., 2004). Previous studies have demonstrated the effectiveness of parental interventions in improving children's responsiveness, expressive language, and functional play as well as significantly reducing children's behavioral difficulties and sleep problems (Anan et al., 2008; Elder et al., 2005; Kasari et al., 2010; Siller et al., 2013; Weiskop et al., 2005). Moreover, parental involvement in the treatment of anxiety in children with ASD has been found to be effective and is considered a core modification when adapting cognitive behavioral therapy (CBT) for children on the autism spectrum (Moree & Davis, 2010; Sofronoff et al., 2005). Other advantages of parental involvement include increased generalization and long-term maintenance of treatment gains, as well as cost-effectiveness and better allocation of resources (Matson et al., 2009; Solomon et al., 2007). Taken together, these findings suggest that parent-mediated interventions could be an efficacious alternative to one-to-one clinician support.

However, the literature suggests that parental capacity to promote the health and overall adjustment of their children may be affected by their own emotional state and well-being. For example, parental stress can compromise parents' and children's coping resources and affect their ability to solve problems (Friedman & Chase-Lansdale, 2002; Vasilopoulou & Nisbet, 2016).

In this context, collaboration has been described as "mutually supportive interaction through which knowledge and skills are shared, mutual understandings occur, and shared decisions are made" (An et al., 2016, p. 1844). Collaboration can be divided into participatory practices and relational practices (Mas et al., 2022). Participatory practices aim to increase active parent engagement and include behavior such as shared goal setting, building on parents' strengths, and promoting the acquisition of new skills (Dunst & Trivette, 2009). An and Palisano (2014) described a four-step process of collaborative service delivery comprising mutually agreed-upon goals, shared planning, shared implementation, shared evaluation, and integrating the child's and family's needs, preferences, and routines.

For parents, relational practices are essential for participation in the therapy process (Klatte et al., 2020; Kokorelias et al., 2019). Relational practices aim to build on the relationship with parents and include aspects such as empathy, active and reflective listening, effective communication, and cultural sensitivity to parental values and needs (Hill, 2001). All collaborative practices should be performed with a two-way interaction style between parents and therapists (An & Palisano, 2014; Melvin et al., 2019). This involves not only informing parents and explaining things to them but also listening to parents' concerns and giving them a voice.

In the theoretical literature, collaboration is clearly explained and its importance for clinical practice is recognized. However, there is a gap between theory and practice. Many therapists find collaboration with parents to be complex and difficult to implement in daily practice (Klatte et al., 2020). Therapists commonly find that parents are disengaged from the therapy and few feel proficient in establishing collaboration with parents (Klatte et al., 2019; Melvin et al., 2019).

No one-size-fits-all approach exists, since therapists and parents must deal with multiple factors. First, all parents and therapists have their own unique set of characteristics, needs, priorities, history, and expectations. Second, each child is unique and needs a personalized approach. Third, therapists and parents have personal preferences and communication styles in their collaborations with each other. Fourth, therapists and parents must deal with local institutional and financial factors (Joseph-Williams et al., 2014; Klatte & Roulstone, 2016; Kokorelias et al., 2019). In addition, the parents' personal characteristics and their objective difficulties may impair their effectiveness in interactions with their child. Parents must develop self-awareness and acquire tools to deal with their difficulties to be more effective.

Parents' Participation in the Treatment

The importance of parent participation in the education of young children with autism spectrum disorder (ASD) is well documented, with research linking parent involvement to a variety of positive child outcomes, including improved skill maintenance and generalization. Research suggests that parent involvement varies greatly in early intervention in special education programs for children with disabilities. In addition to difficulties linked to their child's disorder, like all parents, the parents of children with ASD must contend with a variety of other demands on their time and energy, including those associated with employment and the care of other children (Benson et al., 2008).

Parental involvement is crucial to the continuity of the treatment at home; the presence of the parents in the treatment allows them to be aware of the therapeutic process, their child's functioning in various play situations, and reactions to the therapeutic intervention. Parents being present is not enough. The parent must be aware of what is happening and be updated regarding the therapeutic goals and what the therapist is doing toward these goals. The parent must understand what the therapist is doing. Once parents connect to the treatment method, they can ensure its continuity at home and in other environments. Several factors, described below, potentially pose issues and impair the progress of the treatment and its effectiveness.

The Parents Are Not Involved: There is no Continuity of Treatment at Home

The presence of the parents in the treatment allows them to be aware of the therapeutic process, their child's functioning in the various play situations, and reactions to the therapeutic intervention. However, the mere presence of the parents is not enough. The parents must be aware of what is happening, be aware of the therapeutic goals, and understand and be updated regarding what the therapist is doing to work on these goals. Once parents connect to the treatment method, they can ensure its continuity at home and in other environments. When the parents are not involved in the treatment, the frequency of opportunities for practice is low, and they are not always used correctly.

The Parents Have Difficulties or Behavioral Patterns Like Those of Their Child

As children undergo change processes during treatment, their communicative and social conduct is influenced by their parents' behavior patterns or personal tendencies, whether these are inherited or passed down in behavioral modeling. For a change in the child to succeed, the parents must be aware that they also must undergo change. For example, it is difficult for a child who is unregulated or disorganized to change if his parents are unregulated or disorganized.

Infrequent Treatment Sessions

Weekly therapy sessions are sufficient for most children, but in certain situations, there is a need to increase the frequency of treatment. This is because the gap between experiences is too great. Repetition is important to give the child tools. Lack of repetition may cause a feeling that the progress is not sufficient.

Lack of Combination Between Complementary Treatments

In certain situations, the child requires treatment by other professionals (occupational therapists, physical therapists, speech therapists, emotional therapists, physicians who can prescribe medication). These complementary treatments help children establish abilities in areas that are objectively difficult for them. The lack of necessary treatment may harm the therapeutic process.

Lack of Contact with Professional Team

Teams of professionals offering complementary treatments must meet frequently (preferably at least once every 3 months) to inform each other of how they each perceive the child's functioning, therapeutic goals, and working methods. Team members coordinate on how to deal with various situations and support each other to help the child progress. If such meetings are not held, treatment effectiveness may be reduced. Each therapist acts according to his or her knowledge. Situations may arise in which therapists use contradictory procedures.

Behavioral Intervention is Necessary

When behavioral problems arise as symptoms of the child's difficulties, there is a need to develop a behavioral intervention plan for the treatment room, home, and school environment. Lack of such a plan results in a situation in which the child undergoes a treatment process, but the problematic behavior continues and is reinforced by the environment.

The Child Does Not Generalize to Play with Peers

Usually, a child seems calmer upon entering treatment and relatively quickly exhibits a change in social behavior that results in getting along better with peers and making more friends. If this does not occur, it becomes necessary to create a play group with peers, offer opportunities for joint play, and ensure that they experience success.

Parental Characteristics and Their Influence on the Child

Like most important topics in psychology, research on parenting styles is not immune to the nature–nurture debate. Researchers who study parent–adolescent relationships are increasingly looking at the importance of the impact of parenting on adolescent development, and how experience in the family and other contexts interact with genetic factors to influence behavioral and developmental outcomes (Collins et al., 2000).

There are four types of parenting styles. These are authoritative parenting (associated with a warm yet firm personality), authoritarian/controlling parenting (minimally warm with a highly controlling personality), permissive/indulgent parenting (amiable and undemanding personality), and uninvolved/neglectful parenting (not warm, does not demand anything). If the mother and father exhibit different parenting styles, such as when one parent is authoritarian and the other is permissive, they should discuss the child's situation and needs. Cooperative, motivated, and responsible children are a result of the authoritative parenting style, while the uncooperative, immature, irresponsible child is elicited by the uninvolved parenting style.

Environmental and behavioral genetic patterns also play roles in children's cognitive development. Parenting style reflects the mother's and father's behavior, including internalizing problems such as sleep difficulties and mood, and externalizing problems such as social stress and job difficulty. Individual adolescent characteristics like temperament and personality also play an essential role in parenting (Altenburger & Schoppe-Sullivan, 2020; Barlow et al., 2016).

Children require positive parenting in painful and difficult situations. Positive parenting helps the child face non-social or social problems. Positive parenting is required for early cognitive development, emotional balance, and the maturation of thought. In contrast, negative, hostile parenting leads to depression and social and cultural problems. Parenting styles (authoritative, authoritarian, permissive, and uninvolved parenting) have a psychological effect on a child's behavior (Lanjekar et al., 2022).

Research focuses on increasing parental support and responsibility to develop children's cognitive abilities. Providing sensitive caregiving and a supportive emotional climate for young children positively affects children's cognitive development. Supportive and sensitive parenting offers children security and confidence; parents promote reasonable regulations and self-initiation in social and non-social experiments. Self-sufficient support and sensitivity, and a caregiving nature, lead to early brain maturation and cognitive development in children. Sensitive parenting shows affective and behavioral development in children; it is characterized by responsiveness, positive encouragement for something, giving approval or thanking and stimulation (Barnett et al., 2008; Burchinal et al., 2008; Mills-Koonce et al., 2015).

Children's health, behavior, development, and style of parenting cause worry for every parent. In such cases, professional help is required to solve this problem. It is related to family care, youth and parenting support, and children's mental health. The media is exclusively used to increase parenting information and awareness. It enhances parenting skills and decreases depression, anxiety, and stress; it also helps the parents improve their skills in the parent–child relationship and supports them to benefit from the child's health and well-being (Aboud & Yousafzai, 2015; Fierloos et al., 2022; Ginsburg, 2007; Milteer et al., 2012).

Collaboration by Parents Addressing Their Own Characteristics

It is often possible to see that parents and children share behavioral patterns and emotional responses. Given the significant relationship between the parent and the child, the parents' behavioral patterns and responses affect the child's progress in treatment.

In many cases, the parents of the children suffer from the same difficulties that the therapist is supposed to treat in the child. It is essential to change the focus of treatment for the parents as well to bring about significant progress in the treatment of the child. The parent must consider that if he does not treat himself, this may harm the effectiveness of the treatment.

Several significant factors enable effective collaboration:

- Identifying focused goals for treatment regarding problematic characteristics that interfere with the child's social functioning. Similar goals for the parents will also be identified if they exhibit the same problematic characteristics.
- Parental awareness that their characteristics may be related to and influence those of the child. Parental understanding that addressing problematic characteristics will enable effective change in the child.
- Parents being treated by a qualified professional at the same time as the child is being treated (for example, coaching, emotional therapy).
- Parents who work toward targeted goals in everyday situations to break fixed patterns of behavior at home.
- Parental awareness of the child's therapeutic goals and understanding what needs to be done to work on these goals. They are responsible for the continuity of

the treatment at home and in other environments. Parents being present during treatment and receive practical tools from the therapist. Regular updates from the therapist regarding the progress of treatment goals are necessary.

- Parents who complement each other as necessary.
- Parents receiving guidance concerning their interactions with the child at home.

Identifying Targeted Goals for Treatment

In this section of the chapter, the Interactive Play Intervention (IPI) model for applied treatment on social skills will be presented (Moyal, 2023). Proper use of the model will enable effective collaboration between the therapist and the parent and maximize progress in therapeutic goals for both the child and the parent.

The IPI model was developed, based on existing therapeutic theories, to deal with communication and social difficulties in children. This model is a combination of the interactive approach and the behavioral approach. The nature of the therapeutic approach is interactive, but it incorporates concepts, procedures, and tools that belong to the behavioral approach. The child leads the interaction, while the adult is an active partner and behaves like a peer, but is, at the same time, a deliberate guide who helps organize and help when necessary.

Learning takes place during an emotional experience that is meaningful for the child. The treatment focuses on specific goals leading to a gradual change in the areas of communication and social behavior. Children differ from each other in terms of the therapeutic goals necessary, so for each child, a personal set of goals is constructed and adapted to the child's personal profile. Working on these goals should consider an integrative vision that includes the child's functions in all areas. The intervention is carried out by experiencing spontaneous and natural situations, usually through semi-structured activities (Moyal, 2023).

The IPI model is presented in the following diagram (Fig. 12.1) and alternatively in Table 12.1, following Fig. 12.1.

The IPI model consists of six areas (shown as circles in Fig. 12.1) of social skills in which the child may be impaired and which affect the child's overall functioning: communication, socializing, intentionality, coping skills, emotional skills, and physiology. Each area contains eight therapeutic goals, for a total of 48 goals.

Therefore, if the child and parents share the same goal, it is important to identify the matter at the beginning of the therapeutic process to simultaneously undergo a process of change. To do this, we must first identify the child's therapeutic goals.

The same work that the child does, and the same process of change, must be gone through by the parent. Of course, an adult has a higher level of awareness and can observe in depth, receive guidance, and converse around the focal points for work. However, parents can undergo training through activities just as the child does. This helps with mental flexibility and internalization of changes in behavioral patterns.

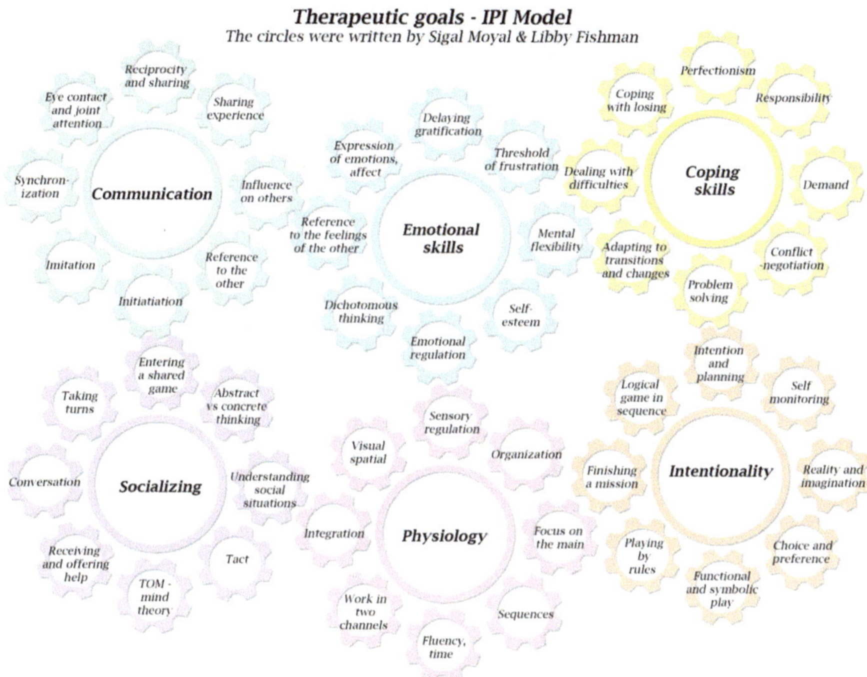

Fig. 12.1 Therapeutic Goals: IPI Model. The model consists of six "circles"—six different areas of social skills in which the child maybe impaired: communication, socializing, intentionality, coping skills, emotional skills and physiology. Each area is called a "circle" and contains eight therapeutic goals

This requires (1) identifying focused goals that are shared by the child and his parents, (2) using external help such as counseling or coaching, (3) playing together with the child, and (4) practicing in a spontaneous environment.

It must be remembered that the meaningful emotional experience for the parent is what creates internalization. It is not enough to memorize cognitive rules for action, but one must find and create opportunities for practice to introduce the change into a permanent pattern (Ozonoff et al., 2005).

Therapeutic Application of Targeted Goals

Below are several therapeutic goals selected from the 48 goals listed in the IPI model above. These goals can be practiced by the child and the parents to improve a specific social skill. Each goal will be presented in a table with application ideas for working with the child through play, and at the same time, application ideas that the parent can practice. To succeed, parents must be aware of their own difficulties, be willing to

Table 12.1 Therapeutic Goals - IPI Model, Tabular Representation

Communication	Socializing	Intentionality	Coping skills	Emotional skills	Physiology
Reciprocity and sharing	Entering a shared game	Intention and planning	Dealing with difficulties	Expression of emotions, affect	Sensory regulation
Eye contact and joint attention	Taking turns	Logical game in sequence	Coping with losing	Reference to the feelings of others	Visual spatial abilities
Reference to the other	Conversation	Finishing a mission	Adapting to transitions and changes	Emotional regulation	Fluency, time
Initiation	Receiving and offering help	Playing by rules	Problem solving	Dichotomous thinking	Work in two channels
Synchronization	TOM—Theory of mind	Functional and symbolic play	Conflict–negotiation	Mental flexibility	Integration
Imitation	Understanding social situations	Choice and preference	Demand	Self-esteem	Sequences
Influence on others	Tact	Reality and imagination	Responsibility	Delaying gratification	Focus on the main
Sharing experience	Abstract thinking	Self-monitoring	Perfectionism	Threshold of frustration	Organization

make changes, and practice the applications that will be presented below daily. The goals that will be presented below are executive function (EF), emotion regulation, mental rigidity, perfectionism, and dealing with difficulties.

Executive Function

Executive function (EF) enables the organization of daily activities toward a goal, sequence planning, and perception. EF is a general term for actions such as planning, prioritization, working memory, control of impulsive behavior, mental flexibility, judgment, and ability to organize (Felsenthal-Berger, 2007; Ozonoff et al., 2005).

EF develops naturally in most people and enables them to manage their lives with long-term thinking, consideration of the viability of activities or behaviors, logical judgment, and rational decision-making (Hill, 2004). Impairment of EF makes it very difficult for children in many areas and directly affects their success as students. Often, a child has difficulty organizing the materials needed to carry out classroom learning activities, plan the preparation of lessons, or complete a class assignment. Despite having good cognitive abilities, they may be unable to manage their life like their peers (Samooha, 2010). EF abilities are important for solving cognitive problems and also have a role in emotional-social behavior, information processing, and adaptive functioning.

The difficulty in switching between activities and over-focusing on one part of an activity leads to a situation in which the child needs mediation to create a sequence of activities and planning. There is a need to explain, organize, and create a set of sequences for different situations, to make order in the child's world, understand rules, and process sequences of parts of situations into a whole concept (Felsenthal-Berger, 2007).

Every activity requires organization. One must be goal-oriented, plan a sequence of activities, take everything that is required to carry out the plan, remember the sequence, and carry it out fluently. Effective organization allows for dealing with tasks calmly, completion of tasks, and moving on to the next task.

Children may show difficulties in executive functioning in various areas.

- Difficulty in designing sequences (e.g., agenda).
  - Difficulty following instructions effectively.
- Difficulty in life skills involving sequences (e.g., getting dressed).
- Difficulty getting organized and completing tasks (e.g., difficulty packing a bag for a trip, difficulty finishing homework).
  - Has difficulty managing tools (e.g., pens, rulers, clothes) or using organizational accessories (e.g., diaries, to-do lists, calendars).
  - Exhibits confusion when getting organized.
  - Takes a long time to do anything, has difficulty moving on to the next activity.
  - Tends to lose things; the child's environment is cluttered.

- Difficulty in judging and making decisions (e.g., how long it takes to complete a task, and determining the priorities in the process).

The Influence of the Parents' EF Characteristics on Those of the Child: The Need for Collaboration

EF is associated with various aspects of school achievement and cognitive development in children and adolescents. There are important connections between parenting behaviors and EF skills in school-age children. It is necessary to show parents the ways in which they can optimally support their children's cognitive development (Sosic-Vasic et al., 2017).

Parents' involvement in their children's education is integral to academic success. EF skills are fluid and influenced by several factors, including parental age, sleep, stress, and mood/affect. Despite possible limitations in parental EF, there are strategies school personnel can employ to strengthen their partnership with parents to support their children's academic success. As reforms in education call for increased customization and collaboration with families, parental EF is an important consideration for school personnel. Awareness and understanding of how parents' EF affects children's learning will help schools better support parents in supporting their children's academic success (Wilson & Gross, 2018) (Table 12.2).

Emotion Regulation

Emotion regulation refers to regulating emotional response, controlling activation of emotions, maintaining an optimal level of arousal, and balancing emotional responses. Emotions navigate our way in the world. It helps us understand the world and orient ourselves, communicate with the environment, convey messages to others, respond to dangers, and help us in intra-psychic processes. Emotions are created in response to external or internal stimuli. These stimuli do not act on us alone but are mediated through the cognitive system—the thoughts; that is, we do not respond to stimuli as they occur in reality, but to stimuli as we perceive them. The way we interpret reality and the stimuli around us create a chemical–electrical reaction in our brain. As a result of this reaction, emotion (physical expression of the emotion) is created, alongside the mental expression of the emotion. The experience of emotion and its physical and mental expressions lead to action. In most cases, emotional experience responses are excellent and helpful; they help us survive and integrate well into the society around us, but there are cases where the responses lose their effectiveness. Although we experience the responses as automatic and uncontrollable, we can activate emotions even in a way that is not automatic. This is done by regulating the emotional response and in a controlled activation of the emotions (Marchewski, 2013).

Table 12.2 Therapeutic Strategies in Treating Executive Functioning

Parent and child during play	The parent in daily activities
Practice organization: In any situation that requires organization in the room, do it with the child. Do not organize the game instead of the child, even if it takes a long time. The emphasis is on the preparation for the game and treating the preparation as an equally important part of the game itself.	**Practice organization:** Tidying up the house or desk, preparing a meal, and doing paperwork.
Think about and plan what is needed before an activity: Before going somewhere or undertaking a complex activity that consists of processes (such as baking a cake) or when not all the materials are in the room, think together about which objects you need to bring from outside, where they are found, and who will be responsible for bringing them. A list can be very helpful. Before the activity, go through the list and make sure you have everything you need.	Think and plan what is needed before an activity that requires preparation: Make a grocery list for preparing food/baking cake, organize a shopping trip.
Give the child an important role: Children like to be given responsible roles. They may be responsible for the money in monopoly, writing down what was bought, and distributing the money. Give them roles that require organization, encourage self-organization, and responsibility.	**Be responsible:** Take responsible roles/ permanent roles at home, such as being responsible for watering potted plants.
Demonstrate and explain techniques for keeping order: Show the child how to organize things to be more comfortable; demonstrate how to arrange things.	**Practice techniques for keeping order:** Put things away. Don't do several things at once. Clean the area before starting and tidy up after finishing an activity.
Help during transitions: Do not wait for the child to fall behind or make mistakes, but suggest to the child to move on to the next activity.	**Make transitions:** Make transitions efficiently and quickly.
Use pictures of sequences of organization: The child can see what needs to be done. After finishing a step, the child marks the picture on the board and moves on to the next step. Teach the child to independently carry out a transition.	Make a list of actions that should be done in order, sequentially.
Use a timer: A timer can be extremely helpful, especially in organizing sequences.	**Use a timer:** Use reminder notes or an alarm clock. Be aware of time management in completing a task.

The ability to regulate emotions allows one to deal with emotions that provoke distress or anger. In situations that evoke such emotions, coping can be through asking an adult for help, by using self-calming actions like finger sucking, or by moving away from the situation that is causing the emotion that is making it difficult. Emotional regulation also helps deal with pleasant emotions or with situations that excite them, such as increasing emotional arousal to make the game more exciting. When emotions can be regulated, the expression of emotions appropriate to the situation can be used to gain the response of others.

Emotion regulation develops with age. In the first half a year of a baby's life, the response to stressful situations is turning their head to the side. At age two, children may be distracted and think of something else. At age three, there is increased reliance on language in trying to control emotion (Greenstein, 2002). As children grow older, they use mental strategies (change of mind, reinterpretation of the situation, use of pretense) and less external strategies (seeking external help, changing the situation, place, or emotional expression.

Emotional regulation, as mentioned, is the ability to regulate emotions and respond to appropriate emotional reactions in a balanced manner. There is a direct connection between sensory regulation and emotional regulation; children differ greatly in the degree of arousal of their nervous system in response to the same stimulus. The meaning of these differences in stimulation is that sensitive children are aware of a level of stimulation that others do not notice. The reason for this is not in a greater sharpness of the sense, but it is that on the way to the brain or in the brain, it goes through a more careful processing of information.

If the arousal of the nervous system is limited, the children may be bored, indifferent, and ineffective. If there is too much stimulation, they have difficulty thinking, their body movements are uncoordinated, they feel as if they have lost control, and they experience stress and distress, clumsiness, and confusion. The optimal degree of arousal is in the middle. Children feel best when they are not apathetic, passive, or in a state of hyper-stimulation. They perform any task well when their nervous system is in a state of moderate stimulation.

Very sensitive children are born with the tendency to notice the small details in their environment and to consider everything in depth before they act. As a result, they tend to be empathetic, clever, intuitive, creative, careful, and conscientious. They are also more easily overwhelmed by loud noises or large amounts of information of any kind. When trying to avoid stimulation, they appear shy or withdrawn. When they cannot avoid overstimulation, they are said to be "easily excited" and "too sensitive" (Aron, 2012).

Children who show difficulties in emotion regulation are often described in the following ways.

- They are easily overwhelmed by loud noises/noisy situations or large amounts of information of any kind, especially when experiencing it for a long period of time (e.g., when in a supermarket or shopping center or at a family gathering).

- They try to avoid overwhelming situations, are shy and withdrawn in certain situations (e.g., the child claims to be tired and does not join an activity with many children and a lot of noise).
  - When calm, they try not to cause problems; they try to obey, hoping not to be noticed.
  - They choose to play alone, watch others quietly from the side, or stay at home doing a familiar activity.
  - They refuse to talk to adults or strangers or in class.
  - They tend to avoid activities.
- In a state of overstimulation and excitement at high intensities, the children tend to be wild, make noises, throw things, or wave their hands (e.g., when there are guests).
- The variety of emotions increases in intensity; the children show difficulty moving from a highly emotional state to a calm state (e.g., when the children are happy, they are wild and it is difficult for them to relax; when the children are angry, their anger increases to the point of severe outbursts).
  - They express emotions in incorrect intensities with no middle ground, and seem out of control.
  - They quickly rise to high intensities and get out of hand.
  - They are prone to tantrums or crying.
  - It takes a while for the children to calm down; they lack strategies to calm down.

Influence of Parents' Emotion Regulation on the Child: The Need for Collaboration

Parent self-regulation is multifaceted, involving emotional, cognitive, and biological processes that support or constrain parenting behavior. It is highly relevant to disciplinary contexts in which parents' regulatory difficulties can contribute to harsh discipline, which is linked to children's maladjustment. Parents' self-regulation is an essential focus for basic and applied research on parental discipline. There is a need to (1) incorporate and test multiple domains of parent self-regulation to understand their respective and interactive contributions and (2) understand how parent self-regulation interfaces with parent–child coregulation. These foci will more fully inform the etiology of children's maladjustment related to harsh discipline and expand knowledge regarding specific, malleable intervention targets aimed at reducing harsh discipline (Lunkenheimer et al., 2023).

Parents' adaptation requires the ability to regulate their own behavior in reaction to their perception and interpretation of the child's behavior. These self-regulation processes are often intertwined with intense emotions that need to be regulated. Parenting attitudes and behaviors cannot be fully understood without considering the parents' emotional dysregulation and their emotional regulation strategies. However, only a few studies focus on the effects of parents' emotional regulation strategies on parenting behavior. Experiential avoidance and overprotection are discussed as extreme cases of parental emotional regulation strategies that may have particularly detrimental effects in child-rearing. Although most parenting interventions already use a self-regulation approach, specific training in adaptive emotional regulation strategies should be included (Barros et al., 2015) (Table 12.3).

Table 12.3 Therapeutic Strategies in Treating Emotion Regulation

Parent and child during play	The parent in daily activities
Speak more calmly when excited, slow down (co-regulation): It is easy to get out of control together with the child. Be careful not to get carried away; stay steady and help the child return to a regulated state. Speak calmly, breathe, and maintain a pace that is not too fast. Pay attention to the stimuli that stress or excite the child during the activity and control the way they are presented.	Speak more calmly when excited; slow down. Observe how others behave and adjust accordingly. When negative emotions are expressed, signal to others in the environment and ask them to stop, take a break, or slow down.
Imagine a "volume" button: Imagine together with the child as if he has a "volume" button that should regulate the intensity of emotions and enthusiasm. Give feedback regarding where the child is on a continuum from 1 to 10. Help the child calm down when excited, such as by saying, "you're currently at 10; go down to 8."	**Imagine a "volume" button:** Practice using the volume button and try to gain control, like in biofeedback. Lower your tone of voice, slow down your pace, control the intensity of your emotions, and reduce strong reactions.
Use codes: Use the "10" code as a continuation of the "volume button." this code helps the child develop awareness when overwhelmed and to practice decreasing the level of enthusiasm. An adult in the vicinity can tell the child "you are at 10" to remind him what has been has practiced.	**Use codes:** Ask others to point out when the pace of speech or level of excitement is unbalanced, try to self-map where I am on the scale, and stay in an optimal state of awareness.
Perform motor activities that require regulation: Sensory regulation is related to emotional regulation. It is important for the child to develop the ability to be attentive to his body, to be regulated and calm, since the physical reactions (arousal level, breathing rate, sensitivity to stimulus) greatly influence emotional reactions.	**Perform motor activities that require regulation:** Practice dancing, going to the mall or grocery store; gradually expose the child to overwhelming situations, don't avoid exciting situations.
Find ways to relax: Think together about ways that can help the child relax. Present examples of how the parents calm down and explain how the child can use the same techniques to calm down. Identify situations in which the child may be uneasy in advance (e.g., when guests come), and find ways to help the child relax in these situations (e.g., go to a room and be alone for a bit, ask for strong hugs with a pillow). Ask the child to tell you later if the relaxation techniques were successful. Help children recognize when they are starting to get out of control and react in the way that was agreed upon before they lose control or are scolded. You can make a list of ideas and refer to it if the child gets out of control.	**Find ways to relax:** Listen to music, wash dishes, walk, or retreat to a closed room. Use them before a flare-up or outburst occurs.

Mental Rigidity

Mental flexibility/dynamic thinking is the ability to improvise between different components and different solution options. Such thinking considers new variables that are added to the activity, either in a planned way or in an unexpected way. Every person is endowed with a different ability to handle accumulated databases, and according to this ability, personal qualities are rated, such as spontaneity, speed of thought, improvisation, flexibility, and adaptation to new situations.

Dynamic thinking includes the following abilities:

- Creativity—the ability to come up with new ideas, deal with hypotheses, and make assumptions about the present and the future.
- Relational thinking—constantly analyze the activity as it occurs and think of solutions regarding the attitude toward the other person, and previous situations.
- Flexibility in cognitive transitions—consider strategies in response to changes when they occur.
- Representation—engaging in imaginary and symbolic play.
- Uncertainty management—regulate emotions and actions jointly, even in situations that are unknown or unexpected (Zohar, 2007).

Mental rigidity/pattern thinking, on the other hand, is built from limited and fixed sequences of information. Such thinking focuses on existing knowledge and is aimed at achieving a defined result. Pattern thinking is characterized by knowing in advance all the actions needed to perform a certain task.

Children exhibiting pattern thinking engage in only one field, even if this field includes the coordination of diverse actions, such as building a train track. The field of activity will be seemingly closed to external intervention, change, or diversification. Also, the transition from a given and defined activity to another is usually difficult, because it requires thinking that includes organization, consideration of a new order of operations, different behavior, and a different set of reactions.

Pattern thinking is caused by three main factors:

- The habit and comfort of processing little information versus the need to consider a lot of data and a fast rate of occurrence.
- The possibility of avoiding sensory or emotional overload and loss of control leading to failure.
- The confidence and control provided by the templates that were built in the past and have been proven, over time, to work.

Pattern thinking affects and harms all areas of life: life skills, independent play, strategies and ways of learning, managerial thinking, the inclusion of others, and social codes. It is important to develop social skills systematically, where primary skills are used as a basis on which more complex skills are built. Once a basic game pattern subject to control is achieved, add nuances and challenges to it (Zohar, 2007).

The repertoire of behaviors recognized by the child (the variety of activities in which he is engaged) may be limited or rich and varied. It is influenced by the child's exposure to his environment, the child's tendency to apply what he sees or learns, and what the child brings from himself. When there is an expansion of the repertoire, there is a diverse and developing activity in a wide range of fields.

Children may show difficulties in mental rigidity such as:

- Insisting that things go according to their plans.
- Losing control if something does not work out according to what they determined.
- Setting rules for the game and changing rules according to their needs.
- Being domineering, deciding things for everyone in the room, announcing their desires, refusing to negotiate, being stubborn, and exhibiting assertiveness.
- Repeating patterns, exhibiting unvaried play, attachment to routines or rituals, and excessive preoccupation with one certain area of interest.
- Refusing to try something unfamiliar (unfamiliar game, new rules in a familiar game).
- Disliking changes (e.g., asking to always get something in a certain color).
- Exhibiting perseveration (repetitive behavior) such as performing the same scenario of the game in a repetitive and patterned manner. This may be expressed by repeating the same passage without reference to its continuation (e.g., explain that if the child gives a doll a bath, it is not necessary to bathe is again; rather, it is possible to feed it or put it to sleep).
- Exhibiting limited reciprocity due to difficulty sharing with others.

Influence of Parents' Characteristics of Mental Rigidity on the Child: The Need for Collaboration

In the past several years, there has been a strong focus on investigating the relationship between psychological flexibility and psychosocial outcomes. Psychological flexibility refers to the ability of an individual to accept aversive emotional experiences while maintaining engagement in value-based behaviors (Hayes et al., 2006). Not surprisingly, greater psychological flexibility is related to a host of positive outcomes, including higher quality of life, greater emotional well-being, and more adaptive psychological functioning (Bond & Bunce, 2003; Hayes et al., 2006). Alternatively, lower levels of psychological flexibility are associated with greater emotional reactivity and increased psychopathology (Tull et al., 2004).

To date, a large portion of research investigating the effects of psychological flexibility has focused on individual outcomes (Hayes et al., 2006). However, there is some evidence to suggest that individual psychological flexibility further affects the broader systems to which the individual belongs. Specifically, research examining individual psychological flexibility within the family context has found a connection between a parent's psychological flexibility and their child's psychological outcomes (e.g., Brassell et al., 2016; Cheron et al., 2009; Williams et al., 2012).

The content of parent–child interactions is often used to predict problem behaviors in early childhood. There is a general agreement that interactions characterized as mutually hostile, harsh, permissive, or over-controlling contribute to a wide spectrum of child psychopathologies. Beyond the individual, it is useful to understand the structure of experience and its contribution to development in a social context. From a systems perspective, developmental trajectories arise from multiple and reciprocally causal interactions. A child's behavior prompts a response from the parent, and this response influences the child's behavior, and so on. Over time, these interactions constrain future behavior to more predictable patterns that, at an extreme, may translate into more specific problems for the child, such as depression or aggression. Thus, it is not only the content but the structure of parent–child behavior over time (i.e., rigidity) that can influence child adjustment. Previous investigations have focused on the negative content of social interaction, but rigidity in structure may apply to interaction content that is positive as well as negative. Flexibility in affective and behavioral states is also likely to better accommodate the variety of typical social tasks encountered by a family.

Children who learn to express a range of emotions also have ample opportunity to modulate those emotions and thus become adept at regulating their social behavior (Gottman et al., 1996). Parents who are less accepting of variety in emotional states do not foster those opportunities and thus limit children's capacities to regulate their own behavior (Eisenberg et al., 1998; Hollenstein et al., 2004; Ramsden & Hubbard, 2002) (Table 12.4).

Perfectionism

Perfectionism is the need to be perfect or to appear as such. Perfectionism may motivate people toward achievement and provide them with motivation to face challenges. The distinction between healthy ambition and perfectionism can be confusing. The normative pursuit of excellence may become a destructive factor that impairs functioning rather than improving it, so that "the pursuit of perfection impairs perfection."

A significant area affected by perfectionism is the interpersonal area. Perfectionism is often accompanied by rigidity and high demands from the environment, which lead to friction, difficulty integrating into teamwork, and hiding information out of fear arising from excessive criticism. Also, many perfectionists find it difficult to admit to mistakes and even resist sharing difficulties and mistakes with those close to them—these factors create discomfort, distance, and conflicts.

Perfectionism also affects the emotional realm. The high standards, the difficulty of dealing with performance that is perceived as less than perfect, and the constant pursuit of excellence lead to procrastination, stress, guilt and disappointment, anxiety, and difficulties in coping with stressful situations and low self-esteem. In addition, it is a risk factor for obsessive-compulsive disorder (OCD), eating disorders, and clinical depression (Benson, 2003).

Hewitt and Flett (1991) devised a 45-item multidimensional perfectionism scale that rates three aspects of perfectionist self-presentation.

Table 12.4 Therapeutic Strategies in Treating Mental Rigidity

Parent and child during play	The parent in daily activities
Diversify between games, expand the child's repertoire of activities: The greater variety of activities that the children know about, the more flexible they will be. It is recommended that the activities be in different fields.	**Expand the repertoire of activities:** Diversify daily activities; do not take the same route all the time; order different dishes at a restaurant.
Teach new things through patterns: Children learn the world through patterns. This makes it easier for them to understand how things work. Therefore, in new situations or new activities, teach them through a pattern. Children are considered rigid when they have few patterns. The more patterns they have, the more options they have for action, and they become more flexible and less dependent on familiar patterns.	**Learn new things through patterns:** Use patterns in new situations, such as when arriving at a new place, until you become accustomed to taking the same route.
Expand within familiar games by different ways of playing the game: Use familiar templates and make slight changes each time. Even if you repeat a familiar game, play it in different ways, and change it in such a way that it is not exactly like the last time you played it. Add or change the rules, despite the difficulty of changing the familiar (e.g., police officers can catch thieves, defuse bombs, find a lost child, direct traffic, and more).	Expand within familiar routines by different ways of playing a familiar game. Diversify everyday life, for example, by using a different tablecloth.
Do familiar everyday things in a different way: All familiar activities in daily life can be kept familiar and constant, while minor changes can be made. The changes must be gradual and not extreme, so that the child can accept them.	**Do familiar everyday things in a different way:** Do not be afraid to do familiar things differently, like improvising while cooking or baking.
"Undoing": Make changes and have the child correct the adults. In the case of a child's resistance, the adult creates a change, and the child corrects it. The adult must repeat the same action about 15 times in a row while being careful not to upset the child. The adult makes a change, the child corrects, and when the child calms down, the adult repeats the same thing. After about 15 times, a new pattern is created for the child, the change bothers the child less, and may even initiate it.	**"Undoing":** Sometimes, adults also get used to new things, like the latest fashion; don't resist.

(continued)

Table 12.4 (continued)

Parent and child during play	The parent in daily activities
Use board games that have changes, introduce luck like throwing dice: Changes are part of some games (e.g., the magical maze). The child must adapt to the change and to the new situation. Practicing changes can also be done in unexpected situations where you depend on luck (i.e., the dice) rather than planning.	Introduce changes instead of familiar activities.
Demonstrate flexibility: Model flexibility and the ability to adapt to a new situation and deal with things that are not planned. Be careful not to be so flexible as to give in to the child all the time, which may reinforce the child's rigidity and habits, and expect others to adjust themselves.	**Demonstrate flexibility**: Adapt to situations where we do not get exactly what we want; compromise for the sake of friendship.
Make changes in the room: Change the location of games; get the child used to changes in the environment.	**Make changes in the room**: Change the location of the games. Rearrange furniture in the home. Travel to a new place.
Overcome controlling: Take turns deciding. Initially, choose a game that the child would choose and gradually move to games that the child prefers less. The child must explain choices and practice negotiation. Do not agree with everything the child decides. Summarize the rules in advance; they cannot be changed during the game. If children change a rule for their benefit, it stays that way for the rest of the game, even when it is beneficial for others.	**Overcome controlling**: It is not always necessary to be in control.

1. Self-oriented perfectionism refers to having unrealistic expectations and standards for oneself that lead to perfectionist motivation.
2. Other-oriented perfectionism is having unrealistic expectations and standards for others that, in turn, pressure them to have perfectionist motivations of their own.
3. Socially prescribed perfectionism is characterized by developing perfectionist motivations due to actual or perceived high expectations of significant others. Parents who push their children to be successful in certain endeavors (such as athletics or academics) provide an example of what often causes this type of perfectionism, as the children feel that they must meet their parents' lofty expectations (Hewitt et al., 1991; Hewitt & Flett, 1991).

Children may show difficulties in perfectionism, such as:

- Presenting themselves as perfect;
- Having a hard time tolerating something that is not perfect;
- Being dissatisfied with what they did, not forgiving their own mistakes, and throwing out their own work;
- Being overly strict about what others do and want to do the work instead of them;
- Giving a lot of instructions when someone is doing something for them;

- Having a hard time losing.

Influence of the Parents' Perfectionism on the Child: The Need for Collaboration

The social expectations model theorizes that parental expectations and parental criticism are integral to the development of perfectionism. Alternatively, the social learning model maintains that children become perfectionistic by observing and imitating parents' perfectionistic behaviors (Smith et al., 2022).

Perfectionism is a significant transdiagnostic process related to the development and maintenance of several psychological disorders. The main models of the development of perfectionism focus on early childhood experiences and postulate that parental relationship is an important factor for understanding this construct in children. The results show a relationship between most of the same parent and child perfectionism dimensions, thus providing supportive evidence for the Social Learning Model. Concerning the analysis of the role of gender in the transmission of perfectionism, observed fathers' perfectionism only relates to the sons' perfectionism, and mothers' perfectionism relates to daughters' perfectionism. The findings allow for a deeper understanding of the role of the perception of an authoritarian parenting style in the development of maladaptive perfectionism. Mothers' and fathers' perceived parenting styles contribute more to perfectionism in the daughter than in the son. Results contribute to expanding the understanding of the role of parental factors in the development of perfectionism (Carmo et al., 2021) (Table 12.5).

Dealing with Difficulties

Dealing with difficulties involves the ability to persevere, not to give up, and to show positivity and persistence, despite the difficulties. Children run into difficulties. Difficulties are an integral part of our day-to-day management and cannot be avoided. Effective dealing with difficulty allows the child to develop and acquire cognitive, motor, and emotional tools. Preventing children from coping by finding easy solutions (giving up, letting someone else do it instead of them) prevents them from acquiring tools for independent coping and makes them dependent on receiving help. The way children perceive difficulty, the degree of success in dealing with it, and the reaction of the environment will greatly influence future experience in similar situations. Children who get along well, have higher self-esteem, believe more in themselves, and are willing to tackle new things, even those they do not know or find difficult. They believe more in their abilities; their frustration threshold rises, and their emotional regulation is more adjusted in situations of difficulty.

Children may show problems in dealing with difficulties:

- Avoid starting activities that seem difficult.
- Choose what they know and are good at.

Table 12.5 Therapeutic Strategies in Treating Perfectionism

Parent and child during play	The parent in daily activities
Demonstrate forgiveness of our own mistakes: Make a mistake on purpose and show that it is not terrible. Treat the mistake as something that can happen. Try to fix it, and if you can, show that it is fine.	**Demonstrate forgiveness of our own mistakes:** Try to forgive others' mistakes. Don't be judgmental about others. Acknowledge that you might not be better than them, even if you think you are.
Show that mistakes can be done "as if on purpose": In some situations, the mistake leads to a better result. For example, if we accidentally painted a painting in the wrong color, paint the same color symmetrically on the other side, and suddenly find that the addition made the painting more beautiful.	**Show that mistakes can be done "as if on purpose":** Some mistakes can be shown as if we did them on purpose; sometimes, the flaw can turn into an advantage.
Show that we are not perfect: Show character traits that are not perfect as part of who we are. (e.g., you can leave the closet messy and show that you do not have to be tidy all the time).	**Admit that you are not perfect:** Show others the things you've done that are not perfect, don't throw them away or hide them.
Choose goals where it is okay for things not to be perfect: A doll's hair may come out of the ponytail and not be neat; one can color out of the lines; put the cards away without sorting them into piles.	**Choose goals where it is okay for things not to be perfect:** Be gradual; you can start with people you don't know, or with people that you feel close to.
Compliment the child even if the child is not happy with what has been done: Indicate what we see and praise the child. Imitate the child, repeat the choices he made, ask him what he did, and do it like him. If the child does not want to take the piece he made, because it is not good enough in his eyes, ask his permission to keep it.	**Compliment yourself even if you are not happy with what you've done:** Compliment small things, such as trying hard or being able to not be perfect.
Pay attention to the whole picture and do not look for what is wrong with it: In everything, it is possible to focus on details and find what is wrong; however, even if there are mistakes, when you look at the whole picture, you do not see the small mistakes.	**Pay attention to the whole picture and do not look for what is wrong with it**: Step back and look at your outcome. Avoid criticism of small details.
You do not have to win: Someone who wins, especially in strategy games, feels capable. Some children are used to winning and being successful. Try to create a situation where the child loses, simply to see that it can happen too.	**You do not have to win:** During arguments, stop criticizing, be more accepting instead of judgmental of others.

(continued)

Table 12.5 (continued)

Parent and child during play	The parent in daily activities
Experience activities in which we are afraid of not being perfect: Choose new activities that the child does not know or is not necessarily the best at. Do not be afraid to try; it is impossible to do new things perfectly without practice. Create an amusing feeling around the experience, instead of getting into the frustration that it is not perfect.	Experience activities in which you are afraid of not being perfect—Try doing things that you are not good at.
Limit the number of tests of what we did: Make a rule, such as that we can only check and correct what we did two times.	**Limit the number of testsof what you did:** When baking a cake, writing a birthday card, or recording a message on the phone.

- When doing a task, they ask others to do what seems difficult.
- They stop in the middle of an activity as soon as it seems challenging.
- They may cry or throw a tantrum when the task is difficult.
- They avoid negative content in a symbolic game.

Influence of Parents' Characteristics in Dealing with Difficulties on Those of the Child: The Need for Collaboration

Children need care that promotes positive emotional health and well-being and that supports their overall mental health, including a positive sense of self, as well as the ability to cope with stressful situations, temper emotional arousal, overcome fears, and accept disappointments and frustrations. Parents and other caregivers are essential resources for children in managing emotional arousal, coping, and behavior. They serve in this role by providing positive affirmations, conveying love and respect, and engendering a sense of security. Provision of support by parents helps minimize the risk of internalizing behaviors, such as those associated with anxiety and depression, which can impair children's adjustment and ability to function well at home, at school, and in the community (Breiner et al., 2016; Osofsky & Fitzgerald, 2000).

Children's beliefs about the contribution of effort and their ability to succeed or fail shape their decisions about whether to persist or to give up on challenging tasks, with consequences for their academic success. But how do children learn about the concept of challenge? Prior work has shown that parents' verbal responses to success and failure shape children's motivational beliefs (Bennett-Pierre et al., 2023) (Table 12.6).

Discussion

Collaboration between therapists and parents is a very significant factor in the success of treatment. In children with ASD, parental involvement in treatment improves its outcomes and speeds up the process. Another aspect of collaboration: the characteristics of the parents. These characteristics can affect the child's characteristics and have a significant impact on the child's communicative and social functioning.

This chapter presented the Interactive Play Intervention (IPI) model for the treatment of communication and social skills. The model contains 48 therapeutic goals, from which the appropriate goals for the child are selected. For each goal, there are applied strategies for treating the child through an interactive game experience.

The innovation in this chapter is the emphasis placed specifically on the parents working on their own characteristics. When therapeutic goals are identified for the child, it is necessary to check whether the parent shares that goal. The parent must go through a process of change, parallel to the process the child goes through.

To demonstrate, several goals were selected. As we have seen in each of the goals, there is a strong connection between the characteristics of the parents and those of the child. Applied strategies were proposed for working on each of the selected goals. Strategies for dyadic treatment of the child and parent were proposed, as well as strategies for daily implementation for the parent. This requires awareness and practice, as well as an understanding of the importance of collaboration.

We must continue to research the influence of the parents' characteristics on those of the child in each of the goals, and continue to raise awareness of the importance of the process of change that the parent must undergo for the child's treatment to be successful.

Table 12.6 Therapeutic Strategies in Dealing with Difficulties

Parent and child during play	The parent in daily activities
Do not allow the child to give up in situations of difficulty: The child must keep trying when things get difficult. Do not panic if the child gets upset when challenged or at failure.	**Do not give up in situations of difficulty:** Keep trying when things get difficult. Even if you are challenged or fail, remember that the effort is what matters.
Demonstrate to the child how to cope and allow him to do so: Show the child slowly what to do and ask the child to do it.	**Cope with difficulties:** Don't be alarmed in difficult situations.
Do not act instead of the child: Help the child succeed. The child must be active and do what is difficult.	**Do not act instead of the child:** Don't ask others to do things for you. You can ask for help and cope.
Give the child a successful experience: After the child has succeeded, especially after saying "I can't," ask, "did you succeed?" the child must answer "I succeeded." get the child used to saying, "it's hard, but I can succeed."	**Successful experience**: Reinforce yourself.
Demonstrate dealing with difficulties: Take advantage of situations where it is difficult for you, show that you are disturbed that you are not succeeding: "Oops, the game piece is not going in!" reflect your emotions excessively; show that you are not giving up if you want to. Characters can be demonstrated in a symbolic game.	**Deal with difficulties:** Don't give up
Adjust the degree of difficulty to the child's abilities: Raise the level of difficulty gradually. When we demand coping from the child, we need to check that the demand is tailored to the child's abilities.	**Adjust the degree of difficulty to your abilities:** Raise the level of difficulty gradually. When we demand of ourselves to cope, we need to check that the demand is tailored to our abilities.
Disassemble a complex mission: A mission with many steps can be disassembled. Do a different part each time until you finish it. Do not forget to finish the task. Make reminders, and continue to do it even if the motivation to perform it has decreased. In such missions, get especially excited when it comes to the end. If the task is too complex or too difficult, the adult can do the main part and leave the child with the end (chaining backwards). Thus, the task seems closer to completion and less threatening. You can repeat the same activity again and gradually reduce the part that the adult performs and increase the part that the child performs, until he performs independently and without help.	**Disassemble a complex mission:** Break down a complex task. A task that consists of many steps can be broken down and done one part at a time until you finish it. Don't forget to finish the task, set reminders, and keep doing it even if your motivation to do it decreases.
Introduce negative content into a symbolic game: If the child avoids negative content, insert it gradually and in a controlled manner, and show the child that the solution to these situations is possible (e.g., check with a doctor and the doctor quickly heals the wound; there is a fire and the firefighters arrive quickly and takes control of it).	**Introduce negative content:** Don't avoid negative content.

References

Aboud, F. E., & Yousafzai, A. K. (2015). Global health and development in early childhood. *Annual Review of Psychology, 66*(1), 433–457. https://doi.org/10.1146/annurev-psych-010814-015128

Altenburger, L. E., & Schoppe-Sullivan, S. J. (2020). New fathers' parenting quality: Personal, contextual, and child precursors. *Journal of Family Psychology, 34*(7), 857–866. https://doi.org/10.1037/fam0000753

An, M., & Palisano, R. J. (2014). Family-professional collaboration in pediatric rehabilitation: A practice model. *Disability and Rehabilitation, 36*(5), 434–440. https://doi.org/10.3109/09638288.2013.797510

An, M., Palisano, R. J., Dunst, C. J., Chiarello, L. A., Yi, C. H., & Gracely, E. J. (2016). Strategies to promote family–professional collaboration: Two case reports. *Disability and Rehabilitation, 38*(18), 1844–1858. https://doi.org/10.3109/09638288.2015.1107763

Anan, R. M., Warner, L. J., McGillivary, J. E., Chong, I. M., & Hines, S. J. (2008). Group intensive family training (GIFT) for preschoolers with autism spectrum disorders. *Behavioral Interventions, 23*(3), 165–180. https://doi.org/10.1002/bin.262

Aron, A. (2012). *The highly sensitive child: Helping our children thrive when the world overwhelms them*. Harmony Publishers.

Barlow, J., Bergman, H., Kornør, H., Wei, Y., & Bennett, C. (2016). Group-based parent training programmes for improving emotional and behavioural adjustment in young children. *Cochrane Database of Systematic Reviews, 8*(CD003680). https://doi.org/10.1002/14651858.CD003680.pub3

Barnett, M. A., Deng, M., Mills-Koonce, W. R., Willoughby, M., & Cox, M. (2008). Interdependence of parenting of mothers and fathers of infants. *Journal of Family Psychology, 22*(4), 561–573. https://doi.org/10.1037/0893-3200.22.3.561

Barros, L., Goes, A. R., & Pereira, A. I. (2015). Parental self-regulation, emotional regulation and temperament: Implications for intervention. *Estudos de Psicologia (Campinas), 32*, 295–306.

Bennett-Pierre, G., Weinraub, M., Newcombe, N. S., & Gunderson, E. A. (2023). "This is hard!" children's and parents' talk about difficulty during dyadic interactions. *Developmental Psychology, 59*(7), 1268–1282. https://doi.org/10.1037/dev0001555

Benson, E. (2003). Intelligent intelligence testing. *Monitor on Psychology, 34*(2), 48–58.

Benson, P., Karlof, K. L., & Siperstein, G. N. (2008). Maternal involvement in the education of young children with autism spectrum disorders. *Autism, 12*(1), 47–63. https://doi.org/10.1177/1362361307085269

Bond, F. W., & Bunce, D. (2003). The role of acceptance and job control in mental health, job satisfaction, and work performance. *Journal of Applied Psychology, 88*(6), 1057–1067. https://doi.org/10.1037/0021-9010.88.6.1057

Brassell, A. A., Rosenberg, E., Parent, J., Rough, J. N., Fondacaro, K., & Seehuus, M. (2016). Parent's psychological flexibility: Associations with parenting and child psychosocial Well-being. *Journal of Contextual Behavioral Science, 5*(2), 111–120. https://doi.org/10.1016/j.jcbs.2016.03.001

Breiner, H., Ford, M., & Gadsden, V. L. (Eds.). (2016). *Parenting matters: Supporting parents of children ages 0–8*. National Academies Press. https://www.ncbi.nlm.nih.gov/books/NBK402020/

Burchinal, M., Vernon-Feagans, L., Cox, M., & Key Family Life Project Investigators. (2008). Cumulative social risk, parenting, and infant development in rural low-income communities. *Parenting: Science and Practice, 8*(1), 41–69. https://doi.org/10.1080/15295190701830672

Carmo, C., Oliveira, D., Brás, M., & Faísca, L. (2021). The influence of parental perfectionism and parenting styles on child perfectionism. *Children, 8*(9), 777. https://doi.org/10.3390/children8090777

Cheron, D. M., Ehrenreich, J. T., & Pincus, D. B. (2009). Assessment of parental experiential avoidance in a clinical sample of children with anxiety disorders. *Child Psychiatry and Human Development, 40*(3), 383–403. https://doi.org/10.1007/s10578-009-0135-z

Collins, W. A., Maccoby, E. E., Steinberg, L. E., Hetherington, M., & Bornstein, M. H. (2000). Contemporary research on parenting: The case for nature and nurture. *American Psychologist, 55*(2), 218–232.

Diggle, T. T., & McConachie, H. (2003). *Parent-mediated early intervention for young children with autism spectrum disorder*. The Cochrane Library.

Dunst, C. J., & Trivette, C. M. (2009). Capacity-building family-systems intervention practices. *Journal of Family Social Work, 12*(2), 119–143. https://doi.org/10.1080/10522150802713322

Eisenberg, N., Cumberland, A., & Spinrad, T. L. (1998). Parental socialization of emotion. *Psychological Inquiry, 9*, 241–273. https://doi.org/10.1207/s15327965pli0904_1

Elder, J. H., Valcante, G., Yarandi, H., White, D., & Elder, T. H. (2005). Evaluating in-home training for fathers of children with autism using single-subject experimentation and group analysis methods. *Nursing Research, 54*(1), 22–32.

Felsenthal-Berger, N. (2007). Gishah ineteraqtivit letippul biyiladim im ASD betifqud gavoah [An interactive approach to the treatment of children with high-functioning ASD]. In S. Lowinger (Ed.), *Tiqshoret: Tippul biyiladim im beayot tiqshoret begilae bet hassefer hayyesodi [Communication: Treating children with communication problems at the elementary school age]* (pp. 225–246). Ach.

Fierloos, I. N., Windhorst, D. A., Fang, Y., Jonkman, H., Crone, M. R., Hosman, C. M. H., Swan Tan, S., & Raat, H. (2022). Socio-demographic characteristics associated with perceived social support among parents of children aged 0–7 years: The CIKEO study. *BMC Public Health, 22*(1), 2441. https://doi.org/10.1186/s12889-022-14830-1

Friedman, R. J., & Chase-Lansdale, P. L. (2002). Chronic adversities. In M. Rutter & E. Taylor (Eds.), *Child and adolescent psychiatry* (4th ed., pp. 261–276). Blackwell Publishing.

Ginsburg, K. R. (2007). The importance of play in promoting healthy child development and maintaining strong parent-child bonds. *Pediatrics, 119*(1), 182–191. https://doi.org/10.1542/peds.2006-2697

Gottman, J. M., Katz, L. F., & Hooven, C. (1996). Parental meta-emotion philosophy and the emotional life of families: Theoretical models and preliminary data. *Journal of Family Psychology, 10*(3), 243–268.

Greenstein, J. (2002). *Social and emotional development*. Tel-Aviv University.

Hayes, S. C., Luoma, J. B., Bond, F. W., Masuda, A., & Lillis, J. (2006). Acceptance and commitment therapy: Model, processes and outcomes. *Behaviour Research and Therapy, 44*(1), 1–25. https://doi.org/10.1016/j.brat.2005.06.006

Hewitt, P. L., & Flett, G. L. (1991). Perfectionism in the self and social contexts: Conceptualization, assessment, and association with psychopathology. *Journal of Personality and Social Psychology, 60*(3), 456–470. https://doi.org/10.1037/0022-3514.60.3.456

Hewitt, P. L., Flett, G. L., Turnbull-Donovan, W., & Mikail, S. F. (1991). The multidimensional perfectionism scale: Reliability, validity, and psychometric properties in psychiatric samples. *Psychological Assessment: A Journal of Consulting and Clinical Psychology, 3*(3), 464–468. https://doi.org/10.1037/1040-3590.3.3.464

Hill, C. E. (2001). *Helping skills: The empirical foundation*. American Psychological Association. https://doi.org/10.1037/10412-000

Hill, E. L. (2004). Executive dysfunction in autism. *Trends in Cognitive Sciences, 8*(1), 26–32. https://doi.org/10.1016/j.tics.2003.11.003

Hollenstein, T., Granic, I., Stoolmiller, M., & Snyder, J. (2004). Rigidity in parent–child interactions and the development of externalizing and internalizing behavior in early childhood. *Journal of Abnormal Child Psychology, 32*(6), 595–607. https://doi.org/10.1023/B:JACP.0000047209.37650.41

Joseph-Williams, N., Elwyn, G., & Edwards, A. (2014). Knowledge is not power for patients: A systematic review and thematic synthesis of patient-reported barriers and facilitators to shared decision making. *Patient Education and Counseling, 94*(3), 291–309. https://doi.org/10.1016/j.pec.2013.10.031

Kasari, C., Gulsrud, A. C., Wong, C., Kwon, S., & Locke, J. (2010). Randomized controlled caregiver-mediated joint engagement intervention for toddlers with autism. *Journal of Autism and Developmental Disorders, 40*(9), 1045–1056. https://doi.org/10.1007/s10803-010-0955-5

Klatte, I. S., Harding, S., & Roulstone, S. (2019). Speech and language therapists' views on parents' engagement in Parent–child interaction therapy (PCIT). *International Journal of Language & Communication Disorders, 54*(4), 553–564. https://doi.org/10.1111/1460-6984.12459

Klatte, I. S., Lyons, R., Davies, K., Harding, S., Marshall, J., McKean, C., & Roulstone, S. (2020). Collaboration between parents and SLTs produces optimal outcomes for children attending speech and language therapy: Gathering the evidence. *International Journal of Language and Communication Disorders, 55*(4), 618–628. https://doi.org/10.1111/1460-6984.12538

Klatte, I. S., & Roulstone, S. (2016). The practical side of working with parent–child interaction therapy with preschool children with language impairments. *Child Language Teaching and Therapy, 32*(3), 345–359. https://doi.org/10.1177/0265659016641999

Kokorelias, K. M., Gignac, M. A. M., Naglie, G., & Cameron, J. (2019). Towards a universal model of family-centered care: A scoping review. *BMC Health Services Research, 19*(1), 564. https://doi.org/10.1186/s12913-019-4394-5

Lanjekar, P. D., Joshi, S. H., Lanjekar, P. D., & Wagh, V. (2022). The effect of parenting and the parent-child relationship on a child's cognitive development: A literature review. *Cureus, 14*(10), e30574. https://doi.org/10.7759/cureus.30574

Lunkenheimer, E., Sturge-Apple, M. L., & Kelm, M. R. (2023). The importance of parent self-regulation and parent–child coregulation in research on parental discipline. *Child Development Perspectives, 17*(1), 25–31. https://doi.org/10.1111/cdep.12470

Marchewski, S. (2013). *Regashot: Maarekhet hafalah [Emotions: An operating system].* Contento De Semrik.

Mas, J. M., Dunst, C. J., Hamby, D. W., Balcells-Balcells, A., García-Ventura, S., Baqués, N., & Giné, C. (2022). Relationships between family-centered practices and parent involvement in early childhood intervention. *European Journal of Special Needs Education, 37*(1), 1–13. https://doi.org/10.1080/08856257.2020.1823165

Matson, M. L., Mahan, S., & Matson, J. L. (2009). Parent training: A review of methods for children with autism spectrum disorders. *Research in Autism Spectrum Disorders, 3*(4), 868–875. https://doi.org/10.1016/j.rasd.2009.02.003

McConachie, H., Randle, V., Hammal, D., & Le Couteur, A. (2005). A controlled trial of a training course for parents of children with suspected autism spectrum disorder. *The Journal of Pediatrics, 147*(3), 335–340. https://doi.org/10.1016/j.jpeds.2005.03.056

Melvin, K., Meyer, C., & Scarinci, N. (2019). What does "engagement" mean in early speech pathology intervention? A qualitative systematised review. *Disability and Rehabilitation, 42*(18), 2665–2678. https://doi.org/10.1080/09638288.2018.1563640

Mills-Koonce, W. R., Willoughby, M. T., Zvara, B., Barnett, M., Gustafsson, H., Cox, M. J., & Family Life Project Key Investigators. (2015). Mothers' and fathers' sensitivity and children's cognitive development in low-income, rural families. *Journal of Applied Developmental Psychology, 38*, 1–10. https://doi.org/10.1016/j.appdev.2015.01.001

Milteer, R. M., Ginsburg, K. R., Council on Communications and Media Committee on Psychosocial Aspects of Child and Family Health, Mulligan, D. A., Ameenuddin, N., Brown, A., Christakis, D. A., Cross, C., Falik, H. L., Hill, D. L., & Hogan, M. J. (2012). The importance of play in promoting healthy child development and maintaining strong parent–child bond: Focus on children in poverty. *Pediatrics, 129*(1), e204–e213. https://doi.org/10.1542/peds.2011-2953

Moree, B. N., & Davis, T. E., III. (2010). Cognitive-behavioral therapy for anxiety in children diagnosed with autism spectrum disorders: Modification trends. *Research in Autism Spectrum Disorders, 4*(3), 346–354. https://doi.org/10.1016/j.rasd.2009.10.015

Moyal, S. (2023). *Hitarevut bemiskhaq ineteraqtivi model IPI leshippur tiqshoret umeyum-manuyot khevratiyyot beemtsaut miskhaq [Interactive game engagement ipi model to improve communication and social skills through play].* Amazon Kindle Publishing.

Osofsky, J. D., & Fitzgerald, H. E. (2000). *WAIMH handbook of infant mental health* (Vol. 1). Wiley.

Ozonoff, S., Goodlin-Jones, B. L., & Solomon, M. (2005). Evidence-based assessment of autism spectrum disorders in children and adolescents. *Journal of Clinical Child and Adolescent Psychology, 34*(3), 523–540. https://doi.org/10.1207/s15374424jccp3403_8

Ramsden, S. R., & Hubbard, J. A. (2002). Family expressiveness and parental emotion coaching: Their role in children's emotion regulation and aggression. *Journal of Abnormal Child Psychology, 30*(6), 657–667. https://doi.org/10.1023/A:1020819915881

Samooha, M. (2010). Horaah muvnet: Sevivah khinnukhit liyiladim im ASD [Structured teaching: Educational environment for children with ASD]. In S. Lowinger (Ed.), *Qishurim: Tippul biyiladim im beayot tiqshoret: Gishot ineteraqtiviyyot [Connections: Interactive approaches to the treatment of children with communication disorders]* (pp. 175–210). Ach.

Siller, M., Hutman, T., & Sigman, M. (2013). A parent-mediated intervention to increase responsive parental behaviors and child communication in children with ASD: A randomized clinical trial. *Journal of Autism and Developmental Disorders, 43*(3), 540–555. https://doi.org/10.1007/s10803-012-1584-y

Smith, M. M., Hewitt, P. L., Sherry, S. B., Flett, G. L., & Ray, C. (2022). Parenting behaviors and trait perfectionism: A meta-analytic test of social expectations and social learning models. *Journal of Research and Personality, 96*, 104180. https://doi.org/10.1016/j.jrp.2021.104180

Sofronoff, K., Attwood, T., & Hinton, S. (2005). A randomised controlled trial of a CBT intervention for anxiety in children with Asperger syndrome. *Journal of Child Psychology and Psychiatry, 46*(11), 1152–1160. https://doi.org/10.1111/j.1469-7610.2005.00411.x

Sofronoff, K., Leslie, A., & Brown, W. (2004). Parent management training and Asperger syndrome: A randomized controlled trial to evaluate a parent-based intervention. *Autism, 8*(3), 301–317. https://doi.org/10.1177/1362361304045215

Solomon, R., Necheles, J., Ferch, C., & Bruckman, D. (2007). Pilot study of a parent training program for young children with autism: The PLAY project home consultation program. *Autism, 11*(3), 205–224. https://doi.org/10.1177/1362361307076842

Sosic-Vasic, Z., Kröner, J., Schneider, S., Vasic, N., Spitzer, M., & Streb, J. (2017). The association between parenting behavior and executive functioning in children and young adolescents. *Frontiers in Psychology, 8*, 472. https://doi.org/10.3389/fpsyg.2017.00472

Tull, M. T., Gratz, K. L., Salters, K., & Roemer, L. (2004). The role of experiential avoidance in posttraumatic stress symptoms and symptoms of depression, anxiety, and somatization. *Journal of Nervous and Mental Disease, 192*(11), 754–761. https://doi.org/10.1097/01.nmd.0000144694.30121.89

Vasilopoulou, E., & Nisbet, J. (2016). The quality of life of parents of children with autism spectrum disorder: A systematic review. *Research in Autism Spectrum Disorders, 23*, 36–49. https://doi.org/10.1016/j.rasd.2015.11.008

Weiskop, S., Richdale, A., & Matthews, J. (2005). Behavioural treatment to reduce sleep problems in children with autism or fragile X syndrome. *Developmental Medicine & Child Neurology, 47*(2), 94–104. https://doi.org/10.1111/j.1469-8749.2005.tb01097.x

Williams, K. E., Ciarrochi, J., & Heaven, P. C. (2012). Inflexible parents, inflexible kids: A 6-year longitudinal study of parenting style and the development of psychological flexibility in adolescents. *Journal of Youth and Adolescence, 41*(8), 1053–1066. https://doi.org/10.1007/s10964-012-9744-0

Wilson, D. M., & Gross, D. (2018). Parents' executive functioning and involvement in their child's education: An integrated literature review. *Journal of School Health, 88*(4), 322–329. https://doi.org/10.1111/josh.12612

Zohar, D. (2007). Signonot khashivah vehashpaotehem al yekhasim khevratiyyim beqerev yeladim al hassepeqterum haotiseti [Thinking styles and their effects on social relationships among children on the autism spectrum]. In S. Lowinger (Ed.), *Qishurim: Tippul biyiladim im beayot tiqshoret: Gishot ineteraqtiviyyot [Connections: Interactive approaches to the treatment of children with communication disorders]* (pp. 161–188). Ach.

Index

S. Lowinger and S. Pearlman-Avnion (eds.), *Collaborative Care and Partnerships in Autism Diagnosis and Treatment*, Autism and Child Psychopathology Series,
https://doi.org/10.1007/978-3-032-07009-8

MIX
Papier aus verantwortungsvollen Quellen
Paper from responsible sources
FSC® C105338

If you have any concerns about our products,
you can contact us on
ProductSafety@springernature.com

In case Publisher is established outside the EU,
the EU authorized representative is:
Springer Nature Customer Service Center GmbH
Europaplatz 3, 69115 Heidelberg, Germany

Printed by Libri Plureos GmbH
in Hamburg, Germany